DIAGNOSTIC ULTRASOUND PHYSICS AND EQUIPMENT

Peter Hoskins BA, MSc, PhD, FIPEM

Senior Research Fellow
Medical Physics Unit
Edinburgh University
Edinburgh, UK

Abigail Thrush BSc, MSc, MIPEM

Principal Medical Physicist
Barts and the London NHS Trust
London, UK

Kevin Martin BSc, PhD, MIPEM

Consultant Medical Physicist
University Hospitals of Leicester NHS Trust
Leicester, UK

Tony Whittingam BSc, MSc, PhD, FInstP, CPhys, FIPEM

Consultant Medical Physicist
Regional Medical Physics Department
Newcastle General Hospital
Newcastle-upon-Tyne, UK

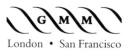

London • San Francisco

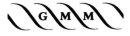

© 2003

Greenwich Medical Media Limited
4th Floor, 137 Euston Road,
London
NW1 2AA

870 Market Street, Ste 720
San Francisco
CA 94109, USA

ISBN 1841100420

First Published 2003

A catalogue record for this book is available from the British Library.

www.greenwich-medical.co.uk

Distributed by Plymbridge Distributors Ltd and in the USA by Jamco Distribution

Typeset by Charon Tec Pvt. Ltd, Chennai, India

Printed in the UK by Ashford Colour Press Ltd, Gosport, Hampshire

DIAGNOSTIC ULTRASOUND
PHYSICS AND EQUIPMENT

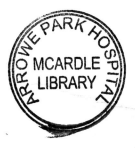

CONTENTS

Appendices

PREFACE

This book is an introductory text in the physics and instrumentation of medical ultrasound imaging. The level is appropriate for sonographers and clinical users in general. This will also serve as a first textbook for physicists and engineers. The text concentrates on explanations of principles which underpin the clinical use of ultrasound systems, with explanations following a "need to know" philosophy. Consequently, complex techniques, such as Doppler frequency estimation using FFT and 2D autocorrelation, are described in terms of their function, but not in terms of their detailed signal processing. The book contains relatively few equations and even fewer derivations. The scope of the book reflects ultrasound instrumentation as it is used at the time of submission to the publishers. Techniques which are still emerging, such as tissue Doppler imaging (TDI) and contrast agents, are covered in a single chapter at the end of the book. Techniques which are even further from commercial implementation, such as vector Doppler, are not covered. We hope this book fills the gap in the market that we perceive from discussions with our clinical colleagues, that of a text which is up to date and at an appropriate level.

Peter Hoskins
Abigail Thrush
Kevin Martin
Tony Whittingham
Summer 2002

CONTRIBUTORS

Mr T. Anderson MSc
Clinical Scientist
Lothian Universities NHS Trust

Ms AL Criton MSc
Ultrasound System Engineer
Philips Ultrasound, Bothell, USA

Prof FA Duck PhD, DSc
Professor of Medical Physics
Royal United Hospital Bath and Bath University

Mr NJ Dudley BSc, MSc, CertMHS, FIPEM
Consultant Medical Physicist
Nottingham City Hospital

Dr AJ Evans BSc, MSc, PhD, CEng
Senior Lecturer in Medical Physics
University of Leeds

Dr PR Hoskins BA, MSc, PhD, FIPEM
Senior Research Fellow
University of Edinburgh

Dr K Martin BSc, PhD, MIPEM
Consultant Medical Physicist
University Hospitals of Leicester NHS Trust

Prof WN McDicken BSc, PhD, FIPEM
Professor of Medical Physics and Medical Engineering
University of Edinburgh

Dr KV Ramnarine BSc, PhD, MIPEM
Principal Medical Physicist
University Hospitals of Leicester NHS Trust

Mr A Shaw BA, MA(Cantab)
Senior Research Scientist
National Physical Laboratory, Middlesex

Ms A Thrush BSc, MSc, MIPEM
Principal Medical Physicist
Barts and the London NHS Trust

Dr TA Whittingham BSc, MSc, PhD, FInstP, CPhys, FIPEM
Consultant Medical Physicist
Newcastle-upon-Tyne Hospital Trust

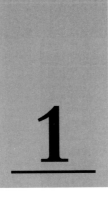

INTRODUCTION

K Martin

Basic principles of ultrasound image formation
B-mode formats
M-mode display
A-mode display

The application of ultrasound to medical diagnosis has seen continuous development and growth over several decades. Early, primitive display modes, such as A-mode and static B-mode, borrowed from metallurgical testing and radar technologies of the time, have given way to high performance, real-time imaging. Moving ultrasound images of babies in the womb are now familiar to most members of the public through personal experience of ante-natal scanning or via television. Modern ultrasound systems do much more than produce images of unborn babies, however. The Doppler effect is used to study motion within the body, particularly that of blood. Modern ultrasound systems are able to make detailed measurements of blood movements in blood vessels as well as show moving two-dimensional (2D) images of flow patterns.

Improvements in technology have been followed by widespread acceptance and use of ultrasound in medical diagnosis. Applications have progressed from simple measurements of anatomical dimensions, such as bi-parietal diameter, to detailed screening for fetal abnormalities, detection of subtle changes in tissue texture and detailed study of blood flow in arteries, including intravascular applications. In many areas, ultrasound is now chosen as the first line of investigation, before alternative imaging techniques.

This book describes the physics and technology of diagnostic ultrasound systems in use at the time of writing. The first part of the book includes a chapter on the physics of ultrasound and its interactions with tissue, but is otherwise devoted mainly to the formation of ultrasound images. Doppler ultrasound techniques, including the original techniques for measuring blood velocity and 2D colour flow mapping, are described in Chapters 7–10. No ultrasound system is complete without some means of recording or storing the image, and Chapter 11 describes the currently available electronic techniques for image storage as well as more traditional hard-copy systems. The safe use of ultrasound includes safe application as well as accurate diagnosis, which requires that the system performs to specification. Techniques for assessing the performance of ultrasound systems are discussed in Chapter 12. The physical safety of diagnostic ultrasound and advice on its safe application are reviewed in Chapter 13. Finally, Chapter 14 explains techniques, which are regarded as new developments. These are techniques that are available, but have not yet become established technologies at the time of writing. These will be incorporated into earlier chapters in the next edition, if they stand the test of time.

Basic principles of ultrasound image formation

We begin the explanation of ultrasound image formation with a description of a B-mode image and the basic principles of its formation. In essence, these principles are still used in modern B-mode systems, although they may be used within more complex arrangements designed to enhance performance. Two other modes, A-mode and M-mode, are introduced here also, as these are techniques that do not involve the Doppler effect.

A B-mode image is a cross-sectional image representing tissues and organ boundaries within the body (Figure 1.1). It is constructed from echoes, which are generated by reflection of ultrasound waves at tissue boundaries, and scattering from small irregularities within tissues. Each echo is displayed at a point in the image, which corresponds to the relative position of its origin within the body cross section, resulting in a scaled map of echo-producing features. The brightness of the image at each point is related to the strength or amplitude of the echo, giving rise to the term B-mode (brightness mode).

Usually, the B-mode image bears a close resemblance to the anatomy, which might be seen by eye, if the body could be cut through in the same plane. Abnormal anatomical boundaries and alterations in the scattering behaviour of tissues can be used to indicate pathology.

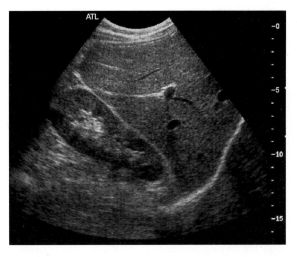

Fig. 1.1 An example of a B-mode image showing reflections from organ and blood vessel boundaries and scattering from tissues.

To form a B-mode image, a source of ultrasound, the transducer, is placed in contact with the skin and short bursts or pulses of ultrasound are sent into the patient. These are directed along narrow beam-shaped paths. As the pulses travel into the tissues of the body, they are reflected and scattered, generating echoes, some of which travel back to the transducer, where they are detected. These echoes are used to form the image.

To display each echo in a position corresponding to that of the interface or feature (known as a target) that caused it, the B-mode system needs two pieces of information. These are

1. the range (distance) of the target from the transducer and

2. the direction of the target from the active part of the transducer, i.e. the position and orientation of the ultrasound beam.

Echo ranging

The range of the target from the transducer is measured using the pulse–echo principle. The same principle is used in echo-sounding equipment in boats to measure the depth of water. Figure 1.2 illustrates the measurement of water depth using the pulse–echo principle. Here, the transducer transmits a short burst or pulse of ultrasound, which travels through water to the seabed below, where it is reflected, i.e. produces an echo. The echo travels back through the water to the transducer,

where it is detected. The distance to the seabed can be worked out, if the speed of sound in water is known and the time between the pulse leaving the transducer and the echo being detected, the "go and return time", is measured.

To measure the go and return time, the transducer transmits a pulse of ultrasound at the same time as a clock is started ($t = 0$). If the speed of sound in water is c and the depth is d, then the pulse reaches the seabed at time $t = d/c$. The returning echo also travels at speed c and takes a further time d/c to reach the transducer, where it is detected. Hence, the echo arrives back at the transducer after a total go and return time $t = 2d/c$. Rearranging this equation, the depth d can be calculated from $d = ct/2$. Thus, the system calculates the target range d by measuring the arrival time t of an echo, assuming a fixed value for the speed of sound c (usually $1540 \, \mathrm{m \, s^{-1}}$ for human tissues).

In the above example, only one reflecting surface was considered, i.e. the interface between the water and the seabed. The water contained no other interfaces or irregularities, which might generate additional echoes. When a pulse travels through the tissues of the body, it encounters many interfaces and scatterers, all of which generate echoes. After transmission of the short pulse, the transducer operates in receive mode, effectively listening for echoes. These begin to return immediately from targets close to the transducer, followed by echoes from greater and greater depths, in a continuous series, to the maximum depth of interest. This is known as the pulse–echo sequence.

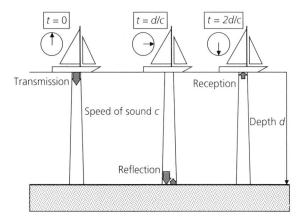

Fig. 1.2 Measurement of water depth using the pulse–echo principle. The depth is worked out by measuring the time from transmission of the pulse to reception of the echo. The speed of sound must be known.

Image formation

The 2D B-mode image is formed from a large number of B-mode lines, where each line in the image is produced by a pulse–echo sequence. In early B-mode systems, the brightness display of these echoes was generated as follows.

As the transducer transmits the pulse, a display spot begins to travel down the screen from a point corresponding to the position of the transducer, in a direction corresponding to the path of the pulse (the ultrasound beam). Echoes from targets near the transducer return first and increase the brightness of the spot. Further echoes, from increasing depths, return at increasing times after transmission as the spot travels down the screen. Hence, the distance down the display at which each echo is displayed is related to its depth below the transducer. The rate at which the display spot travels

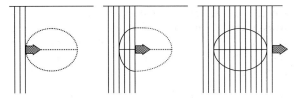

Fig. 1.3 Formation of a 2D B-mode image. The image is built up line by line as the beam is stepped along the transducer array.

down the screen determines the scale of the image. A rapidly moving spot produces a magnified image.

The pulse–echo sequence, described above, resulted in the display of one line of information on the B-mode image. A complete B-mode image, such as that in Figure 1.1, is made up typically of 100 or more B-mode lines.

Let us consider a linear array probe, as described in Chapter 3, where the image is formed as illustrated in Figure 1.3. During the first pulse–echo sequence, an image line is formed, say on the left of the display. The active area of the transducer, and hence the beam, is then moved along the array to the adjacent beam position. Here a new pulse–echo sequence produces a new image line of echoes, with a position on the display corresponding to that of the new beam. The beam is progressively stepped along the array with a new pulse–echo sequence generating a new image line at each position.

One complete sweep may take perhaps 1/30th of a second. This would mean that 30 complete images could be formed in 1 s, allowing real-time display of the B-mode image. That is, the image is displayed with negligible delay as the information is acquired, rather than recorded and then viewed, as with a radiograph or CT scan.

B-mode formats

The B-mode image, just described, was produced by a linear transducer array, i.e. a large number of small transducers arranged in a straight line (see Chapter 3). The ultrasound beams, and hence the B-mode lines, were all perpendicular to the line of transducers, and hence parallel to each other (Figure 1.4a). The resulting rectangular field of view is useful in applications, where there is a need to image superficial areas of the body at the same time as organs at a deeper level.

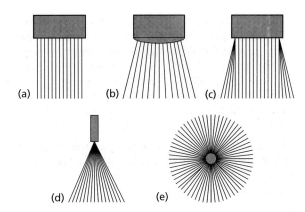

Fig. 1.4 Scan line arrangements for the most common B-mode formats. These are (a) linear, (b) curvilinear, (c) trapezoidal, (d) sector and (e) radial.

Other scan formats are often used for other applications. For instance, a curvilinear transducer (Figure 1.4b) gives a wide field of view near the transducer and an even wider field at deeper levels. This is also achieved by the trapezoidal field of view (Figure 1.4c). Curvilinear and trapezoidal fields of view are widely used in obstetric scanning to allow imaging of more superficial targets, such as the placenta, while giving the greatest coverage at the depth of the baby. The sector field of view (Figure 1.4d) is preferred for imaging of the heart, where access is normally through a narrow acoustic window between the ribs. In the sector format, all the B-mode lines are close together near the transducer and pass through the narrow gap, but diverge after that to give a wide field of view at the depth of the heart.

Transducers designed to be used internally, such as intravascular or rectal probes, often use the radial format (Figure 1.4e). The beam distribution is similar to that of beams of light from a lighthouse. This format is obtained by rotating the transducer on the end of a catheter or rigid tube, which can be inserted into the body. Hence, the B-mode lines all radiate out from the centre of the field of view.

M-mode display

The B-mode display formats, as just described, are designed to give a 2D-anatomical section through the body. The real-time nature of the display means that motion of tissues can be observed, and in some applications, used to obtain diagnostic information. In cardiology studies, there is often a need to measure the rate and

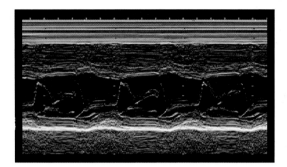

Fig. 1.5 An M-mode display, showing non-moving interfaces as straight horizontal lines, and the pattern of movement of the mitral valve leaflets.

timing of movements of the heart. The M-mode display (motion mode) allows such measurements to be made.

To produce an M-mode display, the ultrasound beam is aligned with the moving target to be studied, and held in position by the operator (i.e. not scanned as in B-mode). Ultrasound pulses are transmitted along the beam and echoes received in a normal pulse–echo sequence as in B-mode. The received echoes are also used to control the brightness of the display line as in B-mode. However, in M-mode, the beam remains fixed, while the display line is stepped across the display after each pulse–echo sequence. Reflecting targets,

which do not move with respect to the transducer, show as straight lines across the display. Targets, which do move towards and away from the transducer, show as a wave pattern, as illustrated in Figure 1.5, where the regular movements of the mitral valve leaflets within the heart can be seen. Diagnostic information relating to the movement of heart valves can be obtained, such as degree, rate and duration of closure.

A-mode display

The A-mode (amplitude mode) display is the simplest form of display of ultrasonic information, but is of historical interest, mainly as it is used now in only a few specialist applications. The A-mode display is not a cross-sectional display. It shows the amplitude of echoes received during each pulse–echo sequence. Following transmission of the ultrasound pulse, the A-mode display line sweeps out horizontally across the display screen. As echoes are received by the transducer, they deflect the display spot upwards according to their strength or amplitude, as in an oscilloscope display. The position of the echo along the horizontal axis of the display is proportional to its time of arrival, and hence the depth of the target. The A-mode display was used in early ultrasound systems to measure the distance between targets by identifying their echoes on the display and measuring their separation in time electronically. It is still used for measurements of eyeball length and skin thickness.

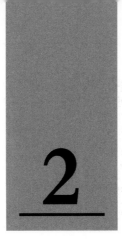

PHYSICS

K Martin and KV Ramnarine

Introduction

Ultrasound is a high frequency sound wave, which can be used to form images of internal body organs, as described briefly in the previous chapter. Ultrasound travels through the body in a way, which makes it possible to form images from echoes from tissues, but gives rise also to imperfections and limitations in the imaging system. In order to be able to use diagnostic ultrasound systems effectively and to be able to distinguish imperfections in the image from genuine diagnostic information, the user must have an appreciation of the basic principles of ultrasound propagation in tissue.

Waves

Transverse waves

A wave is a disturbance with a regularly repeating pattern, which travels from one point to another. A simple and familiar example is a wave on the surface of a pond caused by a stone being thrown into water (Figure 2.1a). Here, water displaced by the stone causes a local change in the height of the water, which travels out from the point of entry of the stone, the change in height at one point causing a change in height in the area of water next to it. An important aspect of the nature of this wave is that it is only the disturbance and not the water, which travels across the pond. The surface of the water at each point in the pond, as shown by a floating object (Figure 2.1b), simply goes up and down like a weight on the end of a spring, giving rise to the oscillating nature of the wave. Energy is transported across the pond from the stone to the shore. This type of wave on the surface of water is described as a transverse wave because the local movement of the water surface is at 90° (transverse) to the direction of travel.

Sound waves

The sound waves used to form medical images are longitudinal waves, which propagate (travel) through a physical medium (usually tissue or liquid). Here, the local movement of the medium is in the direction of propagation (see Figure 2.2). The particles of the medium oscillate backwards and forwards. Where particles in adjacent regions have moved towards each other, a region of compression (increased pressure) results, but where particles have moved apart, a region of rarefaction (reduced pressure) results. As in the transverse wave case, there is no net movement of the medium. Only the disturbance and its associated energy are transported.

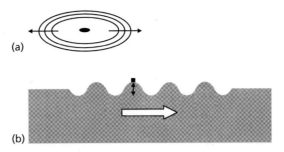

Fig. 2.1 Waves on the surface of a pond: (a) waves on the surface of a pond travel out from the point of entry of a stone; (b) only the disturbance travels across the pond. The water surface simply goes up and down.

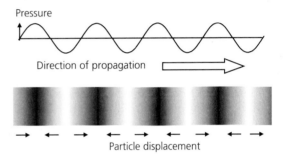

Fig. 2.2 In a longitudinal wave, particle motion is aligned with the direction of travel, resulting in bands of high and low pressure.

The most familiar sound waves are those that travel in air from sources of sound, e.g. a musical instrument or a bell, to the human ear. The surface of a bell vibrates when it is struck. The oscillating motion of the surface pushes and pulls against the adjacent air molecules. Neighbouring air molecules are then set in motion, which displace their neighbours and so the disturbance travels through the air as a sound wave. When the sound wave reaches the listener's ear, it causes the eardrum to vibrate, giving the sensation of sound. Energy from the bell is transported by the wave to the eardrum causing it to move.

Frequency, speed and wavelength

Frequency

When the bell above is struck, its surface vibrates backwards and forwards at a certain frequency (number of

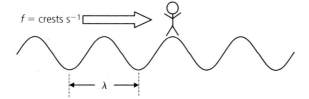

Fig. 2.3   The frequency f of a wave is the number of wave crests passing a given point per second. The wavelength λ is the distance between wave crests.

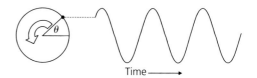

Fig. 2.4   Phase describes the position within a cycle of oscillation and is measured in degrees.

Phase

As a sound wave passes through a medium, the particles are displaced backwards and forwards from their rest positions in a repeating cycle. The motion may be that of a sine wave, as described by a point on the edge of a rotating disc when viewed end on (e.g. the pedals of a bicycle when viewed from behind). Identical points in the wave cycle are said to have the same phase. Because of the association with circular motion, the unit of phase is given as an angle, one complete cycle of a wave being considered as one complete rotation of 360° (see Figure 2.4). Half a cycle corresponds to 180°. The difference between the relative cycles of two waves of the same frequency thus may be expressed in terms of their phase difference in degrees.

Pressure, intensity and power

As explained earlier, a sound wave passing through a medium causes the particles of the medium to oscillate back and forth in the direction of propagation (i.e. longitudinally). The maximum distance moved by a particle from its normal rest position is a measure of the amplitude (or strength) of the wave. This is referred to as the displacement amplitude. The longitudinal motion of the particles results in regions of compression and rarefaction so that at each point in the medium, the pressure oscillates between maximum and minimum values as the wave passes. The difference between this actual pressure and the normal rest pressure in the medium is called the excess pressure p, which is measured in pascals ($1\,\text{Pa} = 1\,\text{N m}^{-2}$). When the medium is compressed, the excess pressure is positive. When the medium undergoes rarefaction, the pressure is less than the normal rest pressure, and so the excess pressure is negative. The amplitude of the wave may also be described by the peak excess pressure, the maximum value during the passage of a wave. Excess pressure is commonly referred to simply as the pressure in the wave.

As described earlier, a sound wave transports energy through a medium from a source. Energy is measured

times per second). An observer listening to the sound at any point nearby will detect the same number of vibrations per second. The frequency of the wave is the number of oscillations or wave crests passing a stationary observer per second (Figure 2.3) and is determined by the source of the sound wave. Frequency is normally given the symbol f and has units of hertz ($1\,\text{Hz} = 1$ cycle per second). Sound waves with frequencies in the approximate range 20 Hz to 20 kHz can be detected by the human ear. Sound waves with frequencies above approximately 20 kHz cannot be heard and are referred to as ultrasound waves.

Speed

As will be shown in more detail later, the speed at which a sound wave travels is determined by the medium in which it is travelling. The speed of sound is normally given the symbol c and has units of m s^{-1} (metres per second). Examples are the speed of sound in air ($330\,\text{m s}^{-1}$) and water ($1480\,\text{m s}^{-1}$).

Wavelength

The wavelength of a wave is the distance between consecutive wave crests or other similar points on the wave, as illustrated in Figure 2.3. Wavelength is normally given the symbol λ (lambda) and has units of metres or millimetres. A wave, whose crests are λ metres apart and pass an observer at a rate of f per second, must be travelling at a speed of $f \times \lambda$ metres per second. That is the speed of sound $c = f\lambda$.

However, it is more accurate physically to say that a wave from a source of frequency f, travelling through a medium whose speed of sound is c, has a wavelength λ, where $\lambda = c/f$. For example, a 30 kHz sound wave travelling through water ($c = 1500\,\text{m s}^{-1}$) has a wavelength of 50 mm whereas a 30 kHz sound wave travelling through air ($c = 330\,\text{m s}^{-1}$) has a wavelength of about 10 mm.

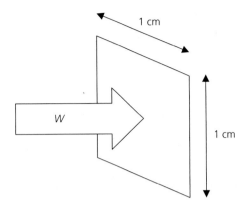

Fig. 2.5 Intensity is the power W flowing through unit area.

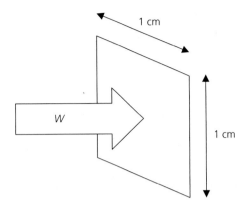

Fig. 2.6 The speed of sound in a medium is determined by its density and stiffness, which can be modelled by a series of masses and springs.

in joules (J). The power produced by a source of sound is a measure of the rate at which it produces energy. Power is measured in watts (W) where $1\,W = 1\,J\,s^{-1}$. The intensity associated with a wave is defined as the power flowing through unit area presented at 90° to the direction of propagation (Figure 2.5). Intensity I is measured in $W\,m^{-2}$ or $mW\,cm^{-2}$.

As one might expect intuitively, the intensity associated with a wave increases with the pressure amplitude of the wave. In fact intensity $I \propto p^2$.

Speed of sound

The speed of propagation of a sound wave is determined by the medium it is travelling in. In gases (e.g. air) the speed of sound is relatively low in relation to values in liquids, which in turn tend to be lower than values in solids. The material properties, which determine the speed of sound, are density (mass per unit volume) and stiffness. Density is normally given the symbol ρ (rho) and is measured in units of $kg\,m^{-3}$. Stiffness is usually denoted by the symbol k (units of Pa). A simple picture of how the density and stiffness of a material determine its speed of sound can be obtained from the model shown in Figure 2.6, which consists of two lines of weights, or more correctly masses, connected by springs. The small masses (m) model a material of low density and the large masses (M) a material of high density. In the two models shown, the small masses are linked by springs of high stiffness K and the large masses by springs of low stiffness k. A longitudinal wave can be propagated along the row of small masses (m) by giving the first mass a momentary push to the right. This movement is coupled to the second small

Table 2.1 Speed of sound in human tissues and liquids (from Duck, 1990).

Material	c $(m\,s^{-1})$
Liver	1578
Kidney	1560
Amniotic fluid	1534
Fat	1430
Average tissue	1540
Water	1480
Bone	3190–3406
Air	333

mass by a stiff spring causing it to accelerate quickly to the right and pass on the movement to the third mass, and so on. As the masses are light (low density), they can be accelerated quickly by the stiff springs (high stiffness) and the disturbance travels rapidly.

In the second case, a momentary movement of the first large mass M to the right is coupled to the second mass by a weak spring (low stiffness). The second large mass will accelerate relatively slowly in response to the small force from the weak spring. Its neighbours to the right also respond slowly so that the disturbance travels relatively slowly.

Hence, low density and high stiffness lead to high speed of sound whereas high density and low stiffness lead to low speed of sound. Mathematically this is expressed in the following equation:

$$\text{Speed of sound } c = \sqrt{\frac{k}{\rho}}.$$

Although gases have low density, they have very low stiffness (high compressibility) leading to relatively low speed of sound compared to liquids and solids.

Table 2.1 shows typical values for the speed of sound in various materials, including a number of different kinds of human tissue. The most important point to note from this table is that the values for the speed of sound in human soft tissues are rather similar. In fact they are sufficiently similar that the B-mode image forming process can assume a single, average value of 1540 m s^{-1} without introducing significant errors or distortions in the image. All the values shown (with the exception of fat) are within 5% of this average value and are not much different from the value in water. The speed of sound in air is relatively low because of its low stiffness, and that in bone is relatively high because of its high stiffness.

Frequencies and wavelengths used in diagnosis

The ultrasound frequencies used most commonly in medical diagnosis are in the range 2–15 MHz, although frequencies up to 40 MHz may be used in special applications and in research. The wavelengths in tissue, which result from these frequencies, can be calculated using the equation given earlier, which relates wavelength λ to the frequency f and speed c of a wave:

$$\lambda = \frac{c}{f}.$$

Assuming the average speed of sound in soft tissues of 1540 m s^{-1}, values are as shown in Table 2.2.

The wavelengths in soft tissues, which result from these frequencies, are within the range 0.1–1 mm. As will be seen later in this chapter and in Chapter 5, the wavelength of the ultrasound wave has an important influence on the ability of the imaging system to resolve fine anatomical detail. Short wavelengths give rise to improved resolution, i.e. the ability to show closely spaced targets separately in the image.

Reflection of ultrasound waves

In Chapter 1, a B-mode image was described as being constructed from echoes, which are generated by reflections of ultrasound waves at tissue boundaries and by scattering from small irregularities within tissue. Reflections occur at tissue boundaries where there is a change in acoustic impedance (see below). When an ultrasound wave travelling through one type of tissue encounters an interface with a tissue with different acoustic impedance, some of its energy is reflected back towards the source of the wave, while the remainder is transmitted into the second tissue.

Table 2.2 Wavelengths used in diagnosis.

f (MHz)	λ (mm)
2	0.77
5	0.31
10	0.15
15	0.1

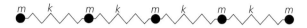
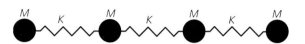

Fig. 2.7 The acoustic impedance of a medium is determined by its density and stiffness, which can be modelled by a series of masses and springs.

Acoustic impedance

The acoustic impedance of a medium z is a measure of the response the particles of the medium, to a wave of a given pressure. It is analogous to electrical impedance (or resistance), which is the ratio of the voltage applied to an electrical component (the electrical driving force or pressure) to the resulting electrical current which passes through it (the response), as expressed in Ohm's Law. Acoustic impedance $z = p/v$, where p is the local pressure and v is the local particle velocity.

The acoustic impedance of a medium is again determined by its density (ρ) and stiffness (k). It can be explained in more detail, as with the speed of sound, by modelling the medium as a row of small or large masses (m) and (M) linked by weak or stiff springs (k) and (K) as shown in Figure 2.7.

In this case however, the small masses m are linked by weak springs k modelling a material with low density and low stiffness. The large masses M are linked by stiff springs K modelling a material with high density and stiffness.

If a given pressure (due to a passing wave) is applied momentarily to the first small mass m, the mass is easily accelerated to the right (reaching increased velocity) and its movement encounters little opposing force from the weak spring k. This material has low acoustic impedance, as particle movements within it (in terms of velocity) in response to a given pressure, are relatively

Table 2.3 Values of acoustic impedance.

Material	z $(\mathrm{kg\,m^{-2}\,s^{-1}})$
Liver	1.66×10^6
Kidney	1.64×10^6
Blood	1.67×10^6
Fat	1.33×10^6
Water	1.48×10^6
Air	430
Bone	6.47×10^6

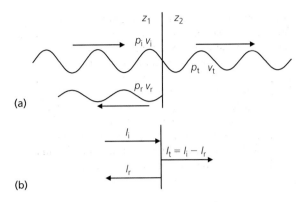

Fig. 2.8 (a) Total particle pressure and velocity cannot change abruptly across an interface. So a reflected wave is formed when there is a change in acoustic impedance; (b) the intensity transmitted across an interface is the incident intensity minus that reflected.

large. In the second case, the larger masses M accelerate less in response to the applied pressure (reaching lower velocity) and their movements are further resisted by the stiff springs. Particle velocity (the response) in this material is lower for a given applied pressure and it has higher acoustic impedance. The acoustic impedance z of a material is given by $z = \sqrt{\rho k}$.

By combining this equation with that for the speed of sound given earlier, it can be shown also that $z = \rho c$. z has units of $\mathrm{kg\,m^{-2}\,s^{-1}}$, but the term rayl is often used to express this unit.

Table 2.3 gives values of z for some common types of human tissue, air and water. Table 2.3 shows that values for z in most human soft tissues are very similar. For air, which has low density and low stiffness, z is very small. For bone, which has high density and high stiffness, z is much higher.

Reflection

When a sound wave travelling through a medium with acoustic impedance z_1 passes into a medium with acoustic impedance z_2 (Figure 2.8a), the pressures and particle velocities in the two media, at points very close together on each side of the boundary, must be the same. However, the change in acoustic impedance across the boundary suggests that the ratio of pressure to particle velocity must change abruptly across the interface. The result of this apparent conflict is the formation of an extra wave, which travels back into medium 1, known as the reflected wave. The sums of the pressures and velocities in the incident and reflected waves in medium 1 are then equal to the pressure and velocity respectively in the transmitted wave in medium 2. From this condition, it can be shown that

$$\frac{p_r}{p_i} = \frac{z_2 - z_1}{z_2 + z_1},$$

where p_i and p_r are the pressure amplitudes of the incident and reflected waves respectively near the boundary.

This ratio of reflected to incident pressure is commonly referred to as the amplitude reflection coefficient R_A. It is very important to ultrasound image formation as it determines the amplitude of echoes produced at boundaries between different types of tissue.

The intensity reflection coefficient describes the ratio of the intensities of the reflected (I_r) and incident waves (I_i). As intensity is proportional to pressure squared, the intensity reflection coefficient

$$\frac{I_r}{I_i} = R_i = R_A^2 = \left(\frac{z_2 - z_1}{z_2 + z_1}\right)^2.$$

As energy flow across the interface must be constant, the intensity, which is transmitted across the interface, must be the difference between the intensity of the incident wave and that of the reflected wave, i.e. $I_t = I_i - I_r$ (Figure 2.8b). From this it follows that the intensity transmission coefficient $T_i = 1 - R_i$. For example, if 0.01 (1%) of the incident intensity is reflected, then the other 0.99 (99%) must be transmitted across the boundary.

Table 2.4 shows values of amplitude reflection coefficient for some interfaces that might be encountered in the body. For most soft tissue to soft tissue interfaces, the amplitude reflection coefficient is less than 0.01 (1%). This is another important characteristic for ultrasound imaging as it means that most of the intensity at soft

Table 2.4 Amplitude reflection coefficients of interfaces.

Interface	R_A
Liver–kidney	0.006
Kidney–spleen	0.003
Blood–kidney	0.009
Liver–fat	0.11
Liver–bone	0.59
Liver–air	0.9995

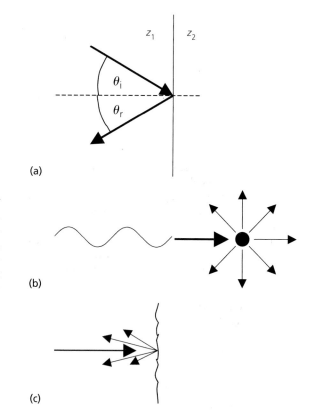

(a)

(b)

(c)

Fig. 2.9 Ultrasound waves are reflected at large interfaces and scattered by small targets: (a) at a large, smooth interface, the angle of reflection is equal to the angle of incidence; (b) small targets scatter the wave over a large angle; (c) a rough surface reflects the wave over a range of angles.

tissue interfaces is transmitted on to produce further echoes at deeper interfaces. The amplitude reflection coefficient at a tissue–fat interface is about 10% due to the low speed of sound in fat. At an interface between soft tissue and air, as might be encountered within the lungs or gas pockets in the gut, the reflection coefficient is 0.999 (99.9%), so no further useful echoes can be obtained from beyond such an interface. For this reason, it is important to exclude air from between the ultrasound source (the transducer) and the patient's skin to ensure effective transmission of ultrasound. At an interface between soft tissue and bone, the reflection coefficient is approximately 0.5 (50%), making it difficult also to obtain echoes from beyond structures such as ribs. Note that the reflection coefficient is not related to the frequency of the wave, it is determined only by the change in z at the interface between the two media.

In this description of reflection, it has been assumed that the interface is large compared to the wavelength of the wave and that the wave approaches the boundary at 90° (normal incidence). Under these circumstances, the reflected and transmitted waves also travel at 90° to the interface. In clinical practice, the wave may approach the interface at any angle and the angle at which it is reflected is governed by the law of reflection. The angle between the direction of propagation and a line at 90° to the interface (the normal) is called the angle of incidence θ_i (which has been 0° so far) as shown in Figure 2.9a. Similarly, the angle between the direction of the reflected wave and the normal is called the angle of reflection θ_r. For a flat, smooth interface, the law of reflection states that the angle of reflection $\theta_r = \theta_i$ the angle of incidence.

Scattering

Reflection, as just described, occurs at large interfaces such as those between organs where there is a change in acoustic impedance. Within the parenchyma of most organs (e.g. liver and pancreas), there are many small scale variations in acoustic properties, which constitute very small-scale reflecting targets (of size comparable to or less than the wavelength). Reflections from such very small targets do not follow the laws of reflection for large interfaces. When an ultrasound wave is incident on such a target, the wave is scattered over a large range of angles (Figure 2.9b). In fact, for a target which is much smaller that the wavelength, the wave may be scattered uniformly in all directions. For targets of the order of a wavelength in size, scattering will not be uniform in all directions but will still be over a wide angle.

The total ultrasound power scattered by a very small target is much less than that for a large interface and is determined by the relationship between the size d of the target and the wavelength λ of the wave. The scattered power is strongly dependent on these dimensions. For targets which are much smaller than a wavelength ($d \ll \lambda$), scattered power

$$W_s \propto \frac{d^6}{\lambda^4} \propto d^6 f^4.$$

This frequency dependence is often referred to as Rayleigh scattering.

Organs such as the liver contain non-uniformities in density and stiffness on scales ranging from the cellular level up to blood vessels, resulting in scattering characteristics, which do not obey such simple rules over all frequencies used in diagnosis. The frequency dependence of scattering in real liver changes with frequency over the diagnostic range (3–10 MHz). The scattered power is proportional to f^m, where m increases with frequency from approximately 1 to 3 over this range (Dickinson, 1986).

There are two important aspects of scattering for ultrasound imaging. Firstly, the ultrasonic power scattered back to the transducer by small targets is small compared to that from a large interface, so the echo level from the parenchyma of organs such as the liver is relatively weak. Secondly, as ultrasound is scattered over a wide angle by small targets, their response, and hence their appearance in the image, does not change significantly with the angle of incidence of the wave. Liver parenchyma looks similar ultrasonically regardless of the direction from which it is imaged.

Tissues such as muscle have long-range structure in one direction, i.e. along the muscle fibres and do not scatter ultrasound uniformly in all directions. Consequently, the appearance of muscle in an ultrasound image may change with the relative orientations of the ultrasound beams and the muscle fibres.

Diffuse reflection

The description of reflection given above assumed a perfectly flat, smooth interface. Some surfaces within the body may be slightly rough on the scale of a wavelength and reflect ultrasound waves over a range of angles, an effect similar to scattering from small targets. This type of reflection is known as diffuse reflection (Figure 2.9c).

Refraction

When the angle of incidence of the wave θ_i is not $0°$ (non-normal incidence), and there is a change in the

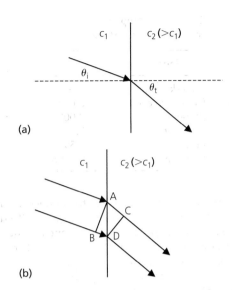

Fig. 2.10 When a wave crosses a boundary at an angle, where there is a change in the speed of sound, the wave is refracted, i.e. there is a change in the direction of travel.

speed of sound c from medium 1 to medium 2, the direction of propagation of the wave changes as it crosses the boundary (Figure 2.10a). This effect is known as refraction. Refraction occurs also with light waves and its effect is seen when an object below the surface of water is looked at from the air above. The speed of light in water is lower than that in air. Light from the object is refracted as it emerges into the air causing the apparent position of the object to be displaced from its real position.

Refraction can be explained as shown in Figure 2.10b. A wave front AB, travelling in medium 1, arrives at an interface with medium 2 where $c_2 > c_1$. The edge of the wave at A then passes into medium 2 where it travels more quickly than the edge at B, which is still in medium 1. By the time the wave edge at B has travelled to the interface (at point D), a wave front from point A will have travelled a greater distance to point C. The new wave front CD is hence deviated away from the normal at angle θ_t. When the wave crosses an interface where the speed of sound increases, the angle to the normal also increases. Conversely, when the wave experiences a reduction in the speed of sound as it crosses the interface, the angle to the normal also decreases. The relationship between the angles θ_i, θ_t, c_1 and c_2 is described by Snell's law:

$$\frac{\sin \theta_i}{\sin \theta_t} = \frac{c_1}{c_2}.$$

Snell's Law shows that for a fixed angle of incidence, the sine of the angle of the transmitted wave is proportional to the ratio of the speeds of sound in the two media. Refraction of ultrasound waves at boundaries where the speed of sound changes, can also cause displacement of the image of a target from its true relative position in the patient as explained in Chapter 5.

Attenuation

When an ultrasound wave propagates through soft tissue, the energy associated with the wave is gradually lost so that its intensity reduces with distance travelled, an effect known as attenuation. For each centimetre travelled into the tissue, the intensity is reduced by the same ratio (Figure 2.11). For example, if the intensity is reduced by a factor of 0.7 in the first centimetre, it will be reduced again by 0.7 in the second and third centimetres. So after 2 cm it will be reduced by 0.49 (0.7×0.7) and after 3 cm by 0.34 ($0.7 \times 0.7 \times 0.7$). Expressed in decibels (Appendix A), the attenuation due to each centimetre travelled can be added rather than multiplied, and we can then measure attenuation in dB per centimetre. In dB the intensity is reduced by 1.5 dB for each centimetre of travel, so after 3 cm it is reduced by 4.5 dB ($1.5 + 1.5 + 1.5$). The rate at which the intensity of the wave is attenuated, in dB cm^{-1} is referred to as the attenuation coefficient.

In most diagnostic systems, ultrasound propagates in the form of a beam, as described later in this chapter. The attenuation of practical interest is the rate at which ultrasound intensity in the beam decreases with distance. This intensity may be reduced due to scattering of ultrasound out of the beam, due to divergence of the beam with distance and due to absorption of ultrasound energy by the medium.

Absorption

Absorption is the process by which ultrasound energy is converted into heat in the medium. When an ultrasound wave passes through a medium, its particles move backwards and forwards in response to the pressure wave as described earlier. At low frequencies, the particles are able to move in step with the passing pressure wave and energy associated with the motion of the particles is effectively passed back to the wave as it moves on. However, the particles of the medium cannot move instantaneously and at high frequencies may be unable to keep up with the rapid fluctuations in pressure. They are unable to pass back all of the energy associated with

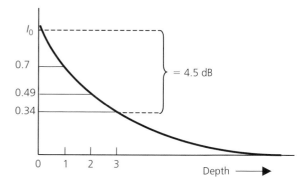

Fig. 2.11 The ultrasound intensity is attenuated (reduced) by the same fraction for each unit of distance travelled into the medium. This equates to attenuation by the same number of dB for each unit of distance.

their movements to the passing wave as they are out of step and some energy is retained by the medium where it appears as heat. Absorption is likely to be strongest at frequencies which excite natural modes of vibration of the particular molecules of the medium as it is at such frequencies that they are most out of step with the passing wave. Understanding of the mechanisms and vibrational modes, which lead to absorption of ultrasound, is still imperfect but absorption has been found to be strongly dependent on tissue composition and structure. For example, tissues with high collagen content such as tendons and cartilage show high absorption, whereas those with high water content show lower absorption. Water and liquids such as urine, amniotic fluid and blood have low absorption and low attenuation. Estimates of the contribution of absorption to attenuation are variable but for many tissues, absorption is the dominant loss mechanism.

Dependence on frequency

Absorption of ultrasound by biological tissues increases with frequency. The attenuation coefficient of most tissues, when expressed in dB cm^{-1} increases approximately linearly with frequency. Hence, for most tissues, it is possible to measure ultrasound attenuation in dB cm^{-1} MHz^{-1}. For example, if a tissue attenuates by 0.7 dB cm^{-1} MHz^{-1}, a 5 MHz ultrasound wave, after travelling a distance of 10 cm, will be attenuated by 5 MHz $\times$ 10 cm $\times$ 0.7 dB cm^{-1} MHz^{-1} = 35 dB.

Table 2.5 shows measured values of attenuation coefficient for some human tissues. Values are typically in the range 0.3–0.6 dB cm^{-1} MHz^{-1} for soft tissues but much

Table 2.5 Values of attenuation coefficient α for some human tissues.

Tissue	α (dB cm^{-1} MHz^{-1})
Liver	0.399
Brain	0.435
Muscle	0.57
Blood	0.15
Water	0.02
Bone	22

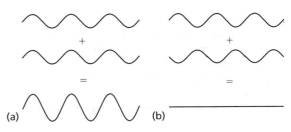

Fig. 2.12 The effects of two waves travelling through the same medium are added, i.e. the waves interfere with each other: (a) waves with the same phase interfere constructively (add); (b) waves with opposite phase interfere destructively (cancel).

lower for water (and watery body fluids). Attenuation in bone is very high and does not increase linearly with frequency as in the case of soft tissues.

When attenuation is large, the echoes returned from deeper targets may be too weak to detect. Hence, for imaging large or deep organs, a low frequency (3–5 MHz) must be used. High frequencies (10–15 MHz) can only be used to image relatively small, superficial targets (e.g. thyroid) as they are attenuated more rapidly. The short wavelengths associated with high frequency ultrasound leads to improved resolution of image detail. The operator must choose the optimum frequency for each particular application. This is a compromise that ensures that the best image resolution is obtained, while allowing echoes to be received from the required depth.

Ultrasound beams

The description of ultrasound wave propagation so far has concentrated mainly on the properties of the wave and how it is affected by the medium in the direction of propagation. The principles outlined apply regardless of the extent of the wave at 90° to this direction, the transverse direction. It is clear from the outline of B-mode image formation given in Chapter 1 that to be able to define where an echo originates from in the imaged cross section, the extent of the wave in the transverse direction must be very limited. That is, the wave must propagate along a narrow corridor or beam. This section describes the formation and properties of ultrasound beams.

Interference of waves

So far, we have considered only a single wave propagating through a medium. When two or more waves from different sources propagate through the same medium, they interfere with each other. That is, the effects of each individual wave are added at each point in the medium. This is to be expected as the pressure at a point in the medium will be the sum of the pressures on it from the different waves. Figure 2.12 shows the simple case of two waves with the same frequency and amplitude propagating in the same direction. In Figure 2.12a, the waves are in phase or in step with each other and the peaks of the two waves coincide, as do the troughs. In this case the resulting wave amplitude is twice than that of the individual waves. This case is referred to as constructive interference, as the resulting amplitude is greater than that of both the individual waves. In Figure 2.12b, the waves are in anti-phase, and the peaks of one wave coincide with the troughs of the other. Hence, at each point in the medium the particles are being pushed in one direction by one wave and by the same pressure in the opposite direction by the second wave. The resulting pressure on the particles is zero and the effects of the waves cancel out. This case is referred to as destructive interference.

Diffraction

When a source generates a sound wave, the way in which the wave spreads out as it moves away from the source is determined by the relationship between the width of the source (the aperture) and the wavelength of the wave. If the aperture is small compared to the wavelength, the wave spreads out as it travels (diverges), an effect known as diffraction. This is rather like the wave on a pond, spreading out from the point of entry of a small stone. For a sound wave from a small point source within a medium, the wave spreads out as an expanding sphere (a spherical wave) rather than a circle as on a water surface. The small scattering targets described earlier effectively act as sources of such spherical waves.

If the width of the source is much greater than the wavelength of the wave, the wave propagates at 90° to

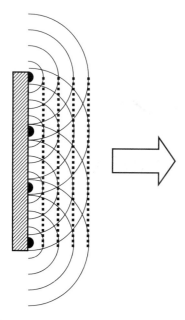

Fig. 2.13 An extended source can be considered as a row of small point sources. Spherical waves from each interfere to form a series of wave fronts.

the surface of the source with relatively little sideways spread, i.e. in the form of a beam. Such a source can be considered to be made up from a long row of small sources as shown in Figure 2.13. Each of the small sources generates a sound wave of the same frequency and amplitude and all are in phase with each other. The curved waves from each propagate outwards and the parts of the wave, which are parallel to the surface of the source, align to form a plane wave front. Other parts of the curved waves interfere destructively and cancel out. This view of the generation of a plane wave from a plane source is put to practical use in forming ultrasound beams from rows of small sources (array transducers) as described in the next chapter.

Ultrasound beams from practical sources

The description of a plane wave being formed from an array of small sources is true only for a very large source (i.e. much greater in size than the wavelength). Although such a large source might generate a very well collimated beam, it would be too wide to be useful in forming images. Real ultrasound sources are designed to give the optimum combination of narrow beam width and minimal divergence or spread.

The plane disc source

One example of a practical source of ultrasound is a plane disc transducer, also referred to as a plane circular piston source. The surface of this source is a flat disc and it is assumed that all parts of the surface move backwards and forwards exactly in phase and with the same amplitude. The basic shape of the ultrasound beam produced by such a source is illustrated in Figure 2.14a. To a first approximation, it can be divided into two parts. These are

1. the near field, which is cylindrical in shape and has approximately the same diameter as the source and

2. the far field, which diverges gradually.

Figure 2.14b shows the real distribution of pressure amplitude within a beam from a plane disc source. Within the near field, the pressure amplitude of the wave is not constant everywhere, but shows many peaks and troughs. As the source is circular, these pressure variations have circular symmetry. That is, the peaks and troughs are in the form of rings centred on the beam axis. This structure can be explained by again considering the source to be made up of many small elements, each of which emits a spherical wave. The pressure amplitude at each point in the near field is determined by the sum of the spherical waves from all of the elements. The different path lengths, from the various elements to the summing point, means that each of the spherical waves has a different phase when it arrives. At some points, this results in overall constructive interference, giving rise to an amplitude maximum. At other points, the overall effect is destructive and a minimum is formed. At points close to the source, the path lengths can be different by several wavelengths. The end of the near field is defined as being the distance from the source at which the maximum path length difference is $\lambda/2$. This distance, the near field length, is given by the expression a^2/λ, where a is the radius of the source (Wells, 1977). Figure 2.14c shows that the pressure amplitude along the beam axis reaches a final maximum value at this point.

In the far field, destructive interference does not occur in the central lobe of the beam, as the path length differences are all less than $\lambda/2$. The resulting beam structure is relatively simple, showing a maximum value on the beam axis, which falls away uniformly with radial distance from the axis. The intensity along the beam axis in the far field falls as the inverse square law, i.e. $I = 1/z^2$, where z is the distance from the transducer. The beam diverges in the far field at an angle given by

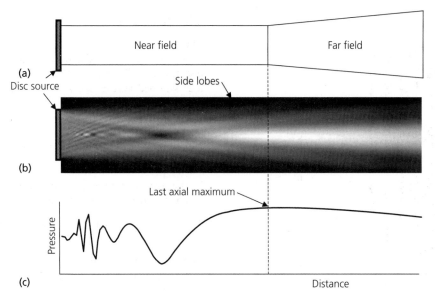

Fig. 2.14 The ultrasound beam from a plane disc source consists of a near field, in which the pressure distribution is complex, and a far field, in which it is more uniform.

$\sin \theta = 0.61 \, (\lambda/a)$, where θ is the angle between the beam axis and the edges of the beam. Hence, when the aperture a is small compared to the wavelength λ, the near field is short and the beam diverges rapidly in the far field, i.e. θ is large. When a is large compared to λ, the near field is long and there is little divergence in the far field, i.e. θ is small. For example, a 3 MHz source with a radius of 0.75 cm has a near field length of 11.25 cm and an angle of divergence of 2.3° in the far field. A 10 MHz source with a radius of 0.25 cm has a near field length of 4.2 cm and an angle of divergence in the far field of 2.1°. Hence, increased frequency allows the source diameter and hence, the beam width to be reduced while maintaining the beam shape in terms of low divergence in the far field.

This description of a beam from a disc source relates to what is called the "main lobe" of the beam. The angle of divergence θ defines the edge of the main lobe in the far field because destructive interference causes a minimum to be formed in the pattern of interference at that angle. At increasing angles to the main lobe greater than θ, alternate maxima and minima are formed, as can be seen in Figure 2.14b. The regions containing these maxima are referred to as side lobes. Side lobes are weaker than the main lobe but can give rise to significant echoes if they are incident on a strongly reflecting target adjacent to the main lobe, resulting in acoustic noise in the image. Manufacturers normally design

their transducers to minimise side lobes. This can be done by applying stronger excitation to the centre of the transducer than at the edges, a technique known as apodisation. Apodisation reduces the amplitude of side lobes but leads to an increase in the width of the main lobe.

This description of the beam from a plane disc-shaped source assumes that the transmitted wave is continuous and hence contains only a single frequency. For imaging purposes, the source must produce a short burst or pulse of ultrasound, which gives distinct echoes from interfaces. As described later, a short pulse contains energy at a range of frequencies rather than just one, each of which produces a slightly different beam. These are effectively added together in the pulsed beam resulting in smearing out of the pressure variations compared to those in the continuous wave beam shown in Figure 2.14.

Focusing

For imaging purposes, a narrow ultrasound beam is desirable as it allows closely spaced targets to be shown separately in the image. Using a small aperture disc source may give a narrow beam close to the source but leads to greater beam divergence and hence greater beam width for deeper targets. A wide disc source gives a well-collimated beam, but it is relatively wide.

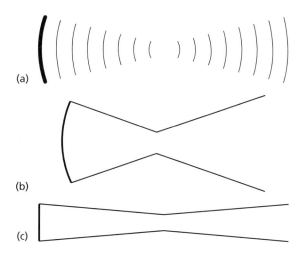

(a)

(b)

(c)

Fig. 2.15 Focusing of ultrasound beams: (a) the wave fronts from a curved source converge towards a focus; (b) the effect is strong if the focus is in the first part of the near field; (c) focusing is weak beyond half the near field length.

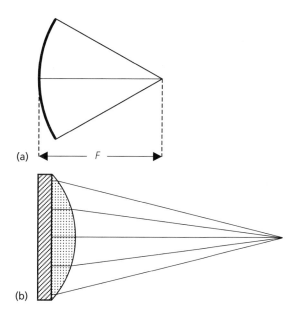

(a)

(b)

Fig. 2.16 Focusing methods: (a) focusing can be achieved by using a curved source; (b) focusing can also be achieved by adding an acoustic lens to a plane source.

A worthwhile improvement to the overall beam width can be obtained by focusing. Here, the source is designed to produce wave fronts, which are curved rather than flat as shown in Figure 2.15a. Each part of the curved wave front travels at right angles to its surface at that point so that the wave fronts converge towards a point in the beam, the focus, where the beam achieves its minimum width. Beyond the focus, the beam diverges again but more rapidly than for an unfocused beam with the same aperture and frequency. The distance from the source to the focus is the focal length F.

The focusing effect on a beam is strongest when the focal length F is short in relation to the near field length of a similar unfocused transducer (Figure 2.15b). Here, the wave fronts converge rapidly to a very narrow beam width at the focus then diverge rapidly again beyond that point. The beam width W at the focus for strong focusing is given approximately by the equation $W = F\lambda/a$. Focusing is weak (Figure 2.15c) when the focal length F is more than half of the near field length (Kossoff, 1979).

For a single element source, focusing is usually achieved in one of two ways. These are by use of

1. a curved source and

2. an acoustic lens.

The curved source (Figure 2.16a) is manufactured with a radius of curvature of F and hence produces curved

wave fronts which converge at a focus F cm from the source. An acoustic lens is attached to the face of a flat source and produces curved wave fronts by refraction at its outer surface as in the case of an optical lens (Figure 2.16b). A convex lens is made from material, which has a lower speed of sound than tissue. Wave fronts from the source pass into the lens at normal incidence and are undeviated. On arrival at the interface between the lens and tissues, the increase in the speed of sound causes the direction of propagation to be deviated away from the normal and a converging wave front is formed.

The ultrasound pulse

As described earlier, a B-mode image is formed from echoes produced by reflection from interfaces and scattering from smaller targets. To produce a distinct echo, which corresponds to a particular interface, ultrasound must be transmitted in the form of a short burst or pulse. To allow echoes from closely spaced interfaces to be resolved separately, the pulse must be short. A typical ultrasound pulse consists of a few cycles of oscillation at the nominal frequency of the wave as illustrated in Figure 2.17a. Typically the wave amplitude increases rapidly at the leading edge, reaches a peak and then decreases more slowly in the trailing edge.

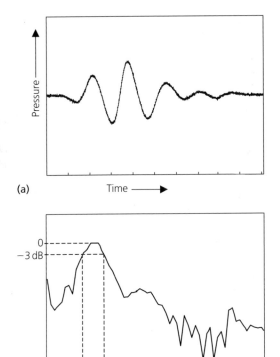

(a) Time ⟶

(b) f_1 f_0 f_2 Frequency ⟶

Fig. 2.17 The pressure waveform and spectrum of a typical ultrasound pulse: (a) a typical ultrasound pulse consists of a few cycles of oscillation; (b) the pulse contains a range of frequencies (a spectrum) dominated by a centre frequency f_0.

The pulse spectrum

When a source is excited continuously to produce a wave whose pressure varies as a pure sine wave, the wave has a specific frequency. A graph of pressure against frequency would show a single value at that frequency and zero at other frequencies. A pulsed wave can be described as being constructed from a range of frequencies centred around the nominal frequency. Interference between the components at the different frequencies effectively results in the formation of a pulse. The graph of pressure versus frequency for a pulse shows a distribution of frequency components centred mainly on the nominal frequency or centre frequency. The frequency content of a pulse has become an important issue in modern imaging systems. A short pulse gives precise time resolution and hence distance resolution and its echoes contain information at a wide range of frequencies.

The information contained in an echo from a long pulse is concentrated near the nominal frequency and gives a stronger signal at that frequency. However, a long pulse results in poor distance resolution.

The graph of amplitude versus frequency for a pulse is termed the pulse spectrum and the range of frequencies it contains is the bandwidth. The width of the spectrum is commonly measured in terms of the -3 dB bandwidth (Figure 2.17b), which is the difference between frequency values above (f_2) and below (f_1) the peak frequency (f_0) at which the amplitude of the spectrum has fallen by 3 dB from its maximum value.

Non-linear propagation

In the description of propagation of sound waves given earlier in this chapter the wave propagated with a fixed speed determined by the properties of the medium. This description is a good approximation to reality when the amplitude of the wave is small. At higher pressure amplitudes (>1 MPa), this simple picture breaks down and the effects of non-linear propagation become noticeable.

The speed at which each part of the wave travels is related to the properties of the medium and to the local particle velocity, which enhances or reduces the speed. In the high pressure (compression) parts of the wave, this results in a slight increase in speed, whereas in the low pressure (rarefaction) parts of the wave, the speed is slightly reduced. As the wave propagates into the medium (see Figure 2.18a), the compression parts of the wave gradually catch up with the rarefaction parts. The compression parts become taller and narrower, while the rarefaction parts become lower in amplitude and longer. The leading edge of the compression parts of the wave become steeper and may form a "shock" front, an instantaneous increase in pressure.

The rapid changes in pressure in the compression part of the wave appear in the pulse spectrum as high frequency components. As shown in Figure 2.18b, these are multiples of the original or fundamental frequency f_0 known as harmonics. A frequency of $2f_0$ is known as the second harmonic, $3f_0$ as the third harmonic and so on. The figure shows that the original pulse spectrum is effectively repeated at these harmonic frequencies. Non-linear propagation results in some of the energy in the pulse being transferred from the fundamental frequency f_0 to its harmonics. As the pulse travels further into the medium, the high frequency components are attenuated more rapidly than the low frequency

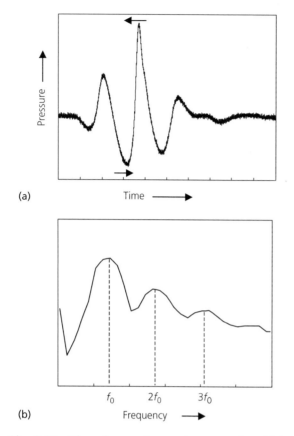

(a)

Pressure →

Time →

(b)

f_0 $2f_0$ $3f_0$

Frequency →

Fig. 2.18 The pulse waveform and spectrum for a high amplitude pulse: (a) at high pressure amplitudes, the pulse waveform becomes distorted due to non-linear propagation; (b) the spectrum of the distorted pulse contains significant components at multiples of the centre frequency (harmonics).

components and the pulse shape becomes more rounded again as the overall amplitude is reduced.

Harmonic imaging

The changes in the pulse spectrum are put to good use in harmonic imaging as described in Chapter 4. In harmonic imaging, a pulse is transmitted with fundamental frequency f_0, but due to non-linear propagation, the echoes returned from within the tissues contain energy at harmonic frequencies $2f_0$, $3f_0$, etc. The imaging system ignores the frequencies in the fundamental part of the spectrum and forms an image using only the 2nd harmonic ($2f_0$) part of the pulse (Desser *et al.*, 2000). The effective ultrasound beam which this produces, the harmonic beam, is narrower than the conventional beam and suppresses artefacts such as side lobes. This is due to the fact that non-linear propagation and hence the formation of harmonics occurs most strongly in the highest amplitude parts of the transmitted beam, i.e. near the beam axis. Weaker parts of the beam such as the side lobes and edges of the main lobe produce little harmonic energy and are suppressed in relation to the central part of the beam. Harmonic imaging can also reduce other forms of acoustic noise such as the weak echoes due to reverberations and multiple path artefacts as described in Chapter 5.

References

Desser TS, Jedrzejewicz T and Bradley C. Native tissue harmonic imaging: Basic principles and clinical applications. *Ultrasound Quart* 2000; **16**: 40–48.

Dickinson RJ. Reflection and scattering. In: CR Hill (Ed.) *Physical Principles of Medical Ultrasonics*. Ellis Horwood, Chichester. 1986.

Duck FA, *Physical Properties of Tissue – A Comprehensive Reference Book*. Academic Press, London. 1990.

Kossoff G. Analysis of focusing action of spherically curved transducers. *Ultrasound Med. Biol.* 1979; **5**: 359–365.

Wells PNT, *Biomedical Ultrasonics*. Academic Press, London. 1977.

3

TRANSDUCERS AND BEAM-FORMING

TA Whittingham

Introduction

The basic principles of B-mode scanning were introduced in Chapter 1. The way the beam is formed and swept through the patient (scanned) in different types of scanner will now be described in more detail.

The *transducer* is the device that actually converts electrical transmission pulses into ultrasonic pulses and, conversely, ultrasonic echo pulses into electrical echo signals. The simplest way to interrogate all the scan lines that make up a B-mode scan is to physically move the transducer from line to line. This is what happens in a *mechanical scanner*, described at the end of this chapter. This was the original method but it has the principal disadvantage that moving parts are involved, and so wear and maintenance become important issues. Most modern scanners avoid this problem by using a probe containing an array of many tiny fixed *transducer elements*, rather than a single moveable transducer. Such array probes allow the beam to be moved electronically, and also give the additional benefit of allowing the shape and size of the beam to be changed to suit the needs of each examination. The *beam-former* is the part of the scanner that determines the shape, size and position of the interrogating beams by controlling signals to and from the transducer array. In transmission, it generates the electronic signals that drive each individual transducer element, and in reception it combines the individual echo sequences from all the transducer elements into a single echo sequence.

The echo sequence produced by the beam-former for each scan line is then amplified and processed in the same way as for a single element mechanical scanner. These processes are the subject of Chapter 4.

Which beam do you mean?

Before discussing transducers and beam-forming further, it will be helpful to consider the idea of beams a little more. In Chapter 2, the shape and size of the beam transmitted by a simple disc transducer was discussed. In most imaging techniques, ultrasound is transmitted in short pulses. The "transmission beam" then represents the "corridor" along which the pulses travel. Whatever the width of the beam at a particular depth, that is the lateral width of the pulse when at that depth.

It is also possible to talk of a "receive beam", which describes the region in which a point source of ultrasound must lie if it is to produce a detectable electrical signal at the receiving transducer. In the case of a single disc transducer, since the same transducer is used for

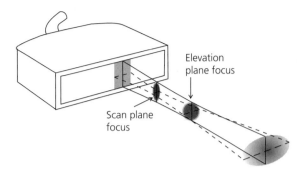

Fig. 3.1 The rectangular beam aperture of an array probe produces a beam with non-circular cross-sections. In this example, the focal beam width in the vertical (elevation) plane is wider and at a greater range than that in the horizontal (scan) plane.

both transmission and reception (at different times, of course), the transmission beam has an identical shape and size to the receive beam. In other words, the points in the transmission beam that have the greatest intensity will also be the points in the receive beam where a point source would produce the greatest electrical signal at the transducer. However, in the case of array transducers, the combination of transducer elements used for transmission can be different to that used for reception, and so the two beams can then be different in shape and size.

In fact, in array probes, the transmitting and receiving apertures are generally rectangular rather than circular. This results in the beams having rectangular cross-sections close to the probe, becoming roughly elliptical towards the focal region and beyond (Figure 3.1). The shape and size of the beam is, therefore, likely to be different in the scan plane to that in the perpendicular "elevation" plane, and it is necessary to be clear which plane is being considered. The beam width in the scan plane determines the lateral resolution of the scanner, whereas that in the elevation plane defines the "slice thickness", and hence the acoustic noise of the image and, to some extent the sensitivity of the scanner. These topics are discussed under the headings of the different types of probe, below. Lateral resolution and slice thickness are also discussed more fully in Chapter 5.

Common features of all transducers and transducer elements

All transducers or transducer elements have the same basic components: a piezoelectric plate, a matching layer and a backing layer, as shown in Figure 3.2. Usually, there is also a lens, but in transducer-array probes it is usual for one large lens to extend across all the transducer elements. There are differences between different types of probes regarding number, size, shape and arrangement of transducer elements, but these will be addressed later, as each probe type is discussed.

Piezoelectric plate

The actual sound generating and detecting component is a thin piezoelectric plate. Piezoelectric materials expand or contract when a positive or negative voltage is applied across them, and, conversely, generate positive or negative voltages when compressed or stretched by an external force (Figure 3.3). Some piezoelectric materials, such as quartz, occur naturally but the piezoelectric material normally used for transducers in medical imaging equipment is a synthetic ceramic material: lead zirconate titanate (PZT). Various versions of PZT can be made, according to the specialist properties required, such as high sensitivity, or the ability to cope with large acoustic powers. Other piezoelectric materials are currently being developed to replace PZT in many applications. These include single crystals of lead titanate (PT) doped with various other elements, such as lead, magnesium and niobium (PMN–PT) or lead, zinc and niobium (PZN–PT). These crystals promise to generate much stronger electrical signals in response to echo pulses

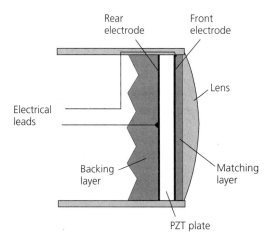

Fig. 3.2 The basic component elements in an imaging ultrasound transducer.

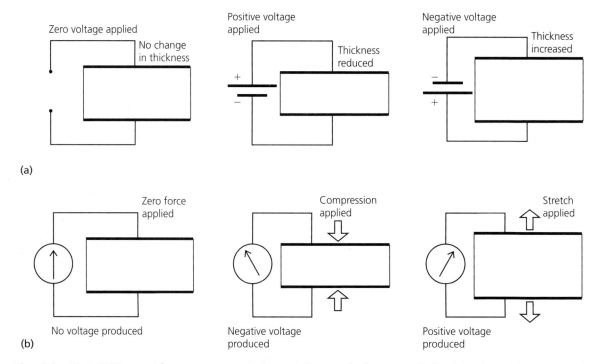

Fig. 3.3 (a) A PZT material contracts or expands according to whether an applied voltage is positive or negative. (b) Conversely, forced expansions or compressions produce positive or negative voltages.

(greater sensitivity and pentration) and larger bandwidths (greater axial resolution). "Composite PZT", made by cutting closely spaced narrow channels through a solid plate of PZT and filling them with an inert polymer, is also being introduced. This has a lower characteristic acoustic impedance than PZT itself, which alleviates the matching problem (discussed next) and thus produces transducers with greater sensitivity and bandwidth. For convenience, the piezoelectric will be referred to henceforth as PZT, but the possibility of other materials being used should be borne in mind.

The thin plate of PZT is coated on both sides with conductive paint, forming electrodes, to which electrical leads are soldered or glued. In order to transmit an ultrasonic pulse, an oscillating voltage of the required frequency is applied across the PZT plate, via these leads, making it expand and contract at this frequency (Figure 3.4). The back and forth movements of the front face send an ultrasonic wave into the patient's tissues. In reception, the pressure variations of returning echoes cause the PZT plate to contract and expand, generating voltage variations across the plate, which are directly proportional to the pressure variations. These voltage variations form the electronic version of the echo signal.

The PZT slab vibrates most strongly at the frequency for which its thickness is half a wavelength, giving rise to the term "half-wave resonance". This resonance occurs because an ultrasound wave propagating across the thickness of the PZT plate will be partially reflected at the front and back faces, and thus continue to travel back and forth (reverberate) within the PZT plate. If the frequency is such that the plate thickness is equal to half the wavelength, it will travel a full wavelength in the PZT before arriving back at its starting point. This means that it will be in phase with the original wave, and add constructively to it to produce a greater output.

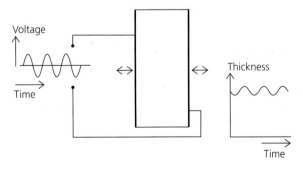

Fig. 3.4 Changes in voltage across a PZT plate produce corresponding changes in thickness.

A PZT plate with a thickness equal to half a wavelength[1] at the required centre frequency is therefore used, as this will resonate and hence produce a large output at this frequency.

Backing layer

PZT has advantages as a transducer material in that it is efficient at converting electrical energy to mechanical energy, and vice versa, and is relatively easy to machine or mould to any required shape or size. However, it has one significant disadvantage in that it has a characteristic acoustic impedance that is about 20 times higher than that of the soft tissue. If the front face of the PZT plate were to be in direct contact with the patient, a large fraction (approximately 80%) of an ultrasound wave's power would be reflected at a PZT–tissue interface (see "Reflection coefficient" in Chapter 2). If nothing were to be done about this, the internal reverberations within the PZT, referred to above, would be very strong and would continue long after the applied driving voltage had finished. Such prolonged internal reverberations (ringing) were a serious problem in early transducers, causing pulses to be too long for good axial resolution.

This unwanted ringing can be much reduced by having a backing (damping) layer behind the PZT, made of a material with both a high characteristic acoustic impedance and the ability to absorb ultrasound. If the impedance of the backing layer were identical to that of PZT, all the sound energy would cross the boundary between the PZT and the backing layer, and none would be reflected back into the PZT. Once in the backing layer the sound would be completely absorbed and converted into heat. This would eliminate ringing, but would be at the expense of sensitivity, as some of the energy of the electrical driving pulse and also of the returning echo sound pulses would be wasted as heat in the backing layer. In modern practice, a backing layer with an impedance somewhat lower than that of the PZT is used. This compromise impedance is chosen to give a useful reduction in reflection without lowering sensitivity too much. The remaining ringing is removed by using matching layers, as discussed next.

Matching layer(s)

Apart from the ringing problem, the fact that only about 20% of the wave's power would be transmitted through the front PZT–patient interface means there is also a potential problem of poor sensitivity. In order to

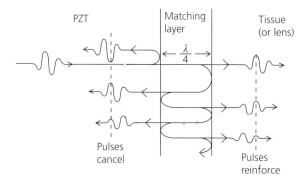

Fig. 3.5 Quarter wave matching layer. Reverberations within the plate produce multiple transmissions into the patient that reinforce each other to give a large amplitude resultant pulse. The resultant of the multiple reflections back into the PZT cancel-out the original (top) reflection back into the backing layer.

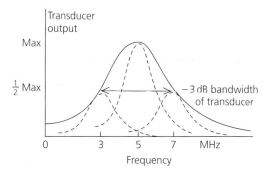

Fig. 3.6 The $-3\,\mathrm{dB}$ bandwidth of a transducer is the range of frequencies over which the output power for a given applied peak-to-peak voltage is within a factor of two of the maximum. A multi-frequency probe must have a large bandwidth, so that it can transmit and receive pulses with several different centre frequencies (pulse spectra shown dashed).

overcome this, at least one "impedance matching layer" is bonded to the front face of the PZT. A single matching layer can increase the transmission across the front face to 100%, provided that two important conditions are met. Firstly, the matching layer should have a thickness equal to a quarter of a wavelength. Secondly, it should have an impedance equal to $\sqrt{(z_{PZT} \cdot z_T)}$, where z_{PZT} is the impedance of PZT and z_T is the impedance of tissue. The explanation behind this remarkable achievement is that the sound reverberates back and forth repeatedly within the matching layer, producing a series of overlapping waves in the patient that are in phase with each other and hence combine to give a large resultant wave. At the same time, another series of waves is sent back into the PZT, which together exactly cancel-out the wave originally reflected at the PZT–matching layer interface (Figure 3.5).

One hundred per cent transmission through the matching layer only occurs at one frequency for which its thickness is exactly one-quarter of a wavelength. It is normal to choose the matching layer thickness to be correct for the centre frequency of the pulse, as there is more energy at this frequency than at any other. Smaller, but nevertheless worthwhile, improvements in transmission will occur at frequencies close to the centre frequency. However, at frequencies well removed from the centre frequency the matching layer will not be very effective. A $-3\,\mathrm{dB}$ transducer bandwidth (Figure 3.6) can be defined, in a similar way to the pulse bandwidth, described in Chapter 2. For a transducer, it is the range of frequencies over which its

efficiency, as a converter of electrical energy to sound energy or vice versa, is more than half its maximum. It is evident that, although the matching layer improves sensitivity at the centre frequency, it also acts as a frequency filter, reducing the bandwidth. For a transducer with a matching layer, a $-3\,\mathrm{dB}$ bandwidth of about 60% of the centre frequency can be achieved. Thus, a $3\,\mathrm{MHz}$ transducer with a matching layer could have a $-3\,\mathrm{dB}$ bandwidth of up to $1.8\,\mathrm{MHz}$.

A large tranducer bandwidth is crucial to good axial resolution, since the latter depends on a large pulse bandwidth (consistent with a short pulse, for example) and the pulse bandwidth cannot be more than that of the transducer producing it. The transducer bandwidth can be increased by using two, or more, matching layers, progressively reducing in characteristic impedance from the PZT to the patient's skin. The reason why this leads to a greater bandwidth is that the impedance change, and hence the reflection coefficient, at the PZT front face is less than that for the case of a single-matching layer. This applies at all frequencies, so there is less difference in the performance at the centre frequency relative to that at other frequencies. Improvements in backing layer and multiple-matching layer technologies have meant that $-3\,\mathrm{dB}$ bandwidths greater than 100% of centre frequency are now available.

A large transducer bandwidth is also needed for harmonic imaging (Chapter 4) and other modern developments. It is also a prerequisite of a "multi-frequency probe". This type of probe allows the operator to select one of a choice of operating frequencies according to the penetration required. Whatever centre frequency is selected, short bursts of oscillating voltage at that frequency are applied across the PZT plate to produce the ultrasound transmission pulses (see the section entitled Beam-former electronics at the end of this chapter). At the same time, the receiving amplifiers (Chapter 4) are tuned to that frequency. In order for a single probe to be able to operate at three frequencies, say 3, 5 and 7 MHz, it would need to have a centre frequency of 5 MHz and a bandwidth of 4 MHz, which is 80% of the centre frequency (Figure 3.6). Note that the bandwidths of the pulses generated at the upper and lower frequencies must be less than that of the transducer itself – this means the axial resolution to be expected from a probe in multi-frequency mode will be less than that which would be possible if the whole transducer bandwidth were used to generate a large bandwidth of 5 MHz pulse.

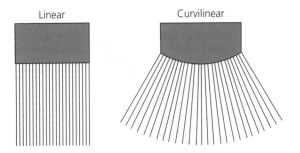

Fig. 3.7 Linear and curvilinear scan formats.

Lens

A lens is usually incorporated after the matching layer. Near the focus of the lens, the width of the beam is least and the transmitted amplitude, or receive sensitivity, is greatest. In linear-array probes, focusing in the scan plane is achieved entirely by electronic means, and so a cylindrical lens, producing focusing only in the plane perpendicular to the scan plane (elevation plane), is used. In phased-array and annular-array probes (see later) the lens may have some curvature (focusing action) in the scan planes as well as in the elevation plane, in order to augment the electronic focusing in the scan plane.

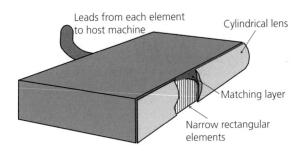

Fig. 3.8 Cut-away view of a linear-array probe, showing the elements, matching layer and lens.

Linear- and curvilinear-array scanners (beam-stepping arrays)

A common type of probe is the linear array, or its curved version – the curvilinear array. Linear arrays offer a rectangular field of view (Figure 3.7) that maintains its width close up to the probe face and is, therefore, particularly suitable when the region of interest extends right up to the surface (e.g. neck or limbs). Curvilinear probes work in the same way as linear arrays, but differ in that the array of elements along the front face forms a curve, rather than a straight line. They share the same benefit of a wide field of view at the surface, but have the additional advantage that the field of view becomes wider with depth. They are, therefore, popular for abdominal applications, including obstetrics. However, in order to maintain full contact, it is necessary to press the convex front face slightly into the patient. This makes the linear array more suitable than the curvilinear array

for applications where superficial structures, such as arteries or veins should not be deformed, or where the skin is sensitive. An answer to this problem is offered by trapezoidal (virtual curvilinear) arrays, discussed later.

From the outside a linear-array probe resembles a basically rectangular block with a rubber lens along the face that makes contact with the patient (Figure 3.8). Behind the lens is a matching layer, and behind this is a line array of typically 128 regularly spaced, narrow, rectangular transducer elements, separated by narrow barriers (kerfs), made of an inert material, usually a polymer or epoxy. Some linear-array probes have as many as 256 elements, but cost considerations and fabrication difficulties mean that 128 is a more common number. Note that these numbers are chosen, rather than say 200 or 100, since they are "round" numbers in binary terms, and hence digital computers find them more convenient to work with.

The width of each element is typically about 1.3 wavelengths (λ), being a compromise that gives a reasonably wide array ($128 \times 1.3\lambda = 83$ mm at 3 MHz), and hence a wide field of view, while still allowing the elements to be narrow enough to radiate over a wide range of angles

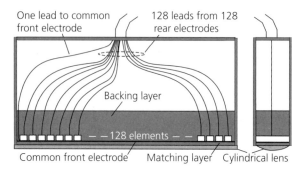

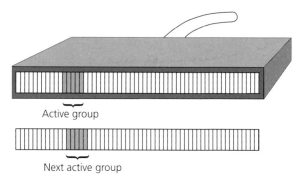

Fig. 3.9 Section through a linear-array probe. For clarity, the sub-dicing of each element is not shown.

Fig. 3.10 The active group is stepped along the array by dropping an element from one end and adding a new on to the other. In reality, the active group would contain at least 20 elements rather than the 5 shown here.

in the scan plane (Chapter 2). The longer side of each element determines the width of the beam in the elevation plane, and a typical value of about 30λ means a weakly focused beam is possible. Weak focusing gives a reasonably narrow width at all depths. Since all probe dimensions are proportional to wavelength, high-frequency probes are smaller than low-frequency ones. Thus, assuming 128 elements, a 3 MHz ($\lambda = 0.5$ mm) probe might typically have a lens face measuring about 85 mm by 15 mm, with each element being about 0.65 mm wide, whereas a 7.5 MHz ($\lambda = 0.2$ mm) probe will have a lens face measuring about 35 mm by 6 mm, with each element being about 0.25 mm wide.

The front electrodes of all the elements are usually connected together, so they share a common electrical lead. However, the rear electrode of each element is provided with a separate electrical lead (Figure 3.9), allowing the signals to and from each element to be individually processed by the beam-former. In practice, each element is usually further "sub-diced" into two or three even narrower elements. This is done because, otherwise, each element would be approximately as wide as it was thick[2] and an undesirable resonant vibration across the element width would accompany, and take energy from, the desired thickness vibration. This mechanical sub-dicing does not affect the number of electrically addressable elements, since the rear electrodes of the two or three sub-diced elements making up the original element are connected together and share a single lead.

Active group of elements

In order to interrogate a particular scan line, an "active group" of adjacent transducer elements, centred on that scan line, is used. While that scan line is being interrogated, all the other elements in the probe are

disconnected and idle. First, a pulse is transmitted, say using the central 20 elements of the group (further details of the transmission process are given at the end of this chapter under the heading "Beam-former electronics"). This pulse travels along the transmission beam, centred on the scan line. As soon as the pulse has been transmitted, a different combination of elements, still centred on the scan line, act together as a receiving transducer, defining the receive beam. The number of elements used for reception is initially less than that used for transmission, but this number is progressively increased as echoes return from deeper and deeper targets until it eventually exceeds that used for transmission (see DYNAMIC FOCUSSING AND APERTURE below). Both the transmission and receive beams can be focused, or otherwise altered, by controlling the signals to or from each of the elements in the active group, as described below.

Once all echoes have been received from one scan line, a new active group of elements, centred on the next scan line, is activated. This is achieved by dropping an element from one end of the old group and adding a new one at the other end (Figure 3.10). This advances the centre of the active group, and hence the scan line, by the width of one element. The new scan line is then interrogated by a new transmission and receive beam, centred on that line. The process is repeated until all the scan lines across the field of view have been interrogated, when a new sweep across the whole array is commenced.

Increasing the line density

Since this procedure produces scan lines spaced at intervals of one element width, an image with only

100 or so scan lines would be produced, assuming an array of 128 elements (the need for elements on both sides of a scan line means that scan lines cannot be located at the very ends of the array, and so there must be fewer scan lines than elements). The distance between scan lines should be less than the width of the beam in the scan plane, otherwise the tissue between scan lines would not be interrogated. Ideally, for good spatial sampling, the distance between scan lines should be about one-quarter of the beam width. In theory, the situation could be improved by using twice as many elements, each of half the width. However, this approach is unattractive to most manufacturers because of the technical difficulties and the cost implications.

In practice, various other methods are used to increase the scan line density. One method is to steer (deflect) all the beams to one side by a very small angle (1° or so) on even numbered sweeps, and by the same angle to the other side on odd numbered sweeps (Figure 3.11a). Beam-steering can be achieved by the technique described later in this chapter for phased-array probes. Normally, no attempt is made to show the small scan line deflections on the display — the display scan lines are simply shown as being perpendicular to the probe face — those for deflections to one side being interlaced between those for the opposite deflection. In effect, the distance between adjacent left- and right-deflected scan lines is taken to be at half the element spacing, even though this is only precisely true at half the depth at which the two sets of scan lines cross.

Another technique involves using an even number of elements in the active group in one sweep and an odd number in the next. For groups with an odd number of elements, the group centre point, and hence the scan line, lies in the middle of an element. For groups with an even number of elements, the scan line lies in the gap between two elements. Thus, over two sweeps, the spacing between scan lines is halved (Figure 3.11b). This method requires correction for the small change in sensitivity in alternate sweeps due to the slightly different beam-forming apertures.

Beam shape control in the scan plane

SCAN PLANE FOCUSING IN TRANSMISSION

Since the cylindrical lens does nothing to reduce the beam width in the scan plane, an electronic method of focusing must be provided for the scan plane, if good lateral resolution is to be achieved. This is controlled by the operator, who sets the transmission focus at the

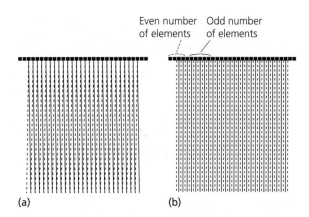

Fig. 3.11   Two ways of increasing line density. (a) Slight angulation of the beams in opposite directions on alternate sweeps. (b) Having an odd number elements in the active group in one sweep, and an even number in the next sweep.

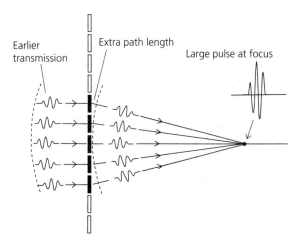

Fig. 3.12   Creating a transmission focus for a linear-array probe. In order to form a large amplitude pulse at the focus, pulses from all elements must arrive there at the same time. This is achieved by transmitting slightly earlier from elements that are further from the centre of the group.

depth for which optimum lateral resolution is desired. This ensures that the transmission beam is as narrow as possible there (the receive beam must also be narrow there, but this is considered next). Usually an arrowhead or other indicator alongside the image indicates the depth at which the transmission focus has been set. Pulses from all the elements in the active group must arrive at the transmission focus simultaneously in order to concentrate the power into a narrow "focal zone"

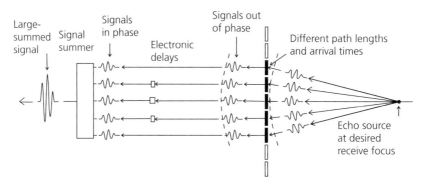

Fig. 3.13 Creating a receive focus for a linear-array probe. In order to obtain a large echo signal from a target at a desired receive focus, contributions from all elements must arrive at the signal summer at the same time. This is achieved by electronic delays that are greater for elements closer to the centre of the group.

there. However, the distance between an element and the focus, which lies on the beam axis passing through the centre of the group, is slightly, but crucially, greater for the outer elements of the group than for more central elements. Pulses from elements further from the centre of the active group must, therefore, be transmitted slightly earlier than those nearer the centre (Figure 3.12). The manufacturer builds a look-up table into the machine for each possible choice of transmission focus depth available to the operator. These tell the controlling computer, the appropriate "early start" for each element. At points outside the required focal zone, the individual pulses from different elements arrive at different times, producing no more than weak acoustic noise.

SCAN PLANE (DYNAMIC) FOCUSING AND APERTURE
IN RECEPTION

Focusing in reception means that, for each scan line, the scanner is made particularly sensitive to echoes originating at a specified depth (the receive focus) on the scan line. This also results in the receive beam being narrowed near this focus, further improving lateral resolution. In order for the sensitivity to be high for an echo coming from, or near, the receive focus, the echo signals produced by all transducer elements in the active group must contribute simultaneously to the resultant electronic echo signal. As in the case of transmission focusing, allowance must be made for the fact that the distance between the required focus and a receiving element is greater for elements situated towards the outside of the group than for those near the centre. This is done by electronically delaying the electrical echo signals produced by all transducer elements except the outermost, before summing them together (Figure 3.13). The

delays are chosen such that the sum of the travel time as a sound wave (from the focus to a particular element) plus the delay imposed on the electrical echo signal, is the same for all elements. This means that the imposed electronic delays are greater for elements closer to the centre of the active group, for which the sound wave travel times are least. In this way, a large-summed signal is obtained for echoes from the desired receive focal zone, but only a weak-summed signal (acoustic noise) results from echoes from elsewhere.

In practice, focusing in reception is automatically controlled by the machine, with no receive focus control available for the operator. This is because the ideal depth for the reception focus at any time is the depth of origin of the echoes arriving at the transducer at that time. This is zero immediately after transmission, becoming progressively greater as echoes return from deeper and deeper targets. Since the time needed for a two-way trip increases by 13 μs for every additional 1 cm of target depth, the machine automatically advances the receive focus at the rate of 1 cm every 13 μs. The continual advancement of the receive focus to greater and greater depths gives rise to the name "dynamic focusing in reception". In fact, high-performance machines advance the reception focus in several hundred tiny steps (as many as one for each image pixel down a scan line), during the echo receiving interval after each transmission. The "effective reception beam" (Figure 3.14) consists of a sequence of closely spaced focal zones, and is, therefore, narrow over a wide range of depths, not just at a single focal zone.

At the same time, as the receive focus is advanced, the number of elements in the active receive group is also

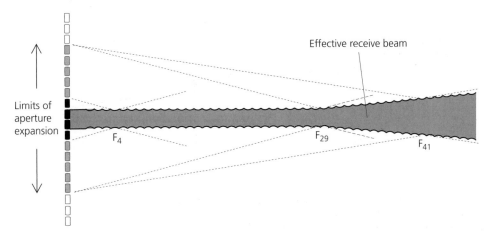

Fig. 3.14 Dynamic focusing and aperture in reception. The machine automatically changes the delays so that the receive focus advances at the rate of 1 cm every 13 μs. At the same time the aperture is expanded, so that the width of the beam at all the foci remains constant (up to the 29th focus in this example). If the aperture stops expanding, the beam widths at deeper foci become progressively greater. The scalloped lines enclosing all the focal zones indicate the "effective receive beam".

increased. The reason for this comes from the fact (Chapter 2) that the beam width at the focus is inversely proportional to the transducer aperture. It is, therefore, desirable that the active receiving group has as many elements (as large an aperture) as possible. However, there is no benefit in using a large group when receiving echoes from close targets since elements far from the centre of the group would not be able to receive echoes from them – these targets would be outside the individual receive beams of the outer elements (Figure 3.15). Such elements would be able to receive echoes from deeper targets, but they would contribute nothing but noise for echoes from close targets. Thus the maximum number of elements, it is worth including in the beam, increases with time after transmission, in proportion to the depth of the reception focus. This means the beam width in the successive focal zones remains fairly constant, keeping lateral resolution as uniformly good as possible at all depths.

Many machines limit the number of elements in the receiving group, on cost grounds, to a maximum of about 30. This means a constant receive beam width is only maintained up to the depth at which the aperture expansion is stopped (Figure 3.14). At greater depths, the beam becomes wider, and lateral resolution becomes noticeably worse. In some more sophisticated (expensive) machines, however, the receiving group continues to expand until all the elements in the array are included. These machines can maintain good lateral resolution to much greater depths.

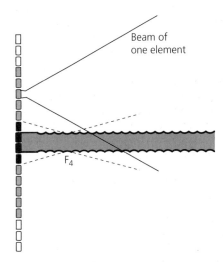

Fig. 3.15 An element can only contribute usefully to the receive active group, if the target lies in the individual beam of that element. Here, elements outside the four elements nearest the scan line cannot receive echoes from focal zone F_4 or nearer. The maximum useful aperture for the active group, increases as the depth of the receive focus increases.

SCAN PLANE APODISATION

Another beam-forming process, known as "apodisation", can also be employed. In transmission, this involves exciting the elements non-uniformly in order to control the intensity profile across the beam. For

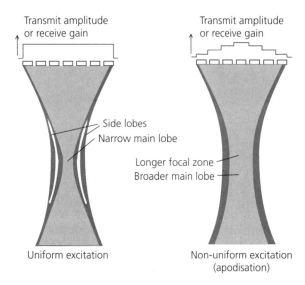

Fig. 3.16 Apodisation. By exciting outer elements less than those in the centre, side lobes can be suppressed and the focal zone extended. However, the width of the main lobe is increased. Non-uniform amplification of echoes from different elements can achieve similar changes in the receive beam.

example, if the inner elements are excited more than the outer elements, side lobes can be reduced in amplitude and the focal zone can be extended. However, as these benefits are at the expense of a broadening of the main lobe (Figure 3.16), a compromise is necessary and this is one judgement in which there is no common view among manufacturers. Apodisation of the receive beam can be achieved by giving different amplifications to the signals from each element. The receive beam apodisation can be changed dynamically to control side lobe characteristics as the receive focus is advanced.

SCAN PLANE MULTIPLE-ZONE FOCUSING

Further improvement in lateral resolution, albeit at the expense of frame rate, is possible by sub-dividing each scan line into two or more sections and interrogating each section with a separate transmission pulse, focused at its centre (Figure 3.17). For example, the operator might select transmission foci at two different depths – F_1 and F_2. These would be indicated by two arrowheads or other focus indicators down the side of the scan. One pulse would be transmitted with a focus at F_1 and echoes from depths up to about half-way between F_1 and F_2 would be captured. Then a second pulse would be transmitted with a focus at F_2 and echoes from all greater depths would be captured. The

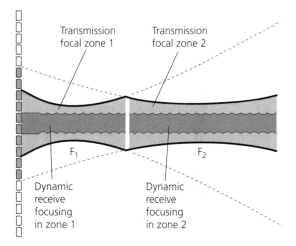

Fig. 3.17 Multiple-zone focusing. The operator has selected two focal zones (F_1 and F_2). Targets lying between the probe and a point about half-way between the two foci are interrogated with a transmission pulse focused at F_1. Targets beyond the half-way point are interrogated by transmitting another pulse along the same scan line, but focused at F_2. The heavy and light scalloped lines indicate the "effective transmission beam", and the "effective receive beam", respectively.

greater the number of transmission focal zones, the greater the depth range over which the "effective transmission beam" is narrow. Unfortunately, the greater the number of focal zones, the longer is spent on each scan line, and so the lower the frame rate.

When using multiple-transmission focal zones, other transmission parameters such as centre frequency, pulse length and shape, aperture, and apodisation may all be optimised independently for each of the focal zones. These changes can take account of the fact that pulses sent out to interrogate deeper regions will experience greater attenuation of the high frequencies in their spectra.

Grating lobes

These can occur with any probe having regularly spaced elements, such as a linear- or curvilinear-array probe or a phased-array probe (discussed later). They are weak replicas of the main beam, at substantial angles (up to 90°) on each side of it (Figure 3.18a). They are named "grating lobes" after the analogous phenomenon that occurs when a light beam passes through a grating of closely and regularly spaced narrow slits (diffraction grating) to form a series of new beams on each side of

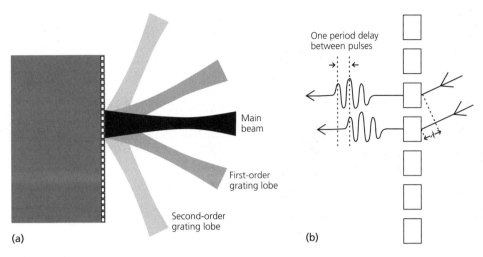

Fig. 3.18 (a) Grating lobes are weak replicas of the main beam, at angles of up to 90°. The greater the angle from the straight ahead direction, the weaker the grating lobe. (b) The first grating lobe occurs at that angle for which the arrival times of an echo at adjacent elements differ by one period.

the original beam. Grating lobes contribute spurious echoes (acoustic noise) and effectively widen the beam in the scan plane, degrading both lateral resolution and contrast resolution.

Consider the arrival of an echo pulse wave from a distant target or a receive focus at an angle to the scan line. The pulse will reach the various transducer elements at slightly different times. As the angle considered increases, the difference in arrival times at a pair of adjacent element will increase. If the distance between adjacent elements is large enough, an angle will exist for which this difference is a full wave period (Figure 3.18b). Thus, when say, the first peak in the pulse is arriving at the more distant element of the pair, the second peak in the pulse will be arriving at the nearer element. When summed in the beam-former, the coincidence of these two peaks (and of other peaks and troughs in the pulse) will lead to the electrical pulses from the two transducer elements reinforcing each other. The regular element spacing means the same thing happens for every pair of elements in the array, so that a large amplitude electronic echo pulse (grating lobe signal) is produced when electrical pulses from all the elements in the active group are combined.

Depending on the spacing of the elements and the number of cycles in the pulse, second- or even third-order grating lobe pairs may exist outside the first grating lobes. For these, the pulse arrives at one element two or three periods, respectively, ahead of at its neighbouring element. However, for a Nth-order grating lobe to exist,

there must be at least N cycles in the pulse; otherwise, there could be no constructive overlap between the signals from two elements. Clearly, the longer pulses and continuous waves used for Doppler techniques are more likely than the 2–3 cycle pulses used for imaging to produce such high-order grating lobes. In all cases, the greater the angle at which a grating lobe occurs, the weaker it will be, since each element is less efficient at transmitting or receiving sound waves in directions at large angles to the straight ahead direction.

The explanation given above has been for reception, but similar arguments apply in transmission by considering the arrival of pulses from pairs of adjacent elements at a distant point in the scan plane.

The smaller the centre-to-centre distance between elements, the larger the angle needed to produce the difference of one period needed for the first grating lobe. If this distance is less than half a wavelength, even a pulse arriving an angle of 90° would produce a time difference less than half a period. This would mean there could be no overlap at all between the first peak in the electrical pulse from one element and the second peak in the electrical pulse from the nearer adjacent element. Consequently, *there can be no grating lobes, if the centre-to-centre distance between elements is half a wavelength or less.*

Applying this rule to clinical linear-array probes with 128 or so elements, grating lobes are always to be expected, since the centre-to-centre distance between elements is then typically about 1.3λ. For the relatively few probes with 256 elements, and thus a centre-to-centre distance of about 0.65λ, grating lobes will still occur but will lie at much greater angles to the intended beam. This results in them being much weaker, due to the fall-off in transmission and reception efficiency with angle, as explained above.

Slice thickness

Since the transmission and receive beams have a certain width in the elevation dimension, echoes may be received from targets situated close to, but not actually in, the intended scan plane. These echoes will constitute acoustical noise and will, therefore, tend to limit penetration and contrast resolution. In effect the image is the result of interrogating a slice of tissue, rather than a plane. At any particular depth, the thickness of the slice is equal to the width of the beam in the elevation plane. The slice thickness is least at the depth at which the cylindrical lens is focused, and hence this is the depth where least acoustic noise can be expected (Figure 3.1). It is also the depth at which the greatest sensitivity can be achieved. The variation of sensitivity with depth depends on the depth at which the operator sets the scan plane transmission focus, but if this coincides with the elevation focus the beam will be at its narrowest in both dimensions and the sensitivity at that depth will be particularly high.

Slice thickness may be improved at other depths by the use of the so-called "1.5D" linear-array probes. These have several rows of elements instead of just one (Figure 3.19).

Electronic delays may be applied to the signals from each row in order to reduce beam width in the elevation dimension, using the electronic focusing techniques (such as transmission focusing and dynamic focusing in reception) described above for the scan plane. The focal length in the elevation plane can thus be automatically changed to match the scan plane focal length. The name is intended to distinguish these arrays from the full two-dimensional (2D) arrays, with equal numbers of elements in both dimensions, that are currently under development, and which will ultimately allow beams to be steered and dynamically focused in all directions.

Strongly convex curvilinear-array probes

These are curvilinear probes with such tight curvature that their field of view becomes sector shaped (Figure 3.20). The advantages of a sector format include a small "acoustic window" at the body surface, and an increasingly wide field of view at depth. Phased-array scanning systems (discussed next) are particularly well suited to sector scanning, but strongly convex curvilinear probes allow manufacturers of linear-array systems to offer sector scanning probes, without having to build in the specialised electronics that phased-array

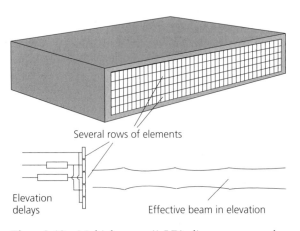

Fig. 3.19 Multiple-row (1.5 D) linear-array probe. Transmission and receive focusing techniques normally used for beam-forming in the scan plane can be used to control focusing in the elevation plane. This means a narrower slice thickness and hence less acoustic noise.

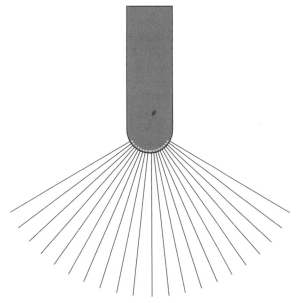

Fig. 3.20 A strongly convex curvilinear-array offers many of the advantages of a sector scan format for linear-array systems.

probes require. However, the convexity of the curvilinear probe face means they are less suitable in situations where the flat face of a phased-array probe is needed.

The maximum useful size of the active group is more limited than in a linear-array probe employing the same sized elements. Consequently, beam width in the focal zone is greater, and lateral resolution is less, than in a comparable linear array. This is primarily due to the fact that, as the number of active elements is increased, the outermost elements point more and more away from the centre line of the group (scan line), until eventually they cannot transmit or receive in that direction at all. Also, the longer paths between the outer elements and a receive focus mean that the problems of providing compensating delays are more challenging.

Phased-array probes (beam-steering probes)

This type of probe produces a "sector" scan format in which the scan lines emanate in a fan-like formation from a point in the centre of the probe face (Figure 3.21). As with all types of scanner, each scan line represents the axis of a transmission–receive beam.

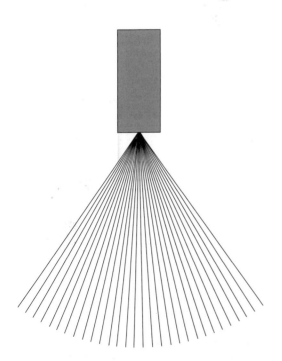

Fig. 3.21 Sector scan format of a phased-array probe.

The construction of a phased-array probe has some similarities to that of a linear-array probe. There are typically 128 rectangular transducer elements sharing a common lead to all their front electrodes, and an individual lead to each of their rear electrodes, as well as matching and backing layers (Figure 3.22). A lens provides fixed weak focusing in the elevation dimension, and in some cases a modest degree of focusing in the scan plane to augment the electronic focusing in that plane. However, the transducer array is much shorter in the scan plane dimension, with an overall aperture of typically 30λ square. The individual elements are much narrower ($\lambda/2$) and one advantage of this is that they do not need to be subdiced, as is the case for the wider elements in a linear array. Unlike the linear-array probe, which uses a different "active group" of elements to interrogate each scan line, all the elements in the array probe are used to form the transmission and receive beams for every scan line. Since the array dimension and method of focusing in the elevation plane (cylindrical lens) is the same as for a linear-array probe, the two types of probe give similar slice thickness.

Electronic beam-steering and focusing in the scan plane

Similar signal delaying techniques to those previously described for the linear-array probe are used to achieve focusing of the transmission and receive beams in the scan plane. However, as well as being focused in the scan plane, the beams must also be steered by up to ±45 in that plane. The principle behind beam-steering is really just an extension of that used for focusing. In fact, it follows automatically from arranging for the transmission focus and the multiple-receive foci to all lie on an oblique scan line.

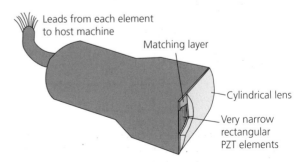

Fig. 3.22 Cut-away view of the elements, matching layer and lens of a phased-array probe.

As described previously for linear-array probes, focusing in transmission requires that pulses from all the elements arrive simultaneously at the transmission focus. The early starts needed by each element can be pre-calculated by the manufacturer for each possible position of the transmission focus along the various scan lines (Figure 3.23). The fact that the transmission focus on a particular scan line is not directly in front of the transmitting elements is of little consequence, provided the transmission beams of

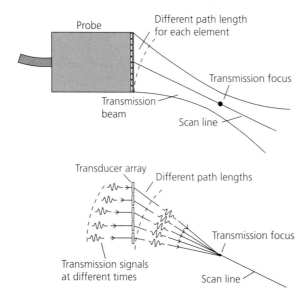

Fig. 3.23 Creating a transmission focus for a phased-array probe. The principle is the same as for a linear-array probe, except that the focus lies on a scan line that is generally oblique.

the individual elements diverge sufficiently to allow the sound from every element to reach it. The use of very narrow elements ensures this, since, as described in Chapter 2, a very narrow element will have an extremely short near field and a far field with a very large angle of divergence.

Similarly, in reception, carefully pre-selected electronic delays are used to ensure that an echo from a desired receive focus takes the same time to reach the signal summer, irrespective of which element is considered (Figure 3.24). As for a linear-array probe, dynamic focusing is used in reception, so again there is no receive focus control available to the operator. The fact that all the receive foci lie along a scan line at some angle to the probe's axis does not matter, provided that each element can receive from ("see") any receive focus. This is ensured by the very narrow width of the elements.

Other techniques for improving lateral resolution, such as apodisation and multiple-zone focusing in transmission are also used in phased-array systems. These techniques are identical to those already described for linear-array systems.

Image quality variation across the field of view

The operator should always angle the probe so that any region of particular interest is in the centre of the probe's field of view. This is where beam deflections are least and, as discussed below, where beam widths are least and signal-to-noise ratio is highest. It will, therefore, be where the best lateral resolution, the highest sensitivity and the best contrast resolution will be obtained.

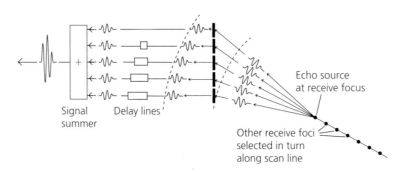

Fig. 3.24 Creating a receive focus for a phased-array probe. The principle is the same as for a linear-array probe, except that the receive foci lie along a scan line that is generally oblique.

DEPENDENCE OF BEAM WIDTH AND SENSITIVITY ON ANGLE

A particular artefact of phased arrays is that the width of the beam, measured at its focus, increases with increasing steering angle (Figure 3.25). Hence lateral resolution becomes poorer towards the sides of the sector-shaped field of view. The width of a strongly focused beam at its focus is inversely proportional to the ratio of transducer aperture to focal length (Chapter 2). Another way of expressing this would be to say it becomes smaller, if the angular width of the transducer, as "seen" from the focus, is large. Just as a door or window looks wider when viewed from directly in front than from somewhat to the side, so the angular width of the transducer aperture is greatest when seen from a point on a scan line at right angles to the probe face, and is less when seen from a scan line steered to a large angle.

Another problem is that, because the individual elements are most efficient when transmitting in, or receiving from, directions close to the "straight ahead" direction, sensitivity decreases with steering angle.

GRATING LOBES

In general, the close spacing of the elements in phased arrays tends to reduce the seriousness of grating lobes compared to those in linear arrays. In view of the "half-wavelength" criterion given earlier when discussing grating lobes for linear arrays, it might be thought that grating lobes should be impossible for phased arrays, since their elements widths are less than half a wavelength ($\lambda/2$). However, wavelength (λ) here refers to that of the centre frequency of the pulse, and it should be remembered that a typical wide-bandwidth pulse will have significant energy at frequencies much higher than this. These higher frequencies have shorter wavelengths and so the $\lambda/2$ condition may not be satisfied for them. Thus weak side lobes at these higher frequencies will, in fact, occur.

Furthermore, such grating lobes will grow stronger at large steering angles (Figure 3.26). As mentioned previously, the individual transducer elements are most efficient when transmitting in, or receiving from, directions close to the "straight ahead" direction. Since beam-steering deflects the grating lobes as well as the intended beam, steering the main lobe to one side will also steer the grating lobe that is following behind it more towards the straight ahead direction. This grating lobe will, therefore, strengthen and generate more acoustic noise, at the same time as the deflected main lobe is weakening.

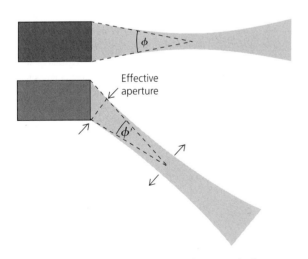

Fig. 3.25 The beam from a phasedarray probe becomes wider as the angle of deflection increases. This is because the angular width of the transducer, as seen from the focus, becomes less ($\phi' < \phi$).

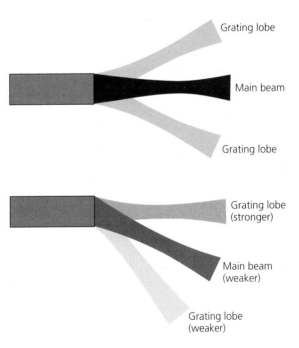

Fig. 3.26 Grating lobes from a phased-array probe are generally weak. As the deflection of the main beam increases, some grating lobes point more ahead and so become stronger. At the same time the main beam becomes weaker.

Hybrid beam-stepping/ beam-steering probes

Some scanning techniques involve steering the beams from a linear- or curvilinear-array probe away from the normal straight ahead direction. One example, previously mentioned, is the use of small deflections to increase line density in linear-array scanners. Another is the need to transmit and receive along an angled "Doppler line" in a duplex linear-array system (see "Mixed mode scanning", later).

Beam-steering in linear arrays is achieved using the combined focusing and steering technique that was described earlier for phased-array scanners. However, the relatively large width of transducer elements in linear-array probes compared to those in phased arrays, leads to greater problems. As the beam is progressively deflected there is greater reduction in sensitivity and greater acoustic noise from grating lobes. Despite these problems, a number of hybrid scan formats have been developed for linear arrays, in which both beam-stepping and beam-steering are used.

Trapezoidal (virtual curvilinear) scanning

Some linear-array systems achieve a trapezoidal field of view by steering the scan lines situated towards the ends of the probe progressively outwards (Figure 3.27). Such probes provide the large field of view advantage of a curvilinear array, without the tissue compression problem that a convex front face generates.

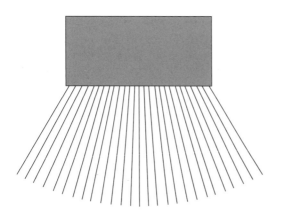

Fig. 3.27 A trapezoidal scanning format is similar to that of a curvilinear probe, but with the practical advantage of a flat probe face.

Steered linear arrays

It is sometimes advantageous to be able to steer the whole field of view of a linear-array probe to one side – to view blood vessels under the angle of the jaw, for example. A number of manufacturers, therefore, provide the option of steering all the transmission and receive beams (i.e. all the scan lines) to left or right, producing a parallelogram-shaped field of view (Figure 3.28).

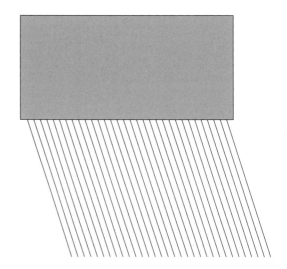

Fig. 3.28 A linear-array probe with beam-steering.

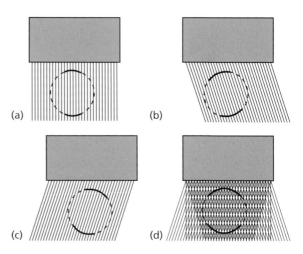

Fig. 3.29 Compound scanning. Several scans from different directions are averaged. This gives more complete delineation of organ boundaries as well as reduced noise and speckle.

Compound scanning

An extension of the steered linear-array technique is to superimpose several such angled views in a single "compound" scan (Figure 3.29). This technique, which is possible for both linear and curvilinear probes, gives more complete delineation of the boundaries of anatomical features, since many such boundaries only give a strong reflection, if the scan lines meet them at perpendicular incidence. Compounding also produces much finer "speckle patterns" (Chapter 5) and reduced acoustic noise. Whereas a genuine tissue target, detected in several different views, will always be shown at the same point in the final image, speckle and noise pattern will be different for each view and will tend to be cancelled out.

Compounding involves a loss of temporal resolution, since each displayed frame is the average of several sweeps. In common with the "frame-averaging" noise reduction technique described in Chapter 4, this introduces a degree of "persistence" to the image. Thus, if each displayed image was the average of the previous nine different sweeps (views), and an organ cross-section were to change instantly from A to B, nine frames would need to pass before all trace of the image of A was lost from the displayed image. Where necessary, a reasonably high-speed compromise is possible by displaying the average of just the last three or so sweeps.

Time-saving techniques for array probes

Real-time operation requires compromises between three competing qualities:

1. temporal resolution;

2. size of the field of view;

3. image quality (e.g. lateral resolution, contrast resolution, dynamic range).

Improvements in any one of these must be at the expense of one or both of the other two. For example, a reduction in frame rate occurs if the maximum depth is increased (more time per scan line) or the width of the field of view is increased (more scan lines). Multiple-zone focusing improves lateral resolution, but this is at the expense of temporal resolution because of the need to remain longer on each scan line while interrogating several zones instead of just one. Compound scanning improves image quality through reduced speckle and

acoustic noise and by better boundary delineation, but reduces temporal resolution. Some of the techniques described in Chapter 4, such as frame averaging and tissue harmonic imaging by pulse inversion improve image quality, but are at the expense of temporal resolution.

If time can be used more efficiently, the time savings can be used to increase one or more of the above three qualities. The following techniques are examples of this.

Write zoom

This technique presents a full-screen real-time image of a restricted area of the normal field of view, selected by the operator (Figure 3.30). Once selected, write zoom restricts the interrogation process to this operator-defined region of interest. One obvious way of using the consequent time savings would be to increase the frame rate. Alternatively, some or all of the time savings could be used to improve lateral resolution, both by narrowing the beam using multiple-zone focusing and by increasing the line density.

Line multiplexing

The frame rate penalty associated with using multiple-zone transmission focusing can be reduced by breaking the usual "rule" that all echoes should have returned from one scan line before transmitting along the next line. Instead, interrogation of each line may be divided over several time periods, interspersed with periods spent interrogating other lines. For example (Figure 3.31), when echoes have been received from the first (most superficial) focal zone on scan line 1, rather than wait for the unwanted echoes from deeper structures to return before transmitting to the second focal zone on line 1, a transmission is sent from another active group centred on a well-removed scan line (e.g. scan line 50) to interrogate the first focal zone of that line. The choice of a distant scan line, in this case about half-way along the probe, ensures that the unwanted echoes from one line do not reach the receiving element group on the other line. As soon as the echoes have arrived from the first zone on line 50, a transmission might then be sent to the first focal zone on scan line 2, etc. Only when the first focal zone on all the scan lines has been interrogated, are the second focal zones on all lines interrogated. These, too, are interrogated in the scan line sequence 1, 50, 2, 51, etc., to save time in the same way. Note that, although more than one transmission pulse is

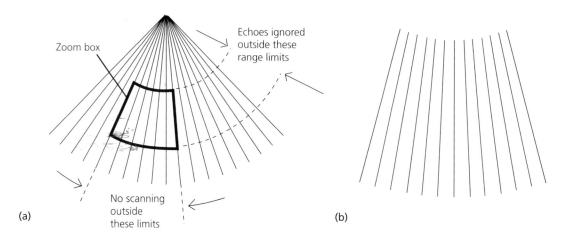

Fig. 3.30 Write zoom. A "zoom box" is defined by the operator. Scanning is then restricted to this area, allowing either a higher-frame rate, or improved lateral resolution by scanning with narrower, more closely spaced beams, or both.

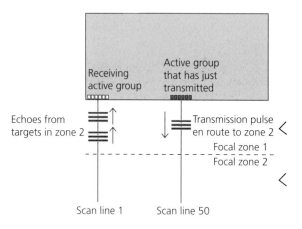

Fig. 3.31 Line multiplexing saves time. A pulse is already on its way to a particular zone on a new line (e.g.line 50), as echoes are being received from that zone on the old line (e.g. line 1).

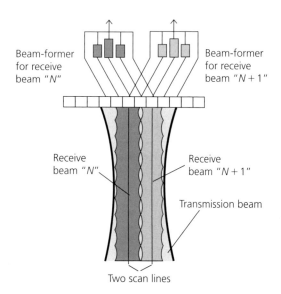

Fig. 3.32 Parallel beam-forming in reception saves time. One pulse is transmitted down a weekly focused transmission beam. Two receive beam-formers act in parallel to simultaneously interrogate two scan lines lying within the transmission beam, using just that one transmission pulse.

in flight at a time, echo reception does not take place on more than one line at a time.

Parallel beam-forming in reception

Since dynamic focusing is used in reception, the effective receive beam is narrower than the weakly focused transmission beam. In fact, it can be arranged for the transmission beam to accommodate two receive beams side by side (Figure 3.32). By sharing the same

transmitted pulse, the echoes from targets located on two adjacent scan lines can be processed simultaneously ("in parallel") in two separate receive beam-formers. The different focusing delays for each receive beam may be in the form of hardware or software. In the former case, each element is connected to two physically separate beam-forming circuits. In the latter case, the two sets of delays are applied on a time-shared basis to digital samples of the echo signal from each element. In some cardiac applications, where high-frame rates can be important, as many as four scan lines are interrogated in parallel ("quad processing"). However, this requires an even broader transmission beam and hence some further compromise in lateral resolution.

Mixed mode scanning

Array scanners make it possible for the operator to highlight a specific scan line on a B-mode image and simultaneously generate a real-time M-mode scan, A-mode scan or a Doppler spectrum for that line on the same display screen.

This is particularly useful in cardiological applications, where a phased-array probe is commonly used because of its ability to fit between ribs. Here, the simultaneous display of a M-mode line and a real-time B-mode (2D) scan allows the operator to check that the M-mode line is placed, and remains, in the correct anatomical position (Figure 3.33). Although the two scans appear to be formed simultaneously, in fact the beam-former rapidly switches back and forth between B-mode and M-mode interrogations. After every few lines of B-mode interrogation, the beam is made to jump to the selected M-mode scan line for one transmission and echo acquisition sequence. It then jumps back to continue the B-mode scan for another few lines; then jumps back to the M-mode line, etc.

"Duplex" Doppler scanning is another example of mixed mode scanning. Here, Doppler measurements are made of blood flow or tissue movements in a "sample volume", whose position is indicated on a "Doppler line" on the B-mode image (Chapter 9). This line can be set by the operator to be either parallel to, or at an angle to, the image scan lines. When set at an angle to the scan lines, the beam-steering and focusing techniques described earlier (see "Phased arrays") are used to interrogate that line. Alternatively, a separate "Doppler" transducer may be built into the probe to one side of the array, angled so that its beam runs diagonally across the field of view.

As explained in Chapter 9, the Doppler line must be interrogated at a high repetition frequency, much higher than would be possible even by jumping to the Doppler line after every B-mode line. The Doppler line is, therefore interrogated without interruption, except for very

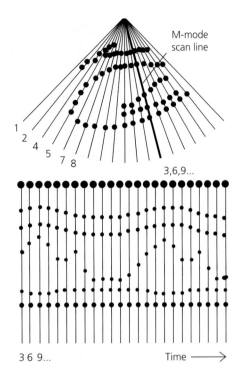

Fig. 3.33 Mixed M-mode and B-mode scanning. The first two transmissions are directed along two lines of the B-mode. The third is transmitted along the M-mode scan line. The fourth and fifth pulses interrogate the next two B-mode scan lines; then the sixth interrogates the M-mode scan line again; etc. Thus the two scans proceed in parallel.

brief periods (about 20 ms) every second or so, as determined by the operator, in which the machine performs one complete "update" frame of the B-mode. Each of these B-mode update images is held frozen on the screen next to the on-going Doppler display until it is automatically replaced by the next one. Note that the pulses transmitted along the Doppler line usually have a lower frequency and greater length than those transmitted along the imaging lines.

Mechanically scanned probes

Mechanical scanning is a popular option for frequencies above around 15–20 MHz, due to the difficulties of fabricating high-frequency linear- or phased-array probes.[3] It was the original scanning method for all applications but, for scans below about 10 MHz, linear- or curvilinear-array probes and phased-array probes are now used much more commonly. Despite the general disadvantages that are commonly associated with the moving components and water baths of mechanical scanners – bulk, vibration, leakage, wear and tear, etc. – a general advantage of all mechanical scanners over linear- or phased-array probes is that they do not suffer from grating lobes, and thus generate less acoustic noise.

Linear mechanical scanners

Mechanical scanners producing rectangular, or trapezoidal, fields of view are used for high-frequency scanning of superficial sites, such as the eye and skin. Here, the transducer is driven back and forth inside an enclosed water bath at the end of a handheld probe (Figure 3.34). The transducer must move in a water-filled bath, rather than in air, since the latter would result in virtually zero transmission across both the transducer–air and the air–skin interfaces (Chapter 2). Part of the wall of this water

bath is made from a thin plastic or rubber membrane, allowing transmission into the patient. Reverberations (Chapter 5) between the transducer and this wall (effectively the patient) can cause a noticeable artefact. The cable between the probe and the machine contains a coaxial cable, carrying signals to and from the transducer, and leads carrying the drive current to the electric motor, and the signal from the position sensor. Linear mechanical scanning is only practical for transducers operating at frequencies above 10 MHz or so, because of the vibration that heavier, lower frequency, transducers would produce when constantly reversing direction.

Mechanical sector scanners

This method is an option where a small "footprint" and a sector-shaped field of view would be advantageous. A sector scan format is the most appropriate mechanical scanning method for lower-frequency transducers, since a linear scan format would involve too much vibration. A schematic diagram of a "rocker" type of mechanical sector scanner is shown in Figure 3.35. The probe contains the same basic features as a linear scanner, but is designed to produce a rocking motion. The probe can be made compact, as shown here, by having the necessary drive components built into and closely around the rocking transducer assembly. Some "mechanical" probes have two transducers of different frequencies or focal lengths, back to back, and a means of flipping the most appropriate one into position.

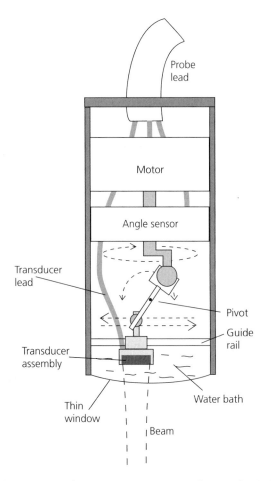

Fig. 3.34 Schematic representation of a mechanical linear scanning probe, as might be used for the eye or skin.

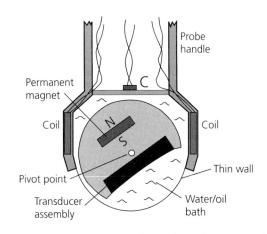

Fig. 3.35 Representation of a mechanical scanner probe in which the coils and magnet of the motor, the position sensor (C) and the transducer are all designed to fit and work together in a compact unit.

Annular-array scanners

These are mechanical scanners in which the single disc transducer is replaced with an *annular-array* transducer (Figure 3.36), consisting of several concentric circular transducer elements. As with other array probes, the front electrodes of all the elements are connected together to a common lead, while there is a separate electrical lead to the rear electrode of each element. This means that each element can be given its own individual electrical transmission pulse, and the echo signals from each element can be individually processed and combined to provide electronic control of focusing and apodisation. Note that the annular transducer is physically moved through its sector sweep by a motor in just the same way as for any mechanical scanner.

Annular-array probes have an advantage over other mechanical scanners in that the operator can improve lateral resolution by using beam-forming techniques similar to those previously described for linear-array scanners. Thus, by transmitting slightly earlier from the outer ring elements, the depth of the transmission focus can be adjusted to match that of a particular target of interest, or multiple-zone transmission focusing can be selected. Dynamic focusing in reception can be achieved by imposing electronic delays on echoes from all but the outermost ring elements. Variable apodisation can also be achieved by applying different drive voltages to the various elements in transmission, or giving different amplifications to signals from each element in reception.

An advantage over both other mechanical scanners and array probe scanners (except the 1.5 D arrays mentioned earlier), is that annular arrays generate a slice thickness that is narrower over a larger depth range. This comes from the fact that the transducer elements are circular. The transmission and receive beams are, therefore, circular in cross section and the use of multiple-zone focusing in transmission, and dynamic focusing in reception, affect the beam equally in the elevation plane and in the scan plane. This contrasts with the situation with linear and phased arrays (except 1.5 D arrays), where electronic focusing only benefits the beam width in the scan plane.

An advantage over array probe scanners is that they suffer much less from grating lobes. This is because the difference in an echo's arrival time at two adjacent elements will not be the same at all points on the array face.

Notwithstanding the practical disadvantages associated with mechanical scanning, annular-array scanners, therefore, have the potential to provide images of superior contrast resolution than those from linear-array or phased-array scanners.

Endo-probes

These are probes intended for insertion into a natural body cavity or surgical wound. A number of different types of endo-probe are represented in Figure 3.37. The ability to place the transducer close to a target organ or mass means that there is less attenuation from intervening tissue, which in turn means a higher frequency may be used and, therefore, superior lateral and axial resolution obtained. The image distortions and artefacts due to any tissue heterogeneity or strongly reflecting or refracting interfaces between the transducer and the target are also reduced.

All the beam-forming techniques previously mentioned are employed in endo-probes, the choice being

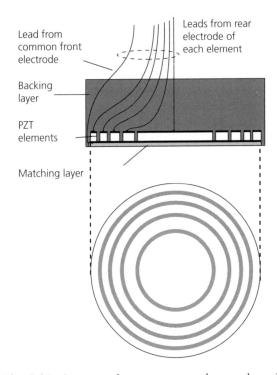

Lead from common front electrode

Leads from rear electrode of each element

Backing layer

PZT elements

Matching layer

Fig. 3.36 In an annular-array scanner, the transducer is composed of several concentric ring transducers, each with its own rear electrode lead. Otherwise, the probe is the same as a mechanical scanner with single element transducer.

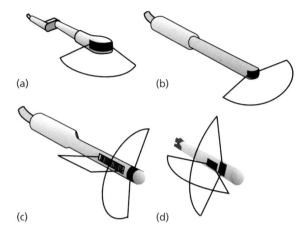

Fig. 3.37 Examples of endo-probes. (a) Curvilinear probe for trans-vaginal scanning. (b) "End-fire" curvilinear-array probe for trans-rectal or trans-vaginal scanning. (c) "Bi-plane" trans-rectal probe with both a linear array and a curvilinear array – allowing both transverse and longitudinal scans of the prostate. (d) Trans-oesophageal probe with two phased arrays set at right angles, giving two orthogonal cross-sections of the heart.

determined primarily by the anatomical features and constraints of the particular application. Thus, a curvilinear array offers a field of view of an appropriate shape for trans-vaginal scanning. The wide field of view close to a linear array is suitable for imaging the prostate from the rectum. Phased arrays give a wide field of view for visualising the left side of the heart from a trans-oesophageal probe.

360° mechanically scanned endo-probes

These rotate a transducer about the axis of a probe so that the beam sweeps through a 360° circle, in a similar way to a light beam-sweeping around a lighthouse. Such probes consist of an outer tube within which is a rotating inner rod, bearing the outwardly pointing transducer. In order for the signals to and from the transducer to cross between the stationary and rotating parts, either slip-rings or a transformer arrangement is used.

The technique can be used with low-frequency transducers, but, because of the size and mass of the transducers, such scanners are likely to be limited to low-frame rates or involve manual rotation of the transducer. A disposable rubber sheath may be clamped to the outer tube, which, when inflated with water,

provides an offset between the rotating transducer and the patient. Applications of this type of probe include scanning the prostate from within the rectum, and imaging the bladder wall with a probe introduced into the bladder via the urethra.

High-frequency versions (e.g. 30 MHz) can be inserted via a catheter into a blood vessel in order to visualise the vessel wall. The transducer is attached to a rotating wire within a non-rotating outer cable. One difficulty with this method is that friction between the rotating wire and the outer cable causes the cable, and hence the transducer, to weave around within the blood vessel. The continual movement of the viewing point with respect to the target leads to difficulties in interpreting the images. The cylindrical-array probes discussed next do not have this problem and are now offering an alternative method for intra-luminal scanning.

Intra-luminal and intra-cardiac catheter probes using transducer arrays

Strongly convex probes were discussed earlier as an exaggerated form of curvilinear array. The ultimate development of this idea is to curve a linear array so tightly that a complete cylindrical array is formed. Such probes offer an alternative to the mechanical 360° scanners mentioned above (Figure 3.38a).

Tiny, high-frequency (e.g. 2 mm diameter, 30 MHz), cylindrical arrays, mounted on catheters, can be inserted into a blood vessel. This gives a direct high-resolution image of the internal wall of the blood vessel. One construction method is to mount the transducer elements, their connecting leads, and other electronic hardware on a flexible printed circuit and then roll this into the required final cylindrical form. Probes made this way have been designed as single use, disposable devices.

Another type of probe designed for intra-cardiac imaging has a 64-element phased array (5–9 MHz) mounted on the side of a 3 mm diameter catheter (Figure 3.38b). The catheter can be introduced into the heart via the femoral or jugular vein.

A problem facing the designers of catheter-mounted arrays is that it is not possible to accommodate 128 or so leads within the narrow catheter. Consequently, the arrays have fewer elements, and in some cases the "synthetic aperture" technique is employed. This allows the number of leads to be a fraction of the number of array elements. Electronic switches are mounted next to the transducer array so that a given lead can be

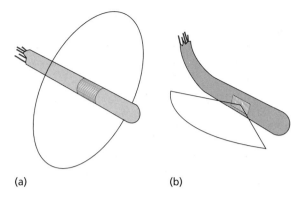

Fig. 3.38 (a) Intra-luminal probe with a cylindrical high-frequency (typically 30 MHz) array, providing 360° transverse images of blood vessel walls. (b) Intra-cardiac phased-array probe mounted on the end of a steerable catheter.

connected to one of several different elements as required. After each transmission the echo sequence from the selected elements are digitised and stored. Several transmissions – reception sequences are carried out, along the same scan line, with the leads being connected to different elements for each one. When all the elements have been selected, all the stored echo sequences are summed together, with each sequence being delayed relative to the others by the appropriate amount. These delay time intervals are just those that would have been used if the echo sequences from all the elements had been available at the same time – as in the electronic focusing techniques described earlier in this chapter.

Beam-former electronics

Transmission

In transmission, electrical drive pulses must be applied to the individual elements at the appropriate times. As explained earlier, these times depend on the depth of the transmission focus selected by the operator and the distance of each element from the centre of the transmitting group. Either a dedicated pulse generator is provided for each element in the probe, or, in the case of a linear-array probe, a smaller number of pulse generators provide pulses for the active group, with electronic switches routing these to the particular elements that form that group at any time.

The electrical drive pulse is applied across the PZT plate of the transducer element, via the signal leads connected to the front and back electrodes. Typically, this will consist of 2–3 cycles of an oscillating voltage, with a peak-to-peak amplitude of as much as 200–300 V. The waveform of the drive pulse may be very similar to that of the required ultrasonic pulse, or simply a series of abrupt rectangular pulses at the appropriate frequency, according to the sophistication of the scanning system. The actual peak-to-peak voltage applied is determined by the setting of the machine's "output power" control, larger voltages producing transmission pulses of greater amplitude. The frequency and duration of this oscillating pulse determine the centre frequency and pulse length of the transmitted ultrasonic pulse, respectively. For pulsed Doppler applications (Chapters 9 and 10), the applied voltage waveform, and hence the transmitted pulse, may have as many as 20 cycles, according to the setting of the "gate width" control.

Different elements in the active group may be driven at different amplitudes, according to the apodisation chosen by the manufacturer. The amplitude, waveform and frequency of the drive pulse to a particular element may all vary according to the depth at which the operator sets the transmission focus (or foci). In general, greater amplitudes and lower frequencies are more suitable for transmissions to deep foci, since propagating through a greater length of tissue involves greater attenuation, particularly for higher frequencies.

Reception

In reception, the echo signal from each element must be amplified, digitised, delayed and summed with those from all the other active elements to form a resultant signal. This is then processed as described in Chapter 4.

There is usually a dedicated "pre-amplifier" for each transducer element, but, in a linear-array probe, it is possible to use electronic switches to route echo signals from the particular elements forming the active receive group to a smaller number of pre-amplifiers. The pre-amplifiers increase the amplitude of the voltage waveform produced between the front and back electrodes of the transducer elements. They are tuned to amplify only the frequencies in the echo spectrum in order to minimise the amplification of electronic noise. They usually have a gain (ratio of voltage out to voltage in) that increases automatically with time after transmission. This "time gain compensation (TGC)" technique is needed to reduce the range of echo amplitudes that the subsequent digitising stage has to deal with. It compensates for the fact that echoes returning late from deeper targets have suffered much more attenuation than those that return early, and, therefore, may be 60 dB or so weaker. Further, operator-set TGC is usually applied after the beam-former stage, as discussed more fully in Chapter 4.

The echo signals from each pre-amplifier are then "digitised". This involves sampling the voltage waveform of each echo many times per cycle and converting the sample voltages to digital numbers. The process of analogue-to-digital conversion is discussed more fully in Chapter 4. Once in digital form, the echo signals from each element (i.e. in each "channel") can be delayed and summed together as required. Being under software control, these digital beam-forming operations can be as complex as required, customised for each probe and mode, and readily updated.

Notes

1. The wavelength here is calculated using the speed with which sound propagates between the two flat faces of the PZT plate. In array probes, discussed later, the plate is made up of PZT elements separated by narrow barriers (kerfs), having a lower speed of sound, so the average speed across the plate is lower than that in pure PZT.

2. Although the typical element width of 1.3λ might seem very different to the element thickness of 0.5λ, the former is for a wave in tissue, while the latter is for a wave in PZT. Since the speed of sound, and hence the wavelength, in PZT is 2–3 times higher than is in the tissue, the two dimensions are, in fact, similar.

3. Rapidly advancing transducer-array technology means that the frequency at which array probes can operate is continually increasing.

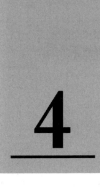

4

B–MODE
INSTRUMENTATION

K Martin

Signal amplitude processing
Amplification
Analogue–to–digital conversion
Amplitude demodulation
Harmonic imaging
Image storage

Signal amplitude processing

The beam-forming techniques described in the previous chapter are used to acquire echo information from different parts of the imaged cross section by selection of the transducer array elements and manipulation of the relative timings of their transmit and receive signals. These yield echo sequences, which represent the B-mode image lines and define the spatial properties of the image. The brightness or amplitude information contained in the B-mode image is also essential to diagnosis, and it is the processing of this aspect of the echo information that we consider mainly in this chapter.

Figure 4.1 illustrates, in block-diagram form, the essential elements of the complete B-mode system, and shows that the B-mode amplitude information is processed in various ways before storage in the image memory, from where the image is displayed. Although it is probably easiest to imagine that, as illustrated, amplitude processing is applied to the B-mode image lines only after the beam-former, in practice some must be applied at an earlier stage to allow the beam-forming processes to be

carried out. Also some processing may be carried out after the image memory to improve the display.

Amplification

The echo signals generated at the transducer elements are generally too small in amplitude to be manipulated and displayed directly and need to be amplified (made bigger). Figure 4.2 shows the conventional symbol for an electronic amplifier. This device in reality consists of numerous transistors and other electronic components, but can be treated as a single entity with an input terminal, and an output terminal. The voltage signal to be amplified (V_{in}) is applied to the input terminal, and the amplified voltage signal (V_{out}) is available at the output terminal. The voltage gain of the amplifier is defined by the ratio V_{out}/V_{in}. Figure 4.2 illustrates the effect that a simple amplifier would have on an imaginary stepped voltage input signal. There are two points to note. First, in the ouput signal, each step is larger by the same ratio. That is, the voltage gain (in this case ×3) is the same for all voltage levels in the input signal. This

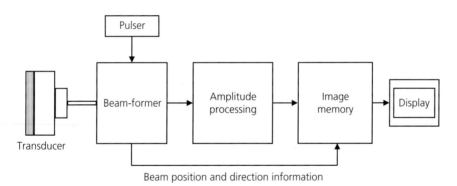

Fig. 4.1 The amplitude of the echo signals must be processed before storage in the image memory. Some amplitude processing also takes place before beam forming.

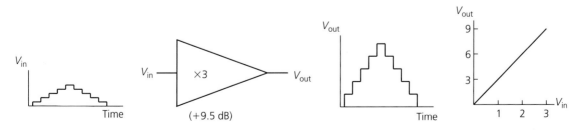

Fig. 4.2 Linear amplification. All signals are multiplied by the same gain factor.

is referred to as linear amplification, because a graph of V_{out} against V_{in} is a straight line. Second, the voltage gain is constant with time. Each of the downward steps in the second half of the signal is amplified to the same extent as the corresponding upward steps in the first half. An amplifier of this type is used to amplify all echo signals equally, irrespective of when they return to the transducer. This type of gain is called overall gain and may be adjusted by the user of the ultrasound system. The effect on the image is to make all echoes brighter or darker, whatever is their depth in the image.

Attenuation

As described in Chapter 2, when an ultrasound pulse propagates through tissue, it is attenuated (made smaller). Echoes returning through tissue to the transducer are also attenuated. Hence, an echo from an interface at a large depth in tissue is much smaller than that from a similar interface close to the transducer (Figure 4.3). The attenuation coefficient of tissues is measured in $dB\,cm^{-1}$. For example, if a particular tissue attenuates an ultrasound pulse by $1.5\,dB\,cm^{-1}$, the amplitude of the pulse will be reduced by $15\,dB$, when it reaches an interface

10 cm from the transducer. The echo from this interface will be attenuated by 15 dB also on its journey back to the transducer, so that compared to an echo from a similar interface close to the transducer, the echo will be 30 dB smaller. In this tissue, echoes received from similar interfaces will be smaller by 3 dB for each centimetre of depth.

Time–gain control

In a B-mode image, the aim is to relate the display brightness to the strength of the reflection at each interface regardless of its depth. However, as we have just noted, echoes from more distant targets are much weaker than those from closer ones. Hence, it is necessary to compensate for this attenuation by amplifying echoes from deep tissues more than those from superficial tissues. As echoes from deep interfaces take longer to arrive after pulse transmission than those from superficial interfaces, this effect can be achieved by increasing the amplification of echo signals with time. The technique is most commonly called time–gain compensation (TGC), but is sometimes referred to as swept gain. It makes use of an amplifier, whose gain may be controlled electronically, so that it can be changed with time. At the start of the pulse–echo sequence, as echoes are being received from more superficial interfaces, the gain is set to a low value (Figure 4.4). It is then increased with time to increase the gain for echoes arriving from greater depths. For the example above, when the pulse and the echo are each attenuated by $1.5\,dB\,cm^{-1}$, the gain must be increased by $3\,dB\,cm^{-1}$. This equates to an increase in gain of 3 dB for every 13 µs, after transmission of the ultrasound pulse (assuming a speed of sound in tissue of $1540\,m\,s^{-1}$).

The actual rate of attenuation of ultrasound with depth is determined by the ultrasound frequency and the type of tissue. The TGC rate (i.e. the number of decibels increase in gain per centimetre) is usually changed automatically by the scanning system, whenever the

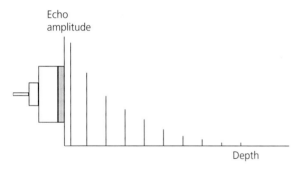

Fig. 4.3 Attenuation results in echoes from interfaces at large depths being smaller than those from similar interfaces near the transducer.

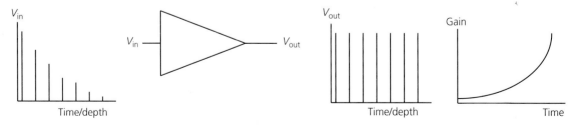

Fig. 4.4 TGC increases the gain with time to compensate for the greater attenuation of echoes from larger depths.

frequency of the transducer is changed. However, it is not possible to set the TGC amplifier to one rate that will compensate for attenuation in all combinations of tissue types, and in practice some manual adjustment is needed by the operator. In adjusting the TGC, the operator seeks to eliminate any trend for the average image brightness to change with depth. There can be no question of making all echoes equal in brightness, of course, nor would this be desirable, since the differences in scattered echo strength between different tissues is crucial to the interpretation of the image.

The most common arrangement for manual TGC controls is illustrated in Figure 4.5. This consists of a set of slider controls, which alter the gain of the TGC amplifier at different times after transmission, i.e. for echoes returning from different depths within the tissue. When all slides are in the central position, an average rate of TGC is applied, related to the frequency of the transducer. Moving the top slide to the right increases the gain applied to echoes from superficial tissues. The bottom slide adjusts the gain applied to the deepest echoes.

Dynamic range of echoes

As discussed in Chapter 2, when an ultrasound pulse is incident on an interface or a scatterer, some of the incident intensity is usually reflected or scattered back to the transducer. For reflection at a large interface, as might be encountered at an organ boundary, the reflected intensity ranges from less than 1% of the incident intensity for a tissue–tissue interface to almost 100% for a tissue–air interface. The intensities of echoes received from small scatterers depend strongly on the size of the scatterer and the ultrasound wavelength, but are usually much smaller than echoes from large interfaces. Hence, the range of echo amplitudes detected from different targets is very large.

Figure 4.6 shows the relative voltages at the transducer produced by typical echoes from different targets. In this figure, the reference used for expressing echo amplitudes in decibels is that from a tissue–air interface (Wells, 1977). Note that because the echoes are all weaker than that from the tissue–air interface, the number of decibels is negative, and that a voltage ratio of 10 between any two amplitudes corresponds to a difference of 20 dB. The figure shows that if the echo from a tissue–air interface gives a transducer voltage of 1 V, that due to echoes from blood will be of the order of $10\,\mu V$. Even smaller signals will be produced by the transducer, but these are likely to be lost in background electrical noise and cannot be detected. The dynamic range of signals at the transducer is defined as the ratio of the largest echo amplitude, which does not cause saturation, to the

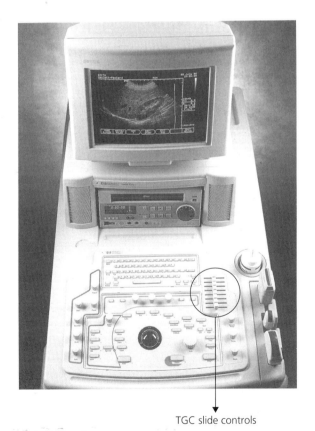

TGC slide controls

Fig. 4.5 TGC is most commonly adjusted using a set of slide controls, each of which affects the gain at a different depth. (Reproduced with permission from Philips Ultrasound.)

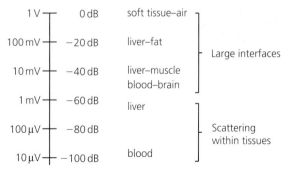

Fig. 4.6 Echoes due to reflection at interfaces and scattering within tissues have a large range of amplitudes.

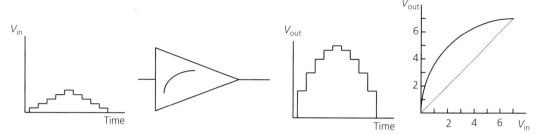

Fig. 4.7 Small echoes can be amplified more than large echoes by using a non-linear amplifier. This results in compression of the dynamic range of echoes.

smallest that can be distinguished from noise. The dynamic range is expressed in decibels.

Weak echoes produced by scattering within tissue give information about organ parenchyma, while strong echoes from large interfaces give information about the size and shape of organs and other tissue features. To be useful diagnostically, a B-mode image should contain both types of echo. Figure 4.6 shows that the range of echo amplitudes displayed needs to be about 60 dB (−20 to −80 dB compared to a soft tissue–air interface) to include echoes from a typical interface (e.g. liver–fat) as well as echoes from tissue scattering.

However, this range of echo amplitudes cannot be displayed without further processing. The ratio of the brightest level that a cathode ray tube screen can display to the darkest is typically about 20 dB. Therefore, if the gain of the B-mode system was adjusted to display an echo signal from a liver–fat interface at peak white level on the display, an echo from a liver–muscle interface would be displayed as the darkest available grey. All weaker echoes from tissue scattering would be displayed as black. Alternatively, if the gain was increased to display weak echoes scattered from tissue (say at the −80 dB level in Figure 4.6) as dark grey, the echoes from within the liver would be near peak white. Echoes with greater amplitudes (e.g. from blood–brain, liver–fat interfaces) would be shown as peak white and could not be distinguished.

Compression

To allow echoes from organ interfaces and organ parenchyma to be displayed simultaneously in a B-mode image, it is necessary to compress the 60 dB range of the echoes of interest into the 20 dB range of brightness levels available at the display. Compression is

achieved using a non-linear amplifier as illustrated in Figure 4.7.

Unlike the linear amplifier described earlier for overall gain, this non-linear amplifier provides more gain for small signals than for large signals. Hence, weak echoes are boosted in relation to large echoes. A graph of the output voltage against input voltage for this amplifier is a curve rather than the straight line of the linear amplifier. In the example shown in Figure 4.7, an input voltage of 2 units gives an output voltage of 4 units (gain of 2), while an input voltage of 6 units gives an output voltage of 6 units (gain of 1). Using this type of amplifier, weak echoes from scattering within the tissue can be boosted more than the large echoes from interfaces, so that they can be displayed at the same time.

In practice, the range of echo amplitudes, which need to be compressed into the display range, depends on the application. For example, when trying to identify local tissue changes in the liver, a wide dynamic range of echoes needs to be displayed, so that these weak echoes are made to appear relatively bright in the image. For obstetric work, interpretation of the shapes in the image may be aided by reducing the displayed dynamic range, so that weak echoes are suppressed and areas of amniotic fluid are clearly identified.

Some commercial B-mode systems provide a dynamic range control (sometimes labelled compression). This control essentially allows adjustment of the curve in Figure 4.7 to alter the dynamic range of echo amplitudes displayed. Figure 4.8 shows the effects of altering the dynamic range control on an image of a liver and right kidney. It can be seen that with the dynamic range set to 80 dB, echoes from within the liver are brighter with respect to those from the diaphram (the bright curved echo in the lower right corner). Irregularities in the liver texture would be easier to detect in this image.

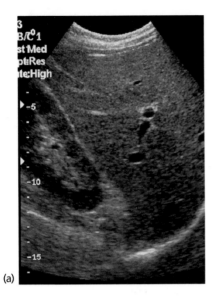
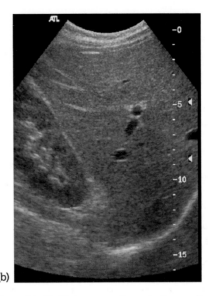

Fig. 4.8 Increasing the dynamic range setting from (a) 40 dB to (b) 80 dB increases the gain for small echoes, making it easier to detect irregularities in the texture of the liver.

Grey-level processing

In addition to controlling the dynamic range as described above, most modern B-mode systems allow further modification of the gain curve that relates echo amplitude to displayed brightness level. The shape of this curve may be altered, e.g. to assign more contrast to low-level echoes from within the liver to aid differentiation of normal from abnormal tissue regions. Alternatively, assigning more grey levels to higher echo levels may aid diagnosis for other organs. Different grey-level processing curves, such as these, are designed into most commercial systems to optimise the system performance for particular parts of the body, such as the abdomen, kidneys, thyroid and breast. When the user selects one of these applications, the optimum processing curve is selected automatically.

Transmit power control

Most B-mode imaging systems allow user control of the amplitude of the pulse transmitted by the transducer. This control is often labelled as "transmit power" and allows the user to reduce the transducer output from its maximum level in steps of several decibels (e.g. 0, −3, −6 dB). The effect is to change the amplitude of the voltage used to drive the transducer, and hence the amplitude of the transmitted pulses. Increasing the amplitude of the transmitted pulses increases the amplitude of all resulting echoes by the same number of decibels

(without increasing the noise level) giving greater penetration. Superficially, the effect on the image is similar to that of the overall gain control. However, the overall gain control applies equal amplification to the echo signals and noise, and does not improve penetration.

Analogue-to-digital conversion

The brightness signal in the early stages of the B-mode system is an analogue signal. That is, its amplitude can vary continuously from the smallest to the largest value. As illustrated in Figure 4.1, the B-mode image is assembled and stored in an image memory before display on the viewing monitor. The brightness information for each echo is stored in the image memory in digital form, i.e. as a sequence of numbers. Hence, at some stage before the image memory, the signal must be converted from analogue to digital form. The process is illustrated in Figure 4.9.

At regular, frequent intervals in time, the amplitude of the echo signal is measured or sampled, producing a sequence of numbers corresponding to amplitude values. If the numbers and the time interval between them are recorded, it is possible to regenerate the signal at a later time by reading them out again at the same rate through a device, which produces a voltage proportional to the stored number (a digital-to-analogue converter).

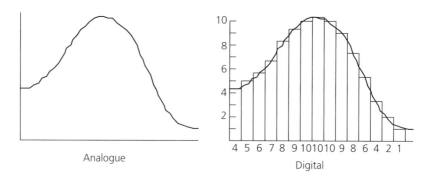

Fig. 4.9 Analogue-to-digital conversion involves measuring the amplitude of the signal at regular intervals in time. The signal can then be stored as a set of numbers.

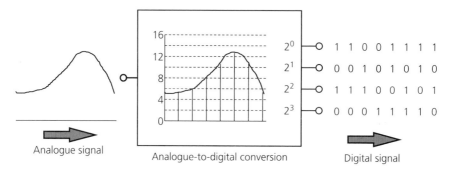

Fig. 4.10 In real ADCs, the continuous analogue signal is converted to a stream of binary numbers.

In digital form, the signal is quantised. That is, it can have only a limited number of values, unlike the analogue signal, which was continuously variable. In the illustration shown, the signal can be quantised into 1 of only 10 different values and the recovered waveform is a relatively crude representation of the original. Apart from zero, the smallest value that can be recorded is 1 and the largest 10, so the maximum dynamic range of echoes that can be recorded is 20 dB (see Appendix A). The analogue-to-digital converters (ADCs) used in modern B-mode systems convert the signal into a much larger number of more closely spaced values, so that the regenerated signal is a much more faithful recording of the original. Also, since the smallest value that can be digitised is smaller, the dynamic range (the ratio of the largest to smallest value) is greater. In Figure 4.9, the signal levels are shown as decimal numbers. In practice, the binary system of counting is used instead (see Appendix B).

Therefore, the input to the ADC is an analogue signal, whose amplitude varies continuously with time, and

Table 4.1 Dynamic ranges for binary systems.

Bits	Max count	DR (dB)
4	15	24
8	255	48
10	1023	60
12	4095	72

the output is a corresponding stream of binary numbers as illustrated in Figure 4.10. The sequence of binary numbers may undergo various digital processing stages before storage in the image memory.

The precision, to which the ADC can measure the amplitude of the signal is normally described by the number of bits (binary digits) available at the output. The 4-bit system illustrated can digitise the signal to 16 different values (including 0). Table 4.1 shows the number of different signal values available with other numbers of bits. The number of bits also determines the dynamic range of signals that can be digitised, since this is equal to the ratio of the largest binary value to the smallest. In the case of a 4-bit number, this is $15 : 1$ giving a dynamic range of approximately 24 dB. Some modern B-mode systems can digitise the echo signal to 12 bits, so that 4096 levels are available, and a dynamic range of approximately 72 dB can be processed and stored. Note that each extra bit of the ADC increases the maximum number of levels by a factor of 2, and hence the dynamic range by an additional 6 dB.

At diagnostic frequencies, the amplitude of the echo signal changes rapidly with time. To preserve detail in the stored image, the ADC must sample the echo signal at a high enough rate to capture these changes. In modern B-mode systems, it is not uncommon to sample at 40 MHz, i.e. 40 million samples per second. To be able to regenerate the signal faithfully after storage, the sample rate must be at least twice the highest frequency present in the analogue signal. A sample rate of 40 MHz fulfils this requirement for most frequencies used for B-mode imaging.

Advantages of digitisation

The echo signal at the transducer is an analogue signal, and for echoes generated by scattering within tissue, is relatively weak. When such signals are processed electronically as analogue signals, they are vulnerable to being degraded by electrical noise and by interference from nearby electrical equipment and from neighbouring parts of the B-mode system. The signal processing techniques available in analogue electronics are relatively limited in their performance. Analogue processing may introduce distortions to the signal, if they are not well designed, and storage of such signals is difficult and can add further noise and distortions. Stored analogue images, e.g. on magnetic tape or discs, may degrade with time due to changes in the storage medium.

Once a signal has been converted into digital form, it consists simply of a set of numbers, which are essentially immune to noise, interference and distortion. Digital information can be stored conveniently in electronic memory or on a magnetic or optical medium without degrading with time. The retrieved image information is identical to the original. The advantages of digital storage are obvious, when the quality of music recordings on CD is compared to that from analogue media, such as audio tape or vinyl records.

Perhaps, the most important advantage of digitisation for B-mode imaging is that it makes digital processing

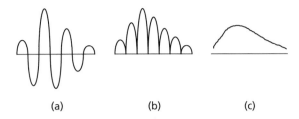

Fig. 4.11 The echo signal is demodulated to remove the variations at the transmit frequency (the radio frequency) and leave just the echo amplitude information. (a) Radio frequency pulse, (b) rectification and (c) low-pass filter.

of echo information possible. Using built in, dedicated computing devices, digital echo information can be processed by powerful mathematical techniques to improve the image quality. While some of these processes may be carried out in real time, others make use of information that has been stored temporarily in a digital memory. For example, information relating to an adjacent part of the image might be used in interpolation (see later).

Amplitude demodulation

The ultrasonic pulse transmitted by the B-mode system consists of several cycles of oscillation at a frequency of a few megahertz. Echoes from reflecting interfaces are of the same form. A typical echo signal due to a reflection at a single interface is illustrated in Figure 4.11a. It consists of oscillations above and below the zero baseline.

The envelope of the signal is described by a pair of curves passing through the peaks above and below the baseline. The strength of the reflection at the interface determines the height or amplitude of the envelope of the pulse (after TGC), and it is this information that is used to control the brightness of the B-mode display. One half of this envelope or amplitude signal is extracted from the high-frequency signal by a process called amplitude demodulation, as illustrated in Figure 4.11.

The signal is first rectified (Figure 4.11b), i.e. one half of the waveform is inverted, so that all half cycles are aligned on the same side of the baseline. The rectified signal is then smoothed by passing it through a low-pass filter, which removes the high-frequency oscillations and retains the slowly varying envelope (Figure 4.11c). Most modern B-mode systems demodulate the echo signal after the ADC. That is, the process is carried out on the stored digital information using fast computing techniques.

Harmonic imaging

As described in Chapter 2, harmonic imaging of tissue is useful in suppressing weak echoes caused by artefacts (see Chapter 5), which cloud the image and can make it difficult for the operator to identify anatomical features with confidence. Such echoes, often referred to as clutter, are particularly noticeable in liquid filled areas, such as the heart or within a cyst and are a common problem when imaging large patients.

As a high-amplitude ultrasound pulse propagates through the tissue, non-linear effects cause energy at the transmitted frequency f_0 to be transferred into the harmonic frequencies $2f_0$, $3f_0$, etc. This effect is strongest for the high-amplitude parts of the beam, i.e. on the beam axis, but weak for small echoes, such as those arising from artefacts. In harmonic imaging, the image is formed by

using only the second-harmonic energy in the returned echoes, suppressing the weak artefactual echoes and enhancing those from the beam axis. This can result in a clearer image, improving the accuracy of diagnosis.

Harmonic imaging can be achieved using a wide bandwidth transducer, which can respond to both the fundamental frequency f_0 and its second harmonic $2f_0$, as illustrated in Figure 4.12. In transmission (Figure 4.12a), the pulse is designed to ensure that its spectrum of frequencies fits into the lower half of the transducer's frequency response. In reception (Figure 4.12b), the received echoes contain information around the transmit frequency f_0 and its second harmonic $2f_0$. To achieve harmonic imaging, these received echoes are passed through a filter, which removes the frequencies around f_0 and allows through only those near to $2f_0$ (Figure 4.12c). As the clutter echoes are mainly at the fundamental frequency, they are suppressed, giving a clearer image.

However, to achieve good separation of the received second-harmonic frequencies from the fundamental frequencies, the frequency spectra of the pulse and the received echoes must be made narrower than for normal imaging. Reduction of the frequency range results in an increase in the length of the pulse in time, reducing the axial resolution of the system as described in Chapter 5.

Image storage

The image memory

The B-mode image is assembled in the image memory using the processed amplitude signal and information from the beam-former on the time since transmission (range), and the position and direction of the ultrasound beam, i.e. the scan line. This process is called writing to the image memory. From the image memory, this echo information is read out to the display monitor. Both writing and reading processes are described in detail later.

The image memory is a digital memory similar to that used in a personal computer. Just as the brightness information of the echo sequence has to be quantised to convert it into digital form before storage in the image memory, the information describing the position of echoes in the image must also be broken into discrete locations to allow storage. The image memory divides the image into a 2D array of picture elements or pixels. These are rather like the 2D grid system of a map or a large set of mail pigeon holes (Figure 4.13).

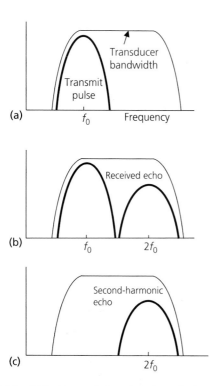

Fig. 4.12 (a) In harmonic imaging, the pulse is transmitted at frequency f_0 using the lower half of the transducer bandwidth. (b) Echoes are received containing information at f_0 and $2f_0$. (c) The frequencies in the echoes around f_0 are filtered out and the image is formed from the $2f_0$ part of the echo.

Each pixel has an address, which is analogous to the grid reference or coordinate system used in maps. Any pixel can be addressed uniquely using its column number, i.e. its position on the horizontal axis, and its row number, i.e. its position on the vertical axis. To allow storage of fine detail, the image is broken into a large number of small pixels, just as in the digitisation of the brightness signal. In a modern B-mode system, the image memory might consist of an array of about 1000×1000 elements. The area of the image within the boundary of one pixel is represented by a single value of brightness. Each memory location corresponding to a pixel stores a binary number corresponding to

the representative echo amplitude or brightness for that pixel. This number is typically 8–12 bits long.

Writing to the image memory

The process of storing B-mode information in the image memory is referred to as writing to the memory. The writing process for each image line begins at a point in the image corresponding to the active part of the transducer face and progresses across the 2D memory array in a direction corresponding to the axis of the ultrasound beam. The process is illustrated in Figure 4.14 for the case of a linear array transducer,

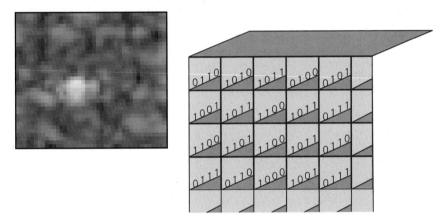

Fig. 4.13 The image consists of a 2D array of picture elements (pixels). The grey level of each pixel is recorded as a number in the corresponding location within the image memory.

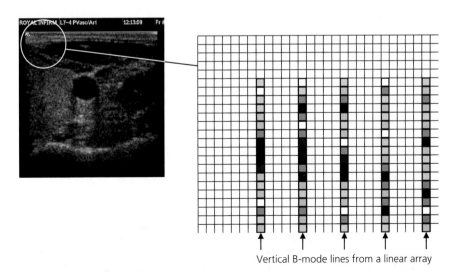

Vertical B-mode lines from a linear array

Fig. 4.14 Image lines are formed by writing to each pixel in turn as echoes arrive from increasing depths.

producing vertical B-mode lines, with the transducer face near the top of the image.

Immediately after transmission of the ultrasound pulse, the system addresses the image pixel corresponding to a position immediately below the centre of the active part of the transducer face. The binary number representing the amplitude of the echo from this point is written to this memory location. The system then addresses the next pixel along the projected track of the image line, writes the representative value of amplitude into that memory location and moves on to address the next pixel. The rate at which this write sequence progresses down the line of image pixels is determined by the field of view selected by the operator.

As described in Chapter 1, the go and return time t for a pulse to reach an interface (at range d) and the echo to return to the transducer, is given by the equation $t = 2d/c$, where c is the speed of sound. At the average speed of sound for soft tissues ($1540\,\mathrm{m\,s^{-1}}$), this equates to approximately $13\,\mu s$ for each centimetre of range from the transducer. Hence, if a maximum imaged depth of 10 cm is chosen, then each line of pixels corresponding to an image line must be addressed and written in a total time of $130\,\mu s$. The spacing of adjacent image lines across the memory is chosen to maintain the scale factor in the horizontal direction.

In the linear array case, the stored ultrasonic line was aligned with a column of pixels, and the system needed only to change the address of the row to write the line into memory. In the case of sector and curvilinear fields, most of the ultrasonic lines cross the memory array at an angle θ to the columns of pixels (Figure 4.15), and the row and column addresses must be changed simultaneously to progress along the correct track.

Interpolation

In linear array systems, the image lines may not always be stored in adjacent columns in the image memory (Figure 4.14). The pixels between are filled by the system's computer using interpolation between values in adjacent filled pixels. The case of linear interpolation in one dimension is illustrated in Figure 4.16. If two adjacent lines are 5 pixels apart and have amplitude values of 5 and 10 at a particular depth, the intervening 4 pixels would be given intermediate values on a linear scale, i.e. 6, 7, 8, 9. In real systems, interpolation is more sophisticated and takes into account the values of neighbouring pixels in 2D and is not necessarily linear.

Interpolation is used extensively in writing sector and curvilinear scanning formats to the image memory. For these formats, the spacing between the lines increases with depth and interpolation is more important.

Write zoom

There are two ways to increase the magnification of part of an image. One is to use the conventional depth control, but this involves losing the deeper parts of the image from the display. Hence, features which are deep within the tissue cannot be magnified by this means. The second method, known as write zoom, was introduced in Chapter 3 and allows the display of a selected region of interest (ROI) remote from the transducer.

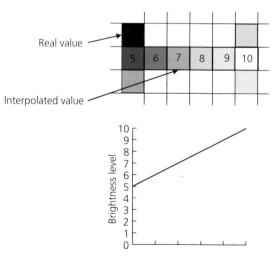

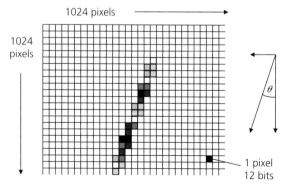

Fig. 4.15 For sector transducers, image lines are written at angle θ by changing row and column addresses.

Fig. 4.16 Pixels, which are not crossed by image lines, are filled in by interpolation between adjacent values. This can be a linear process.

The user outlines the ROI by adjusting the position and dimensions of an on-screen display box, with the image set to a relatively large depth. When ROI display mode is activated, the B-mode system interrogates only those lines, which pass through the ROI. For each of these lines, echoes originating from between the transducer and the near side of the ROI box are ignored. In each pulse—echo sequence, the system waits until echoes arrive from the depth marked by the near side of the box, and writes the subsequent echo amplitude information into the memory on a large scale. Information from within the ROI then fills the image memory.

Reading from the image memory

When brightness information is written to the image memory, the pixel address sequence follows the course of the ultrasonic line in the imaged tissue. To view the image, it must be read out to a display device in a sequence, which is compatible with the display format. The standard display format is the video display raster, as used in current television systems (see Figure 4.17). A display dot is scanned in a sequence of horizontal display lines (a raster) starting at the top left of the screen and finishing at the bottom right. The read process addresses each pixel in turn in synchronism with the display raster. The stored binary values are converted to an analogue level to control the brightness of the display. The process does not degrade the information stored in the memory and can be repeated indefinitely, if required. Hence, the image memory performs the function of scan conversion from ultrasonic line format to TV display format.

Read zoom

Read zoom is another way of magnifying part of the image. During normal read-out, the display raster

Image memory   Display

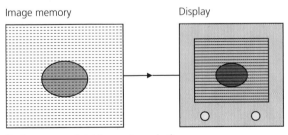

Raster scan read-out (scan conversion)

Fig. 4.17 Grey-level values are read out from the memory in a raster scan synchronised to the display monitor.

interrogates the whole area of the image memory. Where the imaged depth is larger than the imaged width, this can result in inefficient use of the screen area, and imaged features appear small on the display, as described under the heading Write zoom. The read zoom function addresses and reads out a selected part of the stored image defined by the user with an on-screen ROI box similar to that used with the write zoom function. The area of the image memory interrogated by the display raster is then just that required to show the selected area.

An advantage of read zoom over write zoom is that read zoom can be applied to a previously stored image of the total area of interest and the zoomed area moved around to examine different parts of the image on an expanded scale. The disadvantage over write zoom is that when a large image magnification is used, the number of image memory pixels being displayed may become so small that individual pixels become obvious. A higher quality image can be obtained by using write zoom, but the echo information for this needs to be acquired after the ROI box is set. Read zoom is rather like taking a photograph of a distant scene and then examining parts of it with a magnifying glass. The details are enlarged, but the imperfections of the photographic process may be obvious. Write zoom is like a close up photograph of one particular part of the scene. The image quality and definition is maximised, but there is no information available from other parts of the scene.

Image update modes

REAL-TIME DISPLAY

In most medical imaging processes (e.g. X-ray, CT and MRI), there is a significant time delay between image acquisition and image display, so that diagnosis is made on data, which may be many minutes old. Formation of a single ultrasound B-mode image in the image memory takes typically of the order of 1/30 s, so that if repeated continuously, 30 images can be formed each second. This rate is referred to as the frame rate and is measured in hertz. Also, the time delay between image acquisition and display is relatively short (a few tens of milliseconds). This leads to the description "real-time" imaging, i.e. images of events within the patient are displayed virtually as they happen. The real-time nature of the process is an important aspect of ultrasound imaging and, coupled with the use of a hand-held probe in contact with the patient, gives a highly interactive form of investigation. Real-time imaging allows the study of the dynamic behaviour of internal anatomy, such as the heart and can aid identification of normal anatomy (e.g. gut from peristalsis) and pathology (e.g. movement of a gallstone).

The display monitor usually displays a complete image in $1/25$ s, giving 25 images s^{-1}. To avoid conflicts between the reading and writing processes, buffer memories are used to store echo data on a temporary basis, so that the two processes can proceed independently of each other.

FREEZE MODE

If the image acquisition process (writing) is stopped, so that data in the image memory remains unchanged, but is still read out repeatedly to the display, the image is said to be frozen. All commercial systems have a freeze button, which activates this mode. Freeze mode is used, while measurements are made on features in the image and hard-copy records made. Normally, the transducer stops transmitting ultrasound pulses in this mode.

FRAME AVERAGING

In writing brightness information to the image memory, it has been assumed so far that the new brightness information from each B-mode sweep completely replaces that from the previous sweep. However, with this approach, small frame-to-frame variations in the image due to imposed electrical noise can be apparent. This random noise effect can be reduced by frame-to-frame averaging of images. Random noise events then tend to be averaged out, while constant image features are reinforced, improving the signal-to-noise ratio of the image. Frame averaging can be achieved either by weighted updating of the image, or by storing multiple images and computing an average value for each pixel. Weighted updating is achieved by storing a weighted average of the old and new data in each pixel. That is, if the old brightness value in memory is B_o, and the value from the current image is B_c, a value $wB_c + (1 - w)B_o$

is stored, where w is the weighting factor (ranging from 0 to 1). If w is 1.0, the current value simply replaces the old. If $w = 0.8$, then a value of $0.8B_c + 0.2B_o$ is stored, and the effect of the old value is quickly diluted with successive frames (short persistence). If $w = 0.2$, then a value of $0.2B_c + 0.8B_o$ is stored, and the image changes relatively slowly from frame to frame, giving long persistence.

Most current B-mode systems have multiple image memories (e.g. 64) in order to provide a cine-loop facility, with each new frame being stored in the next available image memory, cycling around to overwrite memory number 1 when 64 is filled. Frame averaging can be achieved by computing an average value for each pixel from several frames. The number of averaged frames is typically in the range 1–5, selected by the user.

Long persistence (5 frames) is useful for optimising the image signal-to-noise ratio for relatively stationary images such as liver, whereas short persistence (zero persistence being 1 frame) must be used to image rapidly moving targets, such as heart valves.

CINE LOOP

As just mentioned, multiple image memories are used also to provide the cine-loop function used for studying the dynamic behaviour of organs, such as the heart. During normal real-time scanning, the active image memory is cycled constantly around the available (say 64) image memories, so that the last 64 frames are always available. The image is frozen at the end of the dynamic event of interest, and the 64 images read out to the display as a cycling sequence, repeating the captured movement.

Reference

Wells PNT. *Biomedical Ultrasonics*. Academic Press, London. 1977.

5

PROPERTIES, LIMITATIONS AND ARTEFACTS OF B-MODE IMAGES

K Martin

Introduction
Imaging system performance
Artefacts

Introduction

The B-mode image-forming processes described so far have assumed an ideal imaging system operating in an ideal medium. As described in Chapter 2, real ultrasound beams have significant width and structure, which change with distance from the transducer, and ultrasound pulses have finite length. The speed of sound and the attenuation coefficient are not the same in all tissues. These real properties give rise to imperfections in the image, which are essentially all artefacts of the imaging process. However, those that are related primarily to the imaging system (beam width, pulse length, etc.) are usually considered as system performance limitations, as they are affected by the design of the system. Those that arise due to properties of the target medium (e.g. changes in attenuation and speed of sound) are considered as artefacts of propagation.

Imaging system performance

The performance of a particular B-mode system can be characterised in terms of image properties which fall into three groups, i.e. spatial, amplitude and temporal. At the simplest level, spatial properties determine the smallest separation of targets, which can be resolved. The amplitude properties determine the smallest and largest changes in scattered or reflected echo amplitude, which can be detected. The temporal properties determine the most rapid movement that can be displayed. However, the ability to differentiate between neighbouring targets, or to display targets clearly, may depend on more that one of these property types.

Spatial properties

Lateral resolution

An ideal-imaging system would display a point target as a point in the image. The image of a point target produced by a real imaging system is spread out due to the finite beam width and pulse length, so that it appears as a blurred dot or streak. Figure 5.1 illustrates the effect of beam width on the image of a point target. Here, a point target is imaged with a linear-array system, which has a practical lateral beam width (Figure 5.1a). Echoes from the point target are returned at each beam position, where the beam overlaps the target. However, the imaging system assumes that the beam has zero width, and so displays each echo on the image line corresponding to the current beam axis.

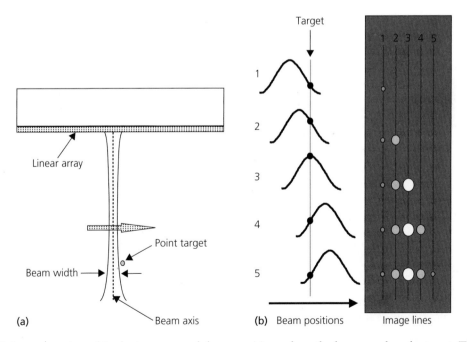

Fig. 5.1 Echoes are registered in the image at each beam position, where the beam overlaps the target. The resulting lateral spread of the image depends on the beam width at the target depth.

At beam position 1 (Figure 5.1b), the right-hand edge of the beam just intercepts the target and a weak echo is produced, but is displayed on image line 1 corresponding to the current position of the beam axis. At beam position 2, the target is still off axis, but in a more intense part of the beam. A larger echo is produced, which is displayed on image line 2. At beam position 3, the target is on axis and the largest echo is produced and displayed on image line 3. At beam positions 4 and 5, the target is in progressively less intense parts of the beam giving weaker echoes, which are displayed on image lines 4 and 5. The resulting brightness profile across the image due to the point target is similar in width and shape to the beam profile at that depth.

As described in Chapter 2, the beam width varies with distance from the transducer. It is narrow in the focal region, but wider at other depths. Small lateral beam width and hence minimal image spread is achieved by using multiple transmit focal zones and swept focus during reception (Chapter 3).

The lateral resolution of an imaging system is usually defined as the smallest separation of a pair of identical point targets at the same range in the image plane, which can be displayed as two separable images. Figure 5.2a shows the brightness profiles along a horizontal line on the image passing through two such point targets. Here, the targets are separated by a distance, which is greater than the beam width, and two distinct images are displayed. As the targets are moved closer together, their brightness profiles meet, when their separation equals the beam width (Figure 5.2b). They then effectively overlap until there is no discernible reduction in brightness between the two and their images are not separable (Figure 5.2d). At a critical separation, the images are just separable (Figure 5.2c). The separation at this point, which is about half the beam width, is a measure of the lateral resolution at that range. Thus, at best, lateral resolution is half the beam width, but can be made worse by other factors.

SLICE THICKNESS

The lateral resolution, just described, refers to pairs of targets within the scan plane. The ultrasound beam has significant width also at right angles to the scan plane, giving rise to the term "slice thickness". Slice thickness is determined by the width of the ultrasound beam at right angles to the scan plane (the elevation plane) and varies with range. Conventional array transducers have fixed focusing in this direction due to a cylindrical acoustic lens next to the transducer face (Figure 5.3).

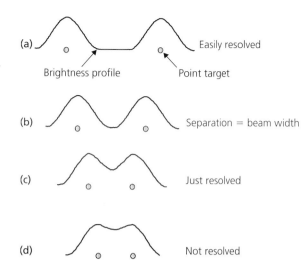

Fig. 5.2 The brightness profiles from laterally spaced targets begin to merge when their spacing is less than the beam width. The targets are just resolved in the image when the spacing is about half the beam width.

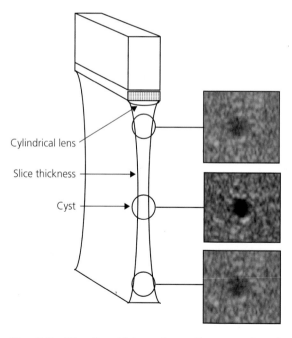

Fig. 5.3 The slice thickness is usually greater than the beam width in the scan plane and can lead to infilling of small cystic structures in the image, especially outside the focal region.

As the transducer aperture is limited in the elevation plane, focusing is relatively weak and so slice thickness is generally greater than the beam width than that can be achieved in the scan plane where wide aperture and electronic focusing is available.

The effect of slice thickness is most noticeable when imaging small liquid areas, such as cysts and longitudinal sections of blood vessels (Figure 5.3). The fluid within a simple cyst is homogeneous and has no features, which can scatter or reflect ultrasound. Hence, it should appear as a black, echo-free area on the image. The surrounding tissues, however, contain numerous small features and boundaries, which generate a continuum of echoes. A small cyst, imaged by an ideal imaging system with zero slice thickness, would appear as a clear black disc within the echoes from the surrounding tissues. However, when a small cyst is imaged by a real imaging system, whose slice thickness is comparable to, or larger than the diameter of the cyst, the slice may overlap adjacent tissues, generating echoes at the same range as the cyst. Such echoes are displayed within the cystic area in the image as if they were from targets, such as debris, within the cyst. The same artefact, often referred to as "slice thickness artefact", is observed in a longitudinal image of a blood vessel, whose diameter is comparable to, or smaller than, the slice thickness.

Until recently, the beam width has been fixed in the elevation direction, and there has been little the operator could do to reduce this artefact. However, some recent probes can be focused electronically in elevation as described in Chapter 3. With these, the operator can adjust the slice thickness focus to be at the range where maximum image detail is required.

AXIAL RESOLUTION

When a point target is imaged by a real imaging system, the spread of the image in the axial direction is determined by the length of the ultrasound pulse. Figure 5.4a illustrates the shape of a typical pulse envelope. It has a short and steep rising edge and a longer falling edge. When an interface is imaged using such a pulse, the echo is much smaller in amplitude, but has a similar shape. Hence, the displayed brightness profile in the axial direction is similar to the shape of the pulse envelope as illustrated.

Axial resolution is defined usually as the smallest separation of a pair of targets on the beam axis, which can be displayed as two separable images. Figure 5.4a shows the brightness profiles from two point targets on the beam axis separated by more than the length L of the

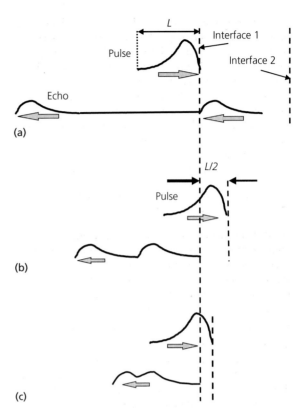

Fig. 5.4 The pulse has to "go and return" from one interface to the next. Hence, the brightness profiles from targets along the beam axis begin to merge when their spacing is less than half the pulse length.

pulse along the beam axis. The profiles do not overlap and the images are separate.

When a pair of interfaces are separated by $L/2$, as in Figure 5.4b, the two-way trip from interface 1 to 2 involves a total distance L. Hence, the axial brightness profiles from reflections at the two interfaces just begin to overlap. As the interfaces are brought closer together (Figure 5.4c), the brightness profiles of the echoes cannot be distinguished in the image. At a critical separation, which is less than $L/2$, the images are just separable. Thus, the axial resolution of a B-mode system is approximately half the pulse length.

Image contrast

The brightness of an echo from a large interface between tissues is determined by the reflection coefficient of the interface as described in Chapter 2. The brightness of echoes representing scatter from within tissues varies according to the tissue type and its state. The absolute value of brightness of such echoes in the display is affected by gain settings, frequency, etc. and is not normally of direct value in diagnosis. However, the use of relative brightness to differentiate tissues within the image is an important aspect of ultrasound diagnosis. The overall relative brightness of echoes within different organs (liver, spleen and kidney) is an aid to identification and can reflect pathological change. Of more importance to diagnosis, small local changes in echo brightness are often related to pathological change in that part of the tissue.

Recognition by the operator, of changes in echo brightness is a relatively complex process, which depends on the characteristics of the imaging system and the human visual system and on the viewing conditions. The smallest change, which can be displayed clearly by the imaging system, is limited by image noise, i.e. random fluctuations in brightness in different parts of the image. For all imaging systems, some noise arises from electronic processes in the image detection and processing circuits. In ultrasound images, there is also acoustic noise, the most prominent type of which is speckle.

Speckle

We have already seen that targets, which are closer together than approximately half a beam width (lateral and elevation) and half a pulse length, cannot be resolved as separate features in the image. Another way of stating this is to say that targets, which lie within a volume, called the sample volume, defined by these three dimensions, cannot be resolved separately. We also know that in the axial direction, the pulse, and hence the sample volume, contains several cycles of the transmitted wave.

Within most tissues, there are numerous features and irregularities within the sample volume at any instant, which scatter ultrasound from the pulse back to the transducer. The scattering strength and distribution of these scatterers within the sample volume are random, so that the echoes they generate vary randomly in amplitude and position (phase), as seen in Figure 5.5. As the voltage generated by the transducer at each point in time can have only a single value, the value registered is the sum of contributions from many scatterers. Echoes, which are in phase, add constructively, while those that are in anti-phase add destructively, leading to random fluctuations in brightness in the displayed image called speckle. The form of the speckle pattern is related to the dimensions of the sample volume. For example, since

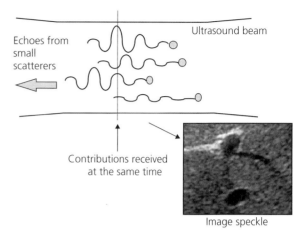

Echoes from small scatterers

Ultrasound beam

Contributions received at the same time

Image speckle

Fig. 5.5 Echoes from small scatterers within the sample volume have random amplitude and relative phase. These add together at the transducer to produce random fluctuations in the image brightness called speckle.

the beam width is generally greater than the pulse length, the pattern includes prominent streaks in the lateral direction, whose lengths are similar to the beam width. In the focal region of the beam, where the beam width is small, such streaks are much shorter.

Some recent developments in ultrasound technology have the effect of reducing image speckle. For example, in real-time compound imaging, the beams from a linear array are deflected to extra positions on each side of the straight-ahead position using phased array techniques. The images obtained from the different beam directions are summed (compounded). The random fluctuations in image brightness due to speckle tend to be averaged out, so that they are less apparent in the image.

Perception of changes in brightness

Perception of changes in image brightness is affected by a number of factors. Clearly, if the difference in average brightness level of two areas in the image is small compared to average fluctuations in brightness due to speckle, the tissues will not appear to be different. If the change in average level is similar to, or greater than, the speckle variations, the difference should be observable.

The perception of differences in image brightness is affected also by the characteristics of the human visual system (Hill, 1986). The visual system is adapted to detect sharp boundaries in an image and is less sensitive to changes in brightness, if the change is gradual. Hence, a small change in overall brightness of the liver compared to that of a neighbouring organ is more difficult to identify than a 1 cm region of reduced echo brightness within the liver. Such small percentage changes in brightness are perceived more easily, if the overall brightness level is high. Hence, if the operator is interested in detecting local changes in echo brightness in the liver, it is beneficial to adjust the gain settings of the system to display these echoes at an above average level of brightness. This can be achieved through adjustment of grey-level processing curves, overall gain and output power.

Movement

Imaging of rapidly moving structures, such as valve leaflets, in the heart requires that the image repetition rate (the frame rate) is high. To show the movement of a valve leaflet smoothly, the system needs to display it in several positions (say 5) between the closed and open positions. As the leaflet takes only about 0.1 s to open, five images are needed in every 0.1 s, a frame rate of 50 Hz.

Tissues, such as the liver and other abdominal organs, can be imaged successfully with much lower frame rates. Here, relative movement between the tissues and the ultrasound transducer is caused mainly by the patient's respiration and by slow operator guided movement of the probe across the patient's skin, both of which can be suspended temporarily. Frame rates of less than 10 Hz can be tolerated, therefore, in the abdomen. Ultrasound image formation in modern equipment involves many complex-processing steps. However, these are performed in a short time by high-speed digital electronics and do not reduce the image repetition rate. However, the travel time of ultrasound to the target and back is a fundamental part of the imaging process and limits the rate at which images can be acquired.

Consider an image from a stepped linear array consisting of N ultrasonic lines interrogating the tissue to a maximum depth D (Figure 5.6a). To form each ultrasound line, the pulse must travel to depth D and echoes return from that depth before the pulse for the next line is transmitted.

If the speed of sound in the tissue is c, the time per line is $2D/c$, i.e. the go and return time to depth D. The total time to form N lines is then $2DN/c$. This is the frame time or time to form one complete B-mode image. The frame rate = 1/frame time. That is, the frame rate = $(c/2DN)$ Hz.

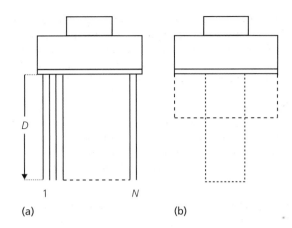

Fig. 5.6 (a) The frame time, and hence the frame rate, is determined by the imaged depth D and the number of lines N. (b) The frame rate can be maximised by reducing the imaged depth or width to the minimum required.

This equation shows that increasing the depth D or the number of lines N reduces the frame rate, whereas decreasing D or N increases it. Hence, reducing the imaged depth to the minimum required to see the tissues of interest will help to avoid low frame rates. Some ultrasound imaging systems allow the operator also to reduce the width of the imaged area (Figure 5.6b). If the spacing between the ultrasound lines is constant, then this reduces the number of lines in the image and increases the frame rate.

The frame rate may be increased also by spacing the image lines further apart, so that the total number in the imaged area is reduced. Some systems have a frame rate control that provides a trade off with line spacing, and thus image quality.

Artefacts

When forming a B-mode image, the imaging system makes a number of assumptions about ultrasound propagation in tissue. These include:

1. the speed of sound is constant,

2. the beam axis is straight,

3. the attenuation in tissue is constant, and

4. the pulse travels only to targets that are on the beam axis and back to the transducer.

Significant variations from these conditions in the target tissues are likely to give rise to visible image artefacts.

Most artefacts may be grouped into speed of sound artefacts, attenuation artefacts or reflection artefacts according to which of the above conditions is violated.

Speed of sound artefacts

RANGE ERRORS

As described earlier, a B-mode image is a scaled map of echo-producing interfaces and scatterers within a slice through the patient, in which each echo signal is displayed at a location related to the position of its origin within the slice. The location of each echo is determined from the position and orientation of the beam and the range of the target from the transducer.

The distance d to the target is derived from its go and return time t, i.e. the time elapsed between transmission of the pulse and receipt of the echo from the target. In making this calculation, the system assumes that $t = 2d/c$, where the speed of sound is constant at $1540\,\mathrm{m\,s^{-1}}$, so that t changes only as a result of changes in d. However, if the speed of sound in the medium between the transducer and the target is greater than $1540\,\mathrm{m\,s^{-1}}$, the echo will arrive back at the transducer earlier than expected for a target of that range (i.e. t is reduced). The system assumes that c is still $1540\,\mathrm{m\,s^{-1}}$ and so displays the echo as if from a target nearer the transducer. Conversely, where c is less than $1540\,\mathrm{m\,s^{-1}}$, the echo arrives relatively late and is displayed as if it originated from a more distant target. Such range errors may result in several variations of image artefacts depending on the pattern of changes in the speed of sound in the tissues between the transducer and the target. These include:

1. misregistration of targets,
2. distortion of interfaces, and
3. errors in size.

Misregistration of targets occurs as illustrated in Figure 5.7a, where the average speed of sound between the transducer and target is greater or less than $1540\,\mathrm{m\,s^{-1}}$. A discrete target will be displayed too near or too far away from the location of the transducer face due to early or late arrival of the echo. In practice, this might be due to a thick layer of fat under the skin surface. The speed of sound in fat could be as low as $1420\,\mathrm{m\,s^{-1}}$, approximately 8% less than the assumed speed of sound of $1540\,\mathrm{m\,s^{-1}}$. For a uniform layer of fat, all targets beyond the fat would be displaced away from the transducer, but this error would not be noticeable, as it would be applied to all targets equally.

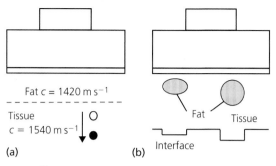

Target O is displayed at ●

Fig. 5.7 (a) The low speed of sound in a superficial fat layer results in the images of all targets beyond it being displaced away from the transducer. (b) Superficial regions of fat can result in visible distortion of smooth interfaces.

BOUNDARY DISTORTION

Range errors due to speed of sound variations may be more obvious in the presence of non-uniform regions of fat superficial to a smooth interface (Figure 5.7b). Here the parts of the interface, which are imaged through a region of fat, will be displaced to greater depths with respect to other parts and the resulting irregularities in the interface can be detected readily by eye.

SIZE ERRORS

Errors in displayed or measured size of a tissue mass may occur, if the speed of sound in the region deviates significantly from $1540\,\mathrm{m\,s^{-1}}$. For example, if the speed of sound in the mass is 5% less than $1540\,\mathrm{m\,s^{-1}}$, the axial dimension of the displayed mass will be 5% too large. For most purposes, an error of 5% in displayed size is not noticeable. However, for measurement purposes, an error of 5% may need to be corrected.

REFRACTION

As described in Chapter 2, an ultrasound wave will be deflected by refraction when it is obliquely incident on an interface, where there is a change in the speed of sound. When an ultrasound wave propagates in the form of a beam, the direction of propagation is the beam axis, which may be deviated by a change in the speed of sound. In writing an ultrasonic line of echoes into the image memory, the B-mode system addresses a line of pixels across the memory assuming that the beam axis is straight, and displays all echoes at points along the assumed scan line at a range corresponding to

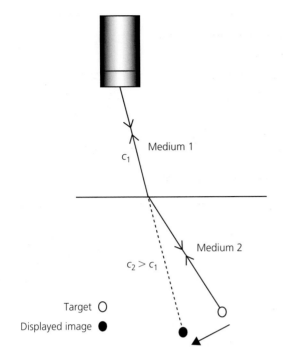

Fig. 5.8 An echo received via a refracted beam is displayed in the image as if originating from a straight beam, and hence is displaced from its correct position.

In the figure: Medium 1, c_1; Medium 2, $c_2 > c_1$; Target; Displayed image.

their time of arrival. Hence, echoes received via a refracted beam will be displayed as if they originated on an undeviated axis (Figure 5.8) and will be displaced from their correct location in the image.

A refraction artefact is seen in some subjects when imaging the aorta in cross section through the superficial abdominal muscles. Here, the ultrasound beams may be refracted towards the centre of the abdomen by the oblique interface at the medial edges of the abdominal muscles. As the muscle structure is symmetrical, two side-by-side images of the aorta may be formed.

Attenuation artefacts

During each pulse–echo cycle of the B-mode imaging sequence, the outgoing pulse and returning echoes are attenuated as they propagate through tissue, so that echoes from deep targets are weaker than those from similar superficial targets. As described in Chapter 4, time–gain compensation (TGC) is applied to correct for such changes in echo amplitude with target depth. Most systems apply a constant rate of compensation (expressed in dB cm^{-1}), designed to correct for attenuation in a typical uniform tissue at the current transmit frequency. Also, the operator can usually make additional adjustments to the compensation via slide controls, which adjust the gain applied to specific depths in the image.

TGC artefacts may appear in the image when the applied compensation does not match the actual attenuation rate in the target tissues. A mismatch may occur due to inappropriate adjustment by the operator or to large deviations in actual attenuation from the constant values assumed. As the same TGC function is normally applied to each line in the B-mode image, inappropriate adjustment of TGC controls would result in bright or dark bands of echoes across the image of a uniform tissue (Figure 5.9a). Under some circumstances, these might be interpreted as abnormalities.

TGC artefacts due to substantial local deviations in tissue attenuation are of more interest as they usually have diagnostic value. Acoustic shadowing occurs distal to a region of increased attenuation, where all echoes in the shadow are reduced compared to those arising lateral to the shadow. This is because the TGC is set to compensate for the lower attenuation in the adjacent tissues, and so does not adequately boost echoes returning from beyond the region of higher attenuation. These undercompensated echoes are displayed at a reduced brightness. The most striking examples of acoustic shadowing are those due to highly reflecting and attenuating calcified lesions, such as gallstones or blood vessel plaque (Figure 5.9b). Shadowing may also occur posterior to some more strongly attenuating tissue lesions, e.g. breast masses.

Post-cystic enhancement, which is the opposite of acoustic shadowing, occurs posterior to regions of low attenuation. Here, compensation is applied to echoes arising from behind the cyst assuming that these echoes have been attenuated by the same depth of tissue as those from regions lateral to the cyst. As the attenuation in the liquid of the cyst is very low compared to that in tissue, the echoes from tissues distal to the cyst are still relatively large and are displayed at a higher brightness level. Post-cystic enhancement (Figure 5.9c) can be a useful diagnostic indication of a liquid-filled lesion.

Reflection artefacts

SPECULAR REFLECTION

In Chapter 2, it was shown that when an ultrasound wave meets a large plane interface between two different media, the percentage of ultrasound intensity reflected is determined by the acoustic impedance values of the

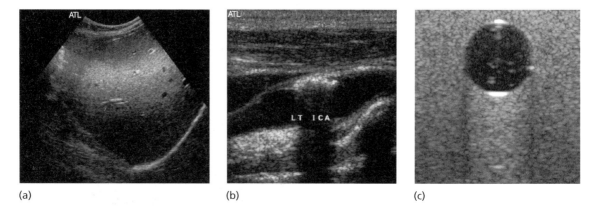

(a)   (b)   (c)

Fig. 5.9 (a) Incorrect setting of the TGC controls can result in non-uniform image brightness. (b) Undercompensation of echoes from beyond highly reflecting or attenuating objects such as plaque in the carotid artery results in acoustic shadowing. (c) Overcompensation of echoes from beyond low attenuation liquid-filled structures results in post-cystic enhancement.

two media. A large change in acoustic impedance gives a strong reflection at the interface. The amplitude of the echo from an interface received back at the transducer is determined not only by the reflection coefficient at the interface and attenuation in the intervening medium, but also by the angle of incidence of the beam at the interface and the smoothness of the surface.

When reflection is from a large, smooth interface, i.e. an interface, which is larger than the beam width, specular reflection occurs. That is, the reflected ultrasound propagates in one direction. When the angle of incidence is zero (normal incidence), the reflected echo from a large, smooth interface travels back along the same line as the incident beam to the transducer where it is detected (Figure 5.10a). When the angle of incidence is not zero, the beam is reflected to the opposite side of the normal at the angle of reflection. The angle of reflection is equal to the angle of incidence. Hence, when a beam is incident on a large, smooth interface at an angle of incidence of 10° or more, the reflected beam misses the transducer and no echo is received.

This specular reflection artefact is seen commonly when imaging through the liver to the diaphragm, a large smooth curved interface. Those parts of the diaphragm, which reflect the beam at near normal incidence, give rise to strong echoes in the image. Other parts of the diaphragm, where the angle of incidence is greater than 10°, are not shown in the image, because the reflected beam misses the transducer.

When the interface is rough or irregular on the scale of the ultrasound wavelength or smaller, diffuse reflection

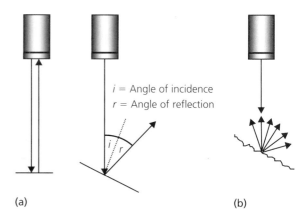

i = Angle of incidence
r = Angle of reflection

(a)   (b)

Fig. 5.10 (a) Specular reflection occurs at a large, smooth interface. A strong echo can only be received at near normal incidence. (b) A large, rough interface gives a diffuse reflection, which may be received over a wider range of angles.

occurs. Here, the incident pulse is reflected over a wide range of angles (scattered), so that echoes may be received back at the transducer even when the angle of incidence is quite large (Figure 5.10b).

MIRROR IMAGE ARTEFACT

Mirror image artefact arises also due to specular reflection of the beam at a large smooth interface. It is most obvious when the reflection coefficient is large (e.g. at a tissue–air interface). If the reflected beam then encounters a scattering target, echoes from that target can be returned along a reciprocal path (i.e. via the

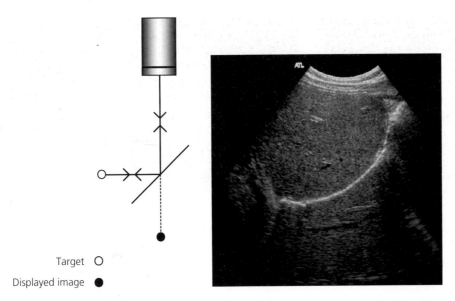

Target   O

Displayed image   ●

Fig. 5.11 Mirror image artefact can occur beyond a strongly reflecting interface. Scattered echoes from targets in front of the interface are received via reflection at the interface. These are displayed in the straight-ahead position behind the interface. The image shows liver echoes displayed behind the diaphragm.

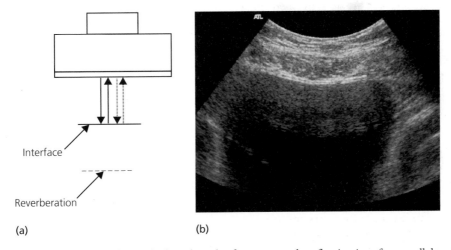

Interface

Reverberation

(a)   (b)

Fig. 5.12 (a) Reverberations are generated when the echo from a strongly reflecting interface parallel to the transducer is partially reflected from the transducer face back to the interface. This generates a second echo, which is displayed at twice the depth of the interface. (b) Reverberations are seen most commonly within liquid–filled areas such as the bladder as shown here.

reflecting interface) back to the transducer, where they are received (Figure 5.11). As in the case of refraction artefact, the B-mode system assumes that all echoes arise from points along a straight beam. Hence, the reflected echoes are displayed in line with the original beam at a point beyond the strongly reflecting interface. The displayed effect is that of a mirror image of the scattering target displayed behind the reflecting surface, as is observed when viewing a conventional optical mirror. Mirror image artefact can often be observed posterior to the diaphragm. Figure 5.11 shows an example of echoes from the liver displayed in this position.

REVERBERATIONS

Reverberations arise also due to reflections of pulses and echoes by strongly reflecting interfaces. However, they occur only for normal incidence of the beam at the interface and can involve multiple reflections. Reverberations occur most commonly where there is a strongly reflecting interface parallel to the transducer face at a relatively small depth. As illustrated in Figure 5.12a, the echo from the interface arrives at the transducer and is displayed in the B-mode image. Some of the energy in the returned echo is then reflected at the transducer face, however, and returns to the reflecting interface as if it was a weak transmitted pulse, returning as a second echo (reverberation). As the time taken for the second echo to arrive is twice that taken by the first echo, the B-mode system displays it at twice the depth of the first echo. This process can continue to give further weak echoes at multiples of the depth of the reflecting interface. The weakness of these echoes is compensated partly by the TGC, which applies increased gain to echoes with longer go and return times.

Reverberations commonly appear in images of liquid-filled areas, such as the bladder, due to multiple reflections between the transducer and the anterior bladder wall (Figure 5.12b). They are more obvious in such liquid-filled regions, which do not normally generate other echoes.

Reference

Hill CR. In: CR Hill (Ed.) *Physical Principles of Medical Ultrasonics.* Ellis Horwood, Chichester. 1986.

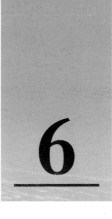

6

B-MODE MEASUREMENTS

NJ Dudley

Introduction

Measurements have a significant role in many areas of ultrasound practice, detailed in many clinical texts. Some of the earliest ultrasound measurements were made in the field of obstetrics, originally in A-mode. A small range of measurements was quickly established in regular practice and this range has been considerably developed over the years. The most frequently performed measurements range from nuchal translucency in detecting abnormalities, through crown-rump-length, biparietal diameter and femur length for dating, to abdominal circumference (AC) and head circumference (HC) for growth assessment. All of these may affect the management of pregnancy and therefore accuracy and reproducibility of measurements are important.

There is also a long history of measurement in echocardiography. Early measurements were made using the M-mode image and this is still used in modern clinical practice. Echocardiography images a dynamic process; the advantage of M-mode is that it contains information on both distance and time, so that changes in dimensions during the cardiac cycle may be measured. Cine-loop displays now provide this temporal information in B-mode in a more accessible form than video recorders.

Most abdominal and small parts examinations are qualitative. Measurements are sometimes used, ranging from the gall bladder wall and common bile duct (a few millimetres) to the kidneys and liver (centimetres).

In vascular ultrasound, vessel diameters have been measured for many years in the diagnosis of, e.g. aneurysms. In modern practice, vascular dimensions are often used in conjunction with Doppler ultrasound in assessing blood flow; accuracy is then more important since small errors in vessel diameter may result in large errors in blood flow estimation, particularly in small vessels (Kiserud and Rasmussen, 1998).

In the following sections the implementation and application of measurement systems will be described. Measurement uncertainty is often overlooked in the development and use of clinical measurements; possible sources of error and practical means for improving accuracy and reproducibility will be discussed.

Measurement systems

Modern measurement systems have the sophistication and flexibility provided by digital electronics and software

control. In the early days of ultrasound, particularly before the advent of digital scan converters, only simple axial measurements were possible on scanners. These were made on the A-mode display by aligning the ultrasound beam with the targets to be measured, and identifying and placing markers on the appropriate signals on the display. The machine took the time interval between these positions on the A-mode display and converted it to distance using the assumed speed of sound. Other measurements, e.g. in the horizontal plane, could be made only on hard copy of the B-mode image using a ruler and scale factors derived from axial distance measurements, or in the case of non-linear measurements using a planimeter or even a piece of string.

These early measurements were difficult and required great care. It is remarkable that early ultrasound practitioners were able to demonstrate the value of measurements. The fact that some of the normal data produced are close to modern values and are still referred to is a testament to the care and dedication of these pioneers (BMUS, 1990; Cosgrove et al., 1993; Feigenbaum, 1993).

Modern calliper systems

Measurements made using ultrasound callipers range from simple linear distance measurements to more complex volume measurements. Scanners may also be able to perform calculations using measurements.

Measurements are made on the image stored in the scan converter and, therefore, depend on the accurate placement of image data in the memory, as described in Chapter 4. Each ultrasound machine will use an assumed ultrasound velocity, e.g. $1540\,\mathrm{m\,s^{-1}}$, to calculate distance along the beam axis and a variety of algorithms, depending on the probe geometry, to calculate the final location of each echo in the image memory.

Distances within the scan converter image memory are then measured from pixel centre to pixel centre using an electronic calliper system. Figure 6.1 shows an image expanded until the individual pixels are seen; the callipers are superimposed and each occupies a group of pixels to form a cross. The measurement will generate a distance in pixels, from the centre of one cross to the centre of the other cross, which is then converted to millimetres or centimetres using a conversion factor. This conversion factor is necessary since the pixel size will depend on selected depth, scale and magnification settings; the conversion factors will be related to these settings.

The most common type of calliper control on modern machines is a track-ball, although some smaller machines

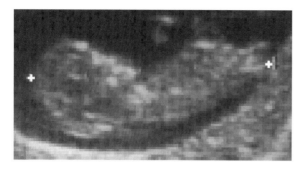

Fig. 6.1 Foetal crown–rump–length image, expanded to show individual pixels, with measurement callipers superimposed.

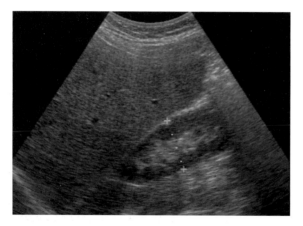

Fig. 6.2 Linear measurement of an adult kidney.

may have a four-way button which is held down to move the calliper in the chosen direction. Older instruments may have a joy-stick. The track-ball is the most user-friendly of these options, as it allows callipers to be placed quickly. Some track-ball systems, however, are very sensitive and difficult to accurately control; for linear measurements, this is irritating but should not compromise accuracy, but for non-linear measurements significant errors may be introduced.

Linear distance, i.e. a measurement in a straight line between two points as shown in Figure 6.2, was the first type of measurement made and is still the most commonly used.

Non-linear distance

This is the distance between two points following the curvature of a structure. It is rarely used, although it

has been suggested for the measurement of embryonic crown–rump–length, where the linear distance may be affected by flexion.

Non-linear distances, including irregular circumferences, must be calculated from a tracing. The calliper is fixed at one end or point on the structure and the outline is traced using the track-ball. During the tracing the system will either plot a line guided by the track-ball movement, or place dots or crosses at intervals of, e.g. 10 mm. The system then calculates the length of the trace, usually by calculating and summing the linear distances between points at intervals along the tracing.

Circumference and area

The circumference of a structure is the distance around the perimeter and is widely used in obstetrics, e.g. fetal AC. There are several possible measurement methods, the choice depending on the regularity of the structure. Circumferences may be traced in the same way as other non-linear distances, fitted or plotted using a number of methods. Figure 6.3 shows traced and fitted circumferences.

Whichever method is used to generate the perimeter of a structure, the area is simply calculated by multiplying the number of pixels enclosed by the area of each pixel. This is not often used, although it has been suggested that it may be more accurate and reproducible than circumference (Rossavik and Deter, 1984). Area measurements are more commonly used in combination to calculate a volume.

Many systems now include ellipse fitting as an option for circumference and area measurement. At least one manufacturer also offers circle fitting. This is a quick and useful method for structures that are truly circular or elliptical. Callipers are initially placed on the extremes of the long or short axis of the ellipse (any diameter for a circle). The length of the other axis is then adjusted using the track-ball, making the ellipse larger or smaller to fit the measured structure. A problem inherent in some of these systems is that if the initial calliper placement is incorrect, i.e. not exactly on an axis of the ellipse, it is impossible to make the ellipse fit the structure. Most manufacturers have overcome this by making both size and position of the ellipse adjustable, so that it may be moved around the screen to match the structure.

Once the size of the ellipse has been fixed, the system calculates the circumference by using a formula. Generally, systems approximate the ellipse to a circle, averaging

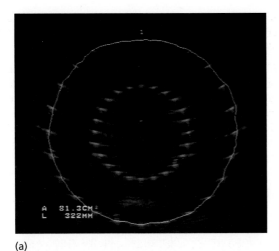

(a)

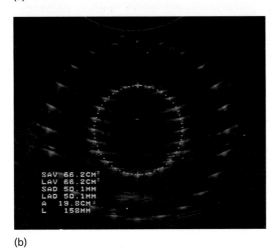

(b)

Fig. 6.3 Image showing measurements made by (a) tracing and (b) ellipse methods.

the long and short axes (d_1 and d_2) and using the equation for the circumference of a circle:

$$\text{circumference} = \frac{\pi \times (d_1 + d_2)}{2}$$
$$= 1.57 \times (d_1 + d_2).$$

This is a good approximation unless the long and short axes are very different, in which case some systems apply a correction factor depending on the difference between the two axes in order to improve the accuracy of the approximation.

Some manufacturers are offering a further alternative, where a series of points is plotted around a structure by

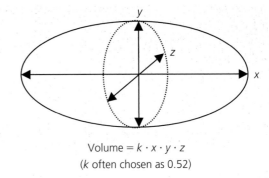

Volume = $k \cdot x \cdot y \cdot z$
(k often chosen as 0.52)

Fig. 6.4 Volume estimation from three orthogonal measurements.

successively moving and fixing the calliper (point-to-point method). The system then joins the points with straight lines or curves, depending on the manufacturer, and calculates the circumference. This is less time consuming than tracing but more so than ellipse fitting, and is useful for measuring non-elliptical structures.

Volume

There are two useful methods for estimating volume from two-dimensional images. Most commonly, a calculation from three linear measurements is used, as shown in Figure 6.4. This method requires two images to be acquired at 90° to each other, e.g. sagittal and transverse images, and three orthogonal diameters to be measured. The volume is calculated by multiplying the diameters together and then multiplying by a constant value, k, appropriate for the shape. The shape is often assumed to be approximate to a sphere, for which the required "k" value is 0.52. Where a sphere is not a good approximation, it may be possible to derive a more appropriate constant from measurements on a number of patients. This requires comparison with an accurate measurement of volume by another means, e.g. in measuring bladder volume the ultrasound measurements can be compared with the volume of urine collected when the bladder is completely emptied. Other structures measured in this way include the gestation sac and cardiac ventricles.

An alternative method is to make area measurements on a series of adjacent slices. The volume of each slice is calculated by multiplying its area by the distance between slices, as shown in Figure 6.5. The slice volumes are added together to obtain the result. This is likely

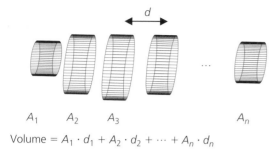

$$\text{Volume} = A_1 \cdot d_1 + A_2 \cdot d_2 + \cdots + A_n \cdot d_n$$

Fig. 6.5 Volume estimation by summing slices.

to be a more accurate method but is more time consuming and is not widely used.

The possibilities for making volume measurements using three-dimensional ultrasound are being explored. Examples include the prediction of birthweight (Lee *et al.*, 1997), assessment of cardiac left ventricular volume and function (Kuhl *et al.*, 1998), and measurement of neonatal cerebral ventricles (Kampmann *et al.*, 1998).

Automatic measurement

Modern image-processing computers provide the opportunity for automating measurements. Although this is not a straightforward process, as the computer must perform some of the operations of the human eye–brain system in determining edges and boundaries, a number of successful systems have been developed.

Boundary detection is a conceptually simple process in cardiology, since the blood–myocardium interface offers high contrast. Methods have been developed in several centres (Perez *et al.*, 1992; Vandenberg *et al.*, 1992).

The most measurement intensive area of ultrasound is obstetrics, where automation offers considerable time saving. The first company to offer automatic measurement facilities in this field was Siemens Medical Systems, Inc. This system requires the operator to identify the structure with a single calliper, then automatically locates the edges or boundaries for measurement. In the case of circumference, the system fits an ellipse to the structure after locating key points on the perimeter. The algorithms that can be used in this type of system were described by Pathak *et al.* (1997).

Calculations

Modern ultrasound scanners have the facility to perform and store measurements. It is, therefore, possible to programme the system to calculate other parameters

from measurements made by the operator. Examples include bladder volume, as described earlier, fetal weight and cardiac volumes.

When a measurement function is selected, the operator must then make the measurements and store them under the appropriate name. The machine may allow for several measurements of each parameter to be made and automatically averaged. Once the measurements have been stored, the result will be calculated using the programmed formula.

Measurement errors

Ultrasound measurements may be different from the true value for a number of reasons. The difference between the observed and true values is called the "error of observation". It is important in any measurement to consider two types of error, viz. random and systematic. Many errors are a combination of these two types, although in different circumstances one or the other may be dominant. Both systematic and random errors affect accuracy. Reproducibility depends largely on random errors.

Random errors

Random errors are accidental in nature and are often due to the observer, either directly or in the use of a system that lacks precision. For example, if the true diameter of a structure is 9.5 mm, and the calliper increment is 1 mm, the observer will never obtain a single true measurement. These errors are often revealed by repeated measurements, where several values above and below the true value are likely to be obtained. Averaging these measurements will reduce the error and produce a result closer to the true value.

A widely used measure of random error is the coefficient of variation (CoV). This is the ratio of the standard deviation to the mean of a series of measurements, expressed in percentage.

Table 6.1 shows two series of traced measurements made on a test object. Note that although the mean values are the same, the two observers have generated different random errors. The CoV reflects the fact that the second observer has made a wider range of measurements. It is also interesting to consider the potential consequences of making only a single measurement in a clinical situation, as there is a 13 mm difference between the first values obtained by the two observers. This shows the importance of making multiple measurements and averaging.

Table 6.1 Ten measurements of the circumference of a test object, made by two observers.

	Observer 1	Observer 2
	317	330
	317	325
	318	323
	321	315
	325	316
	321	318
	323	318
	319	322
	318	321
	322	314
Mean	320	320
CoV	0.9%	1.6%

Systematic errors

Systematic errors are generally consistent in direction and relative size. Both observer- and instrument-related systematic errors are possible in ultrasound as illustrated by the following examples:

1. A sonographer consistently placing callipers just inside the edges of a structure will generate a systematically smaller result than colleagues placing callipers exactly on the edges.

2. If an ultrasound machine is incorrectly calibrated to $1600\,\mathrm{m\,s^{-1}}$, all axial measurements made in a medium with velocity $1540\,\mathrm{m\,s^{-1}}$ will be systematically larger by approximately 4%.

Systematic errors are not revealed by repeated measurements, but may be found by comparison between observers or by measurement of appropriate test objects, depending on the source of error. This is illustrated by Table 6.1, where the true circumference of the test object was 314 mm; there was a systematic error of 6 mm in both series of measurements.

Some degree of systematic error related to the imaging process is inevitable in ultrasound, but it is possible to reduce it to low levels by careful choice of scanner and methods.

Compound errors

Where measurements are combined in some way, e.g. as a ratio or in a volume estimation, the errors in the individual measurements are compounded, leading to a larger error in the result. The error in a product or ratio is approximately equal to the sum of the fractional errors in each variable. For example, if the error in fetal AC and HC measurements is 3%, the error in the AC/HC ratio is approximately 6%.

Sources of errors in ultrasound systems

Human error

There are many possible causes of human error, including inadequate or inappropriate training, inexperience, lack of locally agreed standards or failure to follow local procedures. These will result in either measurement of inappropriate images or incorrect calliper placement. A common source of error is in the measurement of oblique, rather than longitudinal or transverse, sections, leading to overestimation. The frequency, magnitude and effect of human error in fetal measurement have been widely explored (Deter et al., 1982; Sarmandal et al., 1989; Chang et al., 1993; Mongelli et al., 1998; Dudley and Chapman, 2002).

Failure to confirm or average measurements by repetition and errors related to the measurement facilities, such as an over-sensitive track-ball, may also be considered as human error. A measurement system that is difficult to use will deter sonographers from making repeat measurements. This will increase the likelihood, and probably the size, of errors.

The use of evidence-based standards and protocols, training, audit and careful selection of equipment can reduce human errors.

Image pixel size and calliper precision

The ultrasound image is made up of pixels, as described in Chapter 4. The smallest distance that can be represented in the image is one pixel and so all distance measurements have an inherent uncertainty of ± 1 pixel. For example, if an image is 512 pixels square and the image depth is set to 20 cm, each pixel represents one-512th of 20 cm, i.e. 0.39 mm.

A further limitation may be the calliper increment. All calliper systems have a limited calliper increment which may be larger than the pixel size, e.g. 1 mm. The true calliper increment is never smaller than the pixel size, as the calliper must move a minimum of 1 pixel at a time.

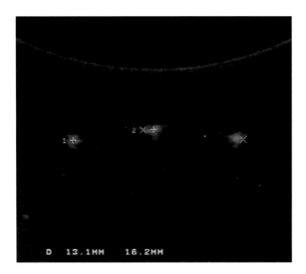

Fig. 6.6 The effect of resolution on measurement accuracy. The difference between centre-to-centre and edge-to-edge measurements on images of point targets is approximately 3 mm in this case.

When measuring small structures, it is, therefore, important to magnify the real-time image using either depth/scale or write zoom controls. The pixel size in the magnified image will be smaller, reducing this uncertainty. These errors are random in nature.

Image resolution

Ultrasound images have a finite spatial resolution, as discussed in Chapter 5. The edges of structures may, therefore, appear blurred or enlarged, and callipers may be placed beyond the true dimensions. Figure 6.6 shows the difference between measurements made from centre to centre and from edge to edge of images of point targets. Errors due to lateral beam width may be minimised by optimising focal settings, so that the resolution is best at the region of measurement.

Resolution may not always present a problem, as measurements are usually compared with a normal range or with previous measurements. If, however, measurements are made on a scanner with performance significantly different to that used to develop reference values, then they may be misleading. An area where this has been evaluated and documented is in the measurement of fetal femur length. Jago *et al.* (1994) demonstrated systematic differences between femur length measurements made with older and more modern machines.

Differences in beam width of about 2 mm generated femur length differences of about 1 mm.

Since lateral resolution is generally inferior to axial resolution, errors are more likely in non-axial measurements. However, the distal margins of structures can be blurred as a result of poor axial resolution or due to reverberation in highly echogenic structures. It is, therefore, important to make axial measurements between the proximal edges of structures (leading edge to leading edge), e.g. when measuring the fetal biparietal diameter.

Gain settings can have a significant effect on resolution, but as the technology develops this has become less of a problem, as gain is more easily managed on modern equipment. Resolution may be generally improved by the use of higher ultrasound frequencies where possible.

Velocity/distance calibration

Since measurements are made on the digitised image in the scan converter memory, it is important that echoes are accurately placed in the image. This depends on the velocity assumed for calculation of the axial origin of echoes and on the algorithms used to calculate the position of scan lines in the image. Any error in echo placement can lead to a measurement error.

Once the image has been frozen, accuracy of any measurement then depends largely on the accuracy of in-built conversion factors to translate the number of pixels between calliper positions into a real distance. A set of factors is required for each probe geometry and a correction factor for scale or depth setting is required. With the increasing range of probes and the availability of continuously variable scale settings, it is important that the electronics or software used to make these conversions is carefully designed and tested.

The consequence of incorrect calibration is a systematic error in all measurements or, more subtly, differences between measurements made on different scale settings. Velocity errors inherent in the equipment can be avoided by rigorously testing calliper accuracy prior to purchase and at commissioning.

Ultrasound propagation

Ultrasound machines are generally designed to assume an ultrasound velocity of $1540 \, \text{m s}^{-1}$. This represents a mean velocity in human soft tissue. True soft tissue velocities vary about this mean by approximately 5% and this may lead to slight distortions in the image and, therefore, to measurement errors. These distortions are described in Chapter 5 and are shown in Figure 5.7.

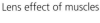

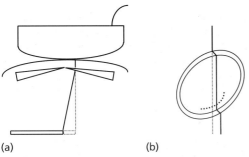

Fig. 6.7 The effect of refraction in (a) surface structures and (b) measured structures. Solid lines show the true position of the structure, dashed lines show the assumed ultrasound path and the refracted position of the structures in the image.

The clinical impact of these distortions will depend on the anatomy under investigation. Measurements of a single organ may be incorrect if the velocity within the organ is not $1540\,\mathrm{m\,s^{-1}}$, but so long as the velocity is the same in other patients there will be no error between patients. Measurements that cross structural boundaries may be adversely affected when compared with normal ranges or between patients, where the contribution of each structure to total distance varies. In most clinical situations, however, a single structure is measured. Where other structures are included, their size and velocity differences are often small, e.g. blood vessels included in an organ diameter measurement.

A further source of distortion is refraction, where the ultrasound beam changes direction as it passes between tissues with different velocities. This has a greater potential clinical impact as distortions may be introduced into a structure by proximal tissues or by the structure itself. Refraction is described in more detail in Chapter 5.

An area where the possibility of measurement errors due to refraction should be, especially, considered is obstetrics. Refraction around the maternal mid-line can lead to apparently stretched objects (Figure 6.7a) and refraction in the fetal skull may shorten biparietal diameter measurements if the measured surfaces are not at 90° to the beam axis (Figure 6.7b). The biparietal diameter should be measured along the beam axis.

Errors in circumference and area

Circumference and area measurements are subject to all of the above errors. Traced measurements are,

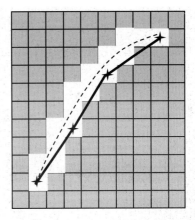

Fig. 6.8 Illustration of the effect of measurement point separation on traced perimeters (point separation of 5 pixels: solid line; pixel-to-pixel: white blocks). For a pixel size of 1 mm, the pixel-to-pixel measurement is 15 mm and the measurement with point separations of 5 pixels is 10.8 mm, compared to the "true" distance (dashed line) of 11 mm.

particularly, sensitive to human error, where calliper controls may be difficult to manipulate in generating an accurate outline. This leads to systematic and random errors, as every deviation is added to the circumference. In clinical practice, structural outlines are not always completely and reliably visualised and this may also lead to errors.

The magnitude of the systematic error in tracing depends on several factors. Difficulty in manipulating the track-ball, accurately, will increase the error, as will any lack of care on the part of the operator. The separation of points on the tracing used by the system to calculate the distance is also important as shown in Figure 6.8. If the points are far apart, this will result in a shortening of the distance and if the points are too close together every small deviation will be included, increasing the measurement. Errors as high as 15% have been documented (Dudley and Griffith, 1996). The optimum number of points depends on the sensitivity of the track-ball and the distance measured; this will be determined in the design of the equipment. For a fetal AC in the third trimester, one point per centimetre might be appropriate.

In the clinical situation, errors will usually be larger than those shown in Table 6.1, as measurements are rarely repeated 10 times and it is more difficult to obtain a good image from a patient than from a test object. Examples of clinical inter-observer CoVs for circumferences and areas of 3% and 5%, respectively, have been reported (Sarmandal *et al.*, 1989; Owen *et al.*, 1996).

Table 6.2   Dependency and errors in each type of measurement.

Type of measurement	Error depends on	Approximate size of error
Linear	Pixel size	0.1–0.5 mm
	Calliper increment	0.1–1 mm
	Resolution	1–5 mm
Ellipse (circumference and area)	Ellipse calculation	1%
Point to point (circumference and area)	Point-to-point calculation	1%
	Number of points	1–5%
Tracing (circumference)	Track-ball sensitivity	2%
Tracing (area)	Operator dexterity	1%

Alternative methods are less prone to errors of operator dexterity. Ellipse fitting provides an accurate and reproducible measurement, provided that the outline of the structure is clearly visualised and is elliptical in shape. The point-to-point methods described earlier can provide accurate and reproducible results, with the advantage that the points may be fitted to any shape. This method is likely to give the most accurate and reproducible results in clinical practice, provided sufficient points are used.

Area measurements are somewhat more reliable where outline tracing is erratic, as small areas are both added to and subtracted from the true area by deviations outside and inside the outline. Mean errors are typically less than 1.5% with CoV of less than 0.5%.

Errors in volume

Since volume estimation methods always use a combination of measurements, they are subject to compound errors as described above. If the volume is the product of three diameters, each with an error of 5%, the error in the volume is approximately 15% (neglecting any assumptions about shape).

The human error may be large, as the method may rely on finding maximum diameters of an irregular structure or measuring multiple areas. In many cases, however, the largest errors may be introduced by assumptions used in calculations. The shape of a structure will vary from patient to patient, reducing the validity of "constants" used in the calculation.

One solution to the problem of variable shape is to develop different constants for the shapes encountered. This has been proposed for the measurement of bladder volume, where Bih *et al.* (1998) have derived constants for a number of shapes.

Summary of errors

In a controlled situation, e.g. test object, with careful measurement, errors can be summarised as shown in Table 6.2. In clinical practice, errors depend on additional factors such as the quality of image acquired, the shape of structures measured and any assumptions used when combining quantities in calculations. With careful imaging, measurement and choice of methods, it is possible to achieve errors similar to those shown in Table 6.2, although some clinical measurements may have errors of two or three times this size. Calculated parameters, such as volume, may have errors of up to 100%.

Interpretation of measurements

Once measurements have been made, they must be interpreted. This requires an understanding of the source and magnitude of any possible errors, an aspect that is often ignored. Measurements that do not rely on operator dexterity or assumptions about shape tend to have the smallest errors. In the clinical situation, errors are influenced by other factors including the ease of obtaining and recognising the correct section for measurement. Where landmarks are well recognised and reproduced in clinical practice, measurements are widely used and are interpreted with confidence. The size of errors must be considered in the context of the normal biological variation of the measurement. A 5 mm measurement uncertainty is insignificant in a 50 mm normal range, but highly significant in a 5 mm normal range. Absolute accuracy is generally more important for small structures than for large structures.

The variation in size of errors between equipment, together with inter-operator and inter-centre variation, may limit the value of clinical ultrasound. Understanding and reducing this variation may allow ultrasound measurement to be used to its full potential. It is important to evaluate and minimise human error in order to achieve the best value from the precision and accuracy of modern equipment.

Use of normal reference data

Interpretation often involves a reference normal range or chart. This introduces a further potential source of human error in the reading of values or transcription of measurements. It is also important to consider how these data were derived. What technique was used? What was the uncertainty in the results? There may have been systematic errors and there are always random errors. Were these addressed?

Systematic errors in the derivation of normal data may be significant compared to the normal ranges, particularly when the equipment used was inferior to that available today. If these errors were not evaluated in the originating centre, this limits the value of the data. The uncertainty this generates is illustrated by the following example.

In measuring the fetal AC, some centres trace directly around the perimeter while others fit an ellipse. In generating normal ranges, Chitty et al. (1994) found the average tracing to be 3.5% greater than the ellipse measurement. This is consistent with the findings of Tamura et al. (1986) who found an average difference of 3.1% between the methods. These measurements were made in the late 1980s and early 1990s. In our centre, we have found a difference of 1.5% between the two methods in a clinical setting (Dudley and Chapman, 2002), but even in a single centre this varied between sonographers, ranging from 0.5% to 2.1%. This difference has been reproduced in test-object measurements (Dudley and Griffith, 1996) and represents the systematic error associated with operator dexterity and the sensitivity of the calliper control.

Normal ranges and charts may be evaluated against local practice and equipment by comparison with results from patient measurements. This is straightforward where large numbers of normal measurements are made, e.g. antenatal screening. A dating chart can be evaluated by plotting a number of measurements, say 20 at each gestational age, and assessing their distribution within the normal range; they should be centred on the mean and the majority should be within the normal range. Where a large amount of normal data is not available the evaluation requires more careful judgement, considering where the measurements should fall with respect

to the normal range based on knowledge of the likely composition of the patient population.

Measurement packages

Most ultrasound machines now arrive equipped with "measurement packages". As well as providing a variety of measurement methods, these packages include programmed charts and automatic calculations to aid interpretation. Examples include fetal growth charts, fetal weight estimation and bladder volume calculation. Although charts and calculations will be based on published data the source may well be the choice of the manufacturer. Many manufacturers offer a selection of pre-installed charts and also provide the facility for users to enter their own preferred data.

Use of such packages removes a potential source of human error, as the sonographer is no longer required to make manual calculations or read from graphs. It is essential, however, that the equipment purchaser makes active decisions in the choice of charts and calculation algorithms, and ensures that these are thoroughly tested before being put into clinical use.

Summary

Measurements are performed in all clinical ultrasound specialities. Although modern calliper systems are generally flexible, offering a range of measurements and calculations, not all systems have the required level of accuracy and reproducibility. In particular, the reliability of circumference measurements on some equipment is unacceptable.

Errors are present, to varying degrees, in most measurements and can arise from the instrumentation, the ultrasound propagation properties of tissue and the equipment operator. These errors can be minimised by adopting good practice at all stages of equipment selection and use.

The choice of equipment is important. Systematic and random errors can be minimised by thorough evaluation of measurement controls and packages prior to purchase, although reliable measurements and the highest quality images may not always be available in the same instrument. At acceptance testing, systematic and random errors should be quantified, so that they may be reflected in the choice of normal reference data and reporting policies. Any programmed charts and calculations should be consistent with locally accepted practice.

Measurement technique is important. All users should understand locally accepted practice, which should be clearly defined in written procedures. Good practice should include the appropriate selection of probe type and frequency, the optimum use of image magnification, setting focal zones at the region of measurement, avoiding image distortion due to refraction whenever possible and the correct and careful placement of callipers. Methods should be appropriate for the selected normal reference data. Random errors can be greatly reduced by performing repeated measurements and using average results.

In interpretation of measurements, clinicians should always be aware of the size of any uncertainty in the result and the size of the normal biological variation. Where these are both small, results may be interpreted with confidence, otherwise a degree of caution is required.

In order to minimise errors, the following steps must be taken:

1. Buy a machine with correct calibration and good reproducibility.

2. Train and assess staff to national standards where available. As a minimum, ensure local consistency by training and audit.

3. Use an appropriate method of measurement.

4. Overcome the limitations of pixel size and resolution by making the best use of scale/depth, magnification and focusing controls, so that the measured structure is large and optimally resolved within the field of view.

5. Repeat measurements to increase certainty. This either gives confidence where the same value is obtained or allows reduction of the random error by averaging.

References

Bih LI, Ho CC, Tsai SJ, Lai YC and Chow W. Bladder shape impact on the accuracy of ultrasonic estimation of bladder volume. *Arch. Phys. Med. Rehabil.* 1998; **79**: 1553–1556.

BMUS Fetal Measurements Working Party. *Clinical Applications of Ultrasonic Fetal Measurements.* British Institute of Radiology, London. 1990.

Chang TC, Robson SC, Spencer JAD and Gallivan S. Ultrasonic fetal weight estimation: analysis of inter- and intra-observer variability. *J. Clin. Ultrasound* 1993; **21**: 515–519.

Chitty LS, Altman DG, Henderson A and Campbell S. Charts of fetal size: 3 Abdominal measurements. *Br. J. Obstet. Gynaecol.* 1994; **101**: 125–131.

Cosgrove D, Meire H, Dewbury K and Farrant P (Eds). *Abdominal and General Ultrasound,* Volume 1. Churchill Livingstone, London. 1993.

Deter RL, Harrist RB and Hadlock FP. Fetal head and abdominal circumference: 1 Evaluation of measurement errors. *J. Clin. Ultrasound* 1982; **10**: 357–363.

Dudley NJ and Chapman E. The importance of quality management in fetal measurement. *Ultrasound Med. Biol.* 2002; **19**: 190–196.

Dudley NJ and Griffith K. The importance of rigorous testing of circumference measuring calipers. *Ultrasound Med. Biol.* 1996; **22**: 1117–1119.

Feigenbaum H. *Echocardiography,* 5th edition. Lea & Febiger, London. 1993.

Jago JR, Whittingham TA and Heslop R. The influence of scanner beam width on femur length measurements. *Ultrasound Med. Biol.* 1994; **20**: 699–703.

Kampmann W, Walka MM, Vogel M and Obladen M. 3-D sonographic volume measurement of the cerebral ventricular system: *in vitro* validation. *Ultrasound Med. Biol.* 1998; **24**: 1169–1174.

Kiserud T and Rasmussen S. How repeat measurements affect the mean diameter of the umbilical vein and the ductus venosus. *Ultrasound Obstet. Gynecol.* 1998; **11**: 419–425.

Kuhl HP, Franke A, Janssens U *et al.* Three-dimensional echocardiographic determination of left ventricular volumes and function by multiplane transesophageal transducer: dynamic *in vitro* validation and *in vivo* comparison with angiography and thermodilution. *J. Am. Soc. Echocardiogr.* 1998; **11**: 1113–1124.

Lee W, Comstock CH, Kirk JS *et al.* Birthweight prediction by three-dimensional ultrasonographic volumes of fetal thigh and abdomen. *J. Ultrasound Med.* 1997; **16**: 799–805.

Mongelli M, Ek S and Tambyrajia R. Screening for growth restriction: a mathematical model of the effect of time interval and ultrasound error. *Obstet. Gynaecol.* 1998; **92**: 908–912.

Owen P, Donnet ML, Ogston SA *et al.* Standards for ultrasound fetal growth velocity. *Br. J. Obstet. Gynecol.* 1996; **103**: 60–69.

Pathak SD, Chalana V and Kim Y. Interactive automatic fetal head measurements from ultrasound images using multimedia computer technology. *Ultrasound Med. Biol.* 1997; **23**: 665–673.

Perez JE, Waggoner AD, Barzilai B, Melton Jr HE, Miller JG and Sobel BE. On-line assessment of ventricular function by automatic boundary detection and ultrasonic backscatter imaging. *J. Am. Coll. Cardiol.* 1992; **19**: 313–320.

Rossavik IK and Deter RL. The effect of abdominal profile shape changes on the estimation of fetal weight. *J. Clin. Ultrasound* 1984; **12**: 57–59.

Sarmandal P, Bailey SM and Grant JM. A comparison of three methods of assessing inter-observer variation applied to ultrasonic fetal measurement in the third trimester. *Br. J. Obstet. Gynaecol.* 1989; **96**: 1261–1265.

Tamura RK, Sabbagha RE, Wen-Harn P and Vaisrub N. Ultrasonic fetal abdominal circumference: Comparison of direct versus calculated measurement. *Am. J. Obstet. Gynaecol.* 1986; **67**: 833–835.

Vandenberg BF, Rath LS, Stuhlmuller P, Melton Jr HE and Skorton DJ. Estimation of left ventricular cavity area with an on-line semiautomated echocardiographic edge detection system. *Circulation* 1992; **86**: 159–166.

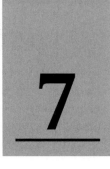

7

PRINCIPLES OF DOPPLER ULTRASOUND

PR Hoskins

The Doppler effect enables ultrasound to be used to detect the motion of blood and tissue. Most Doppler ultrasound systems provide both spectral Doppler displays and colour Doppler images. Many of the features of these two modalities are common, and are described in this chapter. Specific details of spectral Doppler and colour Doppler systems are given in the chapters following this.

The descriptions that follow in this chapter refer to the detection and display of blood flow, as this is the most common application of Doppler techniques at the time of writing. Chapter 14 describes the use of Doppler in detection of tissue motion.

Doppler ultrasound systems

The Doppler effect

The Doppler effect is observed regularly in our daily lives. For example, it can be heard as the changing pitch of an ambulance siren as it passes by. The Doppler effect is the change in the observed frequency of the sound wave (f_r) compared to the emitted frequency (f_t) which occurs due to the relative motion between the observer and the source, as shown in Figure 7.1. In Figure 7.1a, both the source and the observer are stationary so the observed sound has the same frequency as the emitted sound. In Figure 7.1b, the source is moving towards the observer as it transmits the sound wave. This causes the wavefronts travelling towards the observer to be more closely packed, so that the observer witnesses a higher frequency wave than that emitted. If, however, the source is moving away from the observer the wavefronts will be more spread out, and the frequency observed will be lower than that emitted (Figure 7.1c). The resulting change in the observed frequency from that transmitted is known as the Doppler shift, and the magnitude of the Doppler shift frequency is proportional to the relative velocity between the source and the observer.

It does not matter if the source or the observer is moving. If either one is moving away from the other, the observer will witness a lower frequency than that emitted. Conversely, if either the source or observer move towards the other, the observer will witness a higher frequency than that emitted.

Ultrasound can be used to assess blood flow by measuring the change in frequency of the ultrasound scattered from the moving blood. Usually the transducer is held stationary and the blood moves with respect to the transducer as shown in Figure 7.2. The ultrasound waves

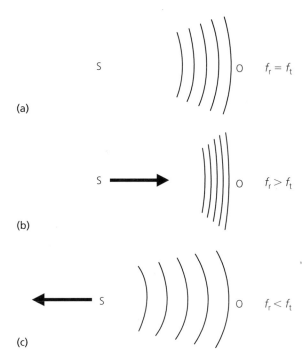

Fig. 7.1 Doppler effect as a result of motion of the source (S) relative to a stationary observer (O). (a) There is no motion and the observer detects sound of frequency equal to the transmitted frequency. (b) The source moves towards the observer and the observer detects sound of a higher frequency than that transmitted. (c) The source moves away from the observer and the observer detects a lower frequency than that transmitted.

transmitted by the transducer strike the moving blood, so the frequency of ultrasound as experienced by the blood is dependent on whether the blood is stationary, moving towards the transducer or moving away from the transducer. The blood then scatters the ultrasound, some of which travels in the direction of the transducer and is detected. The scattered ultrasound is Doppler frequency shifted again as a result of the motion of the blood, which now acts as a moving source. Therefore, a Doppler shift has occurred twice between the ultrasound being transmitted and received back at the transducer (hence the presence of the "2" in Equation (7.1)).

The detected Doppler shift frequency (f_d) is the difference between the transmitted frequency (f_t) and the received frequency (f_r). The Doppler shift frequency f_d depends on the frequency of the transmitted ultrasound, the speed of the ultrasound as it passes through the tissue (c) and the velocity of the blood (v)

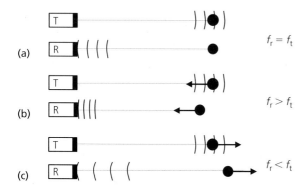

Fig. 7.2 The Doppler effect occurring due to motion of blood. In each case the probe transmits ultrasound which strikes the blood. Separate elements are shown for transmission (T) and reception (R). Ultrasound is scattered by the region of blood, some of which returns to the transducer. (a) The probe and blood are not moving, the frequency of the ultrasound received by the transducer is equal to the transmitted frequency. (b) The blood is moving towards the probe; the blood encounters more wavefronts and the frequency of the ultrasound received by the transducer is greater than the transmitted frequency. (c) The blood is moving away from the probe; the blood encounters fewer wavefronts and the frequency of the ultrasound received by the transducer is less than the transmitted frequency.

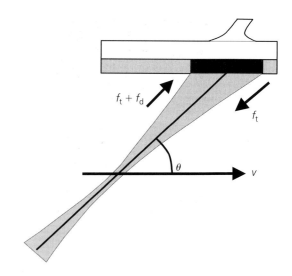

Fig. 7.3 A beam of ultrasound is produced by a linear array in which the active elements are shown in black. Ultrasound is transmitted whose centre frequency is f_t. This strikes blood moving at velocity v. The angle between the beam and the direction of motion is θ. The received ultrasound frequency has been Doppler shifted by an amount f_d, so that the detected frequency is $f_t + f_d$.

(Figure 7.3). This relationship can be expressed by the Doppler equation:

$$f_d = f_r - f_t = \frac{2 f_t v \cos \theta}{c}. \qquad (7.1)$$

The detected Doppler shift also depends on the cosine of the angle θ between the path of the ultrasound beam and the direction of the blood flow. This angle is known as the angle of insonation. The angle of insonation can change as a result of variations in the orientation of the vessel or the probe. Many vessels in the upper and lower limbs run roughly parallel to the skin, although if the vessel is tortuous the angle of insonation will alter. In the abdomen there is considerable variation in the orientation of vessels which will result in many different angles of insonation. The operator is also able to alter the angle of insonation by adjustment of the orientation of the probe on the surface of the skin. The relationship between an angle and the value of its cosine is shown in Figure 7.4. It is often desirable that the operator can adjust the angle of insonation to obtain the highest Doppler frequency shift possible. The highest Doppler frequency shift from any specific vessel occurs when the vessel and the beam are aligned; that is when the angle of

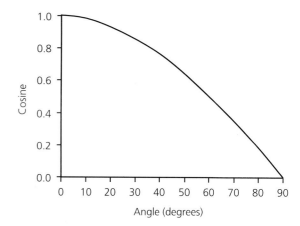

Fig. 7.4 The cosine function. This has a maximum value of 1.0 when the angle is 0°, and a value of 0 when the angle is 90°.

insonation is zero and the cosine function has the value of 1.0. The least desirable situation occurs when the angle approaches 90° as then the Doppler frequency shift will be minimum. In clinical practice it is often not possible to align the beam and the vessel. As a rule, provided the

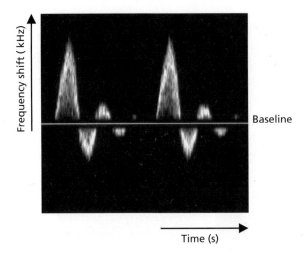

Fig. 7.5 Spectral display. This is a display of the Doppler frequency shift versus time. The Doppler waveform from the femoral artery is shown. Vertical distance from the baseline corresponds to Doppler shift, while the greyscale indicates the amplitude of the detected ultrasound with that particular frequency.

angle is less than about 60°, good quality spectral waveforms can be obtained.

If the angle of insonation of the ultrasound beam is known it is possible to use the Doppler shift frequency to estimate the velocity of the blood using the Doppler equation. This requires rearrangement of Equation (7.1) to give

$$v = \frac{c\,f_d}{2 f_t \cos\theta}. \tag{7.2}$$

In diseased arteries the lumen will narrow and the blood velocity will increase. This provides the means by which the lumen diameter may be estimated using Doppler ultrasound. The blood velocity is estimated within the narrowed region, and converted into a percentage stenosis using standard tables.

Doppler displays

The main display modes used in a modern Doppler system are described below.

- *Spectral Doppler.* All the velocity information detected from a single location within the blood vessel is displayed in the form of a frequency shift–time plot (Figure 7.5). Vertical distance from the baseline

corresponds to Doppler shift, while the greyscale indicates the amplitude of the detected ultrasound with that particular frequency.

- *2D Colour flow imaging.* The Doppler signal is displayed in the form of a 2D colour image superimposed on the B-scan image (Figure 7.6). Colour represents the Doppler shift for each pixel, averaged over the area of the pixel.

The advantage of the 2D colour display is that it allows the user to observe the presence of blood flow within a large area of the tissue. The spectral Doppler display allows closer inspection of the changes in velocity over time within a single small area. Both colour flow and spectral Doppler systems use the Doppler effect to obtain blood flow information. In this respect they are both Doppler systems. The two modalities compliment each other, providing the user with a wide range of useful information.

Continuous wave and pulsed wave Doppler

There is not the restriction in Doppler systems as there is for B-mode devices that the ultrasound must be transmitted in the form of pulses. Some Doppler ultrasound systems, known as continuous wave (CW) systems, transmit ultrasound continuously. Other Doppler systems, known as pulsed wave (PW) systems, transmit short pulses of ultrasound. The main advantage of PW Doppler is that Doppler signals can be acquired from a known depth. The main disadvantage is that there is an upper limit to the Doppler frequency shift which can be detected, making the estimation of high velocities more challenging.

In a CW Doppler system there must be separate transmission and reception of ultrasound (Figure 7.7a). In the pencil probe this is achieved using two elements, one which transmits continuously and one which receives continuously. The region from which Doppler signals are obtained is determined by the overlap of the transmit and receive ultrasound beams. In a PW system it is possible to use the same elements for both the transmit and receive (Figure 7.7b). In the pencil probe only one element is needed, serving both the transmit and receive functions. The region from which Doppler signals are obtained is determined by the depth of the gate and the length of the gate, which can both be controlled by the operator.

The received ultrasound signal is processed by the Doppler signal processor to extract the Doppler

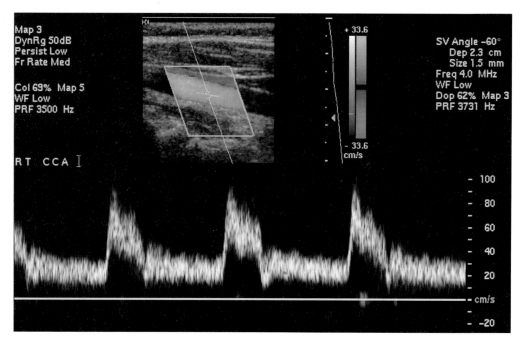

Fig. 7.6 Colour Doppler display. This is a display of the mean (or average) Doppler frequency, at each point in a 2D slice of the tissue from blood, superimposed on the B-mode display. The example also shows simultaneous display of spectral Doppler.

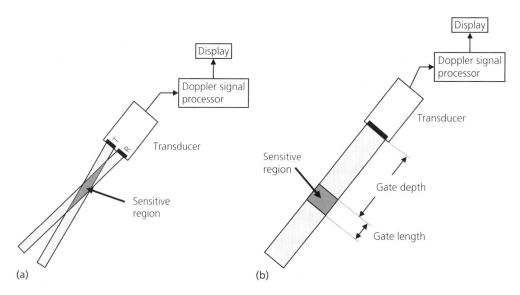

Fig. 7.7 Schematic of CW and PW Doppler system consisting of the transducer, the Doppler signal processor and the display. (a) In a CW Doppler system there must be separate transmission and reception of ultrasound. In the pencil probe this is achieved using two elements, one which transmits continuously and one which receives continuously. The region from which Doppler signals are obtained is determined by the overlap of the transmit and receive ultrasound beams. (b) In a PW system it is possible to use the same element or elements for both transmit and receive. In the pencil probe only one element is needed, serving both the transmit and receive functions. The region from which Doppler signals are obtained is determined by the depth and length of the gate, which are both controlled by the operator.

frequency shifts, which are then displayed in the form of spectral Doppler or colour Doppler.

The ultrasound signal received by the transducer

Before considering in detail the Doppler signal processor, the nature of the ultrasound signal received at the transducer must be considered, as this will determine the subsequent signal processing that is performed.

When ultrasound is emitted from the transducer it will pass through regions of tissue and regions of blood contained in veins and arteries. The blood will almost certainly be moving, but some of the tissue may also be moving. For example, the arteries move during the cardiac cycle, the heart moves as a result of contraction, and tissues in contact with the arteries and with the heart will also move. The received ultrasound signal consists of the following four types of signal:

- echoes from stationary tissue,
- echoes from moving tissue,
- echoes from stationary blood,
- echoes from moving blood.

The task for a Doppler system is to isolate and display the Doppler signals from blood, and remove those from stationary tissue and from moving tissue. Table 7.1 shows the amplitude of signals from blood and tissue, and it is clear that the signal from blood is extremely small compared to tissue; typically 40 dB smaller (Table 7.1). The maximum blood velocity occurs when disease is present, and is about $6 \, \text{m s}^{-1}$. The maximum tissue velocity occurs during the systolic phase of the heart where the myocardium attains a velocity of up to $10 \, \text{cm s}^{-1}$. In general, Doppler signals from blood are of low amplitude and high-frequency shift, whereas those from tissue are of high amplitude and low-frequency shift. These differences provide the means by which signals from true blood flow signal may be separated from those produced by the surrounding tissue.

Table 7.1 Typical velocities and signal intensities.

	Velocity range	Signal intensity
Blood	$0–600 \, \text{cm s}^{-1}$	Low
Tissue	$0–10 \, \text{cm s}^{-1}$	40 dB higher than blood

The CW Doppler signal processor

Dedicated signal processing algorithms are used to produce the Doppler signals from the received ultrasound signal. There are three steps in the process (Figure 7.8): "demodulation" is the separation of the Doppler frequencies from the underlying transmitted signal, "high-pass filtering" is the removal of the tissue signal, "frequency estimation" is where the Doppler frequencies and amplitudes are calculated. There are important differences between the CW and the PW Doppler signal processor which are described in the next section.

Demodulation

The Doppler frequencies produced by moving blood are a tiny fraction of the transmitted ultrasound frequency. Equation (7.1) shows that, if the transmitted frequency is 4 MHz, a motion of $1 \, \text{m s}^{-1}$ will produce a Doppler shift of 5.2 kHz, which is less than 0.1% of the transmitted frequency. Extraction of the Doppler frequency shift information from the ultrasound signal received from tissue and blood is called "demodulation". This process is generally invisible to the user as there are no controls which the user can adjust to alter this process. The process of demodulation consists of

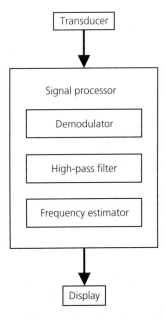

Fig. 7.8 The Doppler signal processor can be considered to be made of three parts; the demodulator, the high-pass filter and the frequency estimator.

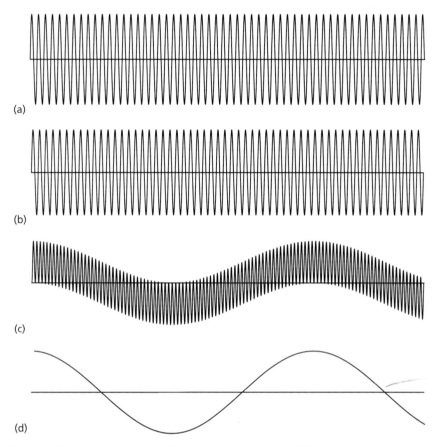

(a)

(b)

(c)

(d)

Fig. 7.9 Doppler demodulation for CW Doppler. (a) Reference signal of frequency f_t. (b) Detected signal which has been Doppler shifted and whose frequency is $f_r = f_t + f_d$. (c) The reference signal is multiplied by the detected signal. (d) The high-frequency oscillations are removed by low-pass filtering. The end result is the Doppler frequency shift signal f_d (the example shown contains no clutter).

comparison of the received ultrasound signal with a "reference" signal which has the same frequency as the transmit echo. This process is illustrated in Figure 7.9, which shows the ultrasound signal obtained from a CW Doppler system being used with a small moving target. The received ultrasound signal has a slightly different frequency compared to the reference signal. The first step of the demodulation process consists of multiplying together the reference signal with the received signal. This process is called "mixing". This produces the signal shown in Figure 7.9c, which consists of a low-frequency component (the Doppler frequency) arising from the moving target, and a high-frequency component arising from the transmit frequency. The high-frequency component can be removed by simple filtering, revealing the Doppler frequency (Figure 7.9d). The end result of demodulation for the example

of Figure 7.9 is the removal of the underlying high-frequency transmit signal, revealing the blood flow Doppler signal.

The example above described demodulation when there was a single moving target present. In reality the sensitive region of the ultrasound system is unlikely to be placed within a region in which all the blood is moving at the same velocity. It is more likely that there will be a range of blood velocities present within the sensitive region, with low velocities present near the vessel wall and higher velocities present near the vessel centre. In addition the sensitive region for a CW system will usually encompass moving tissue. When there are signals from both blood and tissue present, and multiple velocities, the process of demodulation is best understood with reference to the detected ultrasound frequency (Figure 7.10). The received signal from a region in which blood is flowing consists of a high amplitude clutter signal from stationary and slowly moving tissue, and Doppler shifted components from the moving blood. Blood moving towards the transducer gives rise to a positive shift, while blood moving away from the transducer gives rise to a negative Doppler shift. Demodulation removes the high frequencies arising from the transmit frequency, leaving both the Doppler shift signal from blood flow and the clutter signal from tissue motion. At this stage in the process it is not possible to differentiate the tissue signal from the blood flow signal. This requires another step (high-pass filtering) as described below.

Another way of viewing the process of demodulation is that it converts a high-frequency signal (MHz, or millions of cycles per second) into a low-frequency signal (kHz, or thousands of cycles per second). It is easier for the ultrasound system to digitise and process signals which are of lower frequency. This is important as computational efficiency is crucial to ultrasound system design. High-speed processing is expensive, and is the main feature that will increase the cost of the system to the user.

High-pass filtering

We saw above that the signal arising from demodulation can contain Doppler frequency shifts arising from both blood flow and tissue motion. If no further processing were performed then the estimated Doppler signals from blood would be overwhelmed by the large amplitude signal from tissue. In order to correctly estimate the Doppler shift frequencies from blood, the Doppler signals from tissue must be removed. This step is referred to as the "wall-thump filter" or "cut-off filter" in spectral Doppler.

The tissue signals are called "clutter". This term originates from radar and refers to stationary objects such as trees and buildings, which interfere with the detection of moving targets such as aeroplanes. Removal of clutter can be performed using a number of methods. The basis for discrimination between the blood signal and the tissue signal is that signals from tissue tend to be low frequency and high amplitude, and those from blood are high frequency and low amplitude. The simplest approach, and that adopted by many Doppler systems, relies on a frequency filter (Figure 7.10). Removal of components below a certain threshold frequency will remove the Doppler shift components arising from the tissue. An unfortunate consequence of this process is that

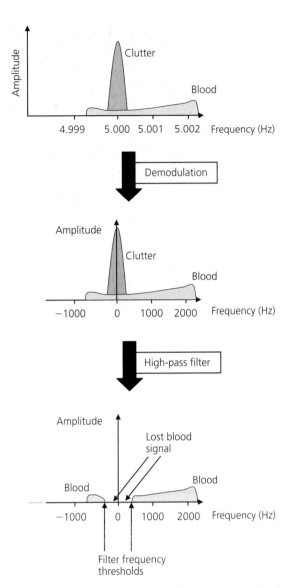

Fig. 7.10 Demodulation and high-pass filtering. Top: The received signal, from a region in which blood is flowing, consists of a high-amplitude clutter signal from stationary and slowly moving tissue, and Doppler shifted components from the moving blood. Blood moving towards the transducer gives rise to a positive shift, while blood moving away from the transducer gives rise to a negative Doppler shift. Middle: Demodulation removes the high-frequency signals arising from the transmit frequency, leaving the Doppler shift signal from both blood flow and the clutter signal from tissue motion. Bottom: The high-pass filter acts to remove the clutter signal. A consequence of this is that the very lowest blood velocities are also removed.

the Doppler frequency shifts from slowly moving blood will also be lost. In general the filter frequency is set by the user to just suppress tissue signals. In cardiology applications a high-filter setting of 300 Hz or more is necessary since myocardium and valves are travelling at high speeds (up to $10 \, \text{cm s}^{-1}$), and the detection of high blood velocities is of interest. In obstetrics, low settings of 50–80 Hz are more typical as it is important to be able to detect the low velocities at end-diastole. After filtering, the Doppler frequency shift data is in a form suitable for the third step in the process, the frequency estimator.

Frequency estimation

When information concerning blood velocity is required then some form of frequency estimator must be used. As CW systems provide no information on the depth from which the blood flow signal has returned, it is not possible to use a colour flow display. CW systems display the time velocity waveform, either in the form of spectral Doppler, or in the form of a single trace.

A spectrum analyser calculates the amplitude of all of the frequencies present within the Doppler signal, typically using a method called the "Fast Fourier Transform (FFT)" in which a complete spectrum is produced every 5–40 ms. In the spectral display the brightness is related to the power or amplitude of the Doppler signal component at that particular frequency. The high speed with which spectra are produced means that detailed and rapidly updated information about the whole range of velocities present within the sample volume can be obtained.

Before the advent of real-time spectrum analysis, it was common to display only a single quantity related in some way to the blood velocity. A relatively simple electronics device known as the "zero-crossing detector" produces an output proportional to the root mean square of the mean frequency. However, the zero-crossing detector is sensitive to noise, and the output depends strongly on the velocity profile within the vessel. Its use in a modern Doppler system is no longer justified.

Origin and processing of the Doppler signal for PW systems

The Doppler signal

There is a crucial difference between CW and PW systems in that for PW systems a received ultrasound signal is not available continuously, as it is for CW systems. This

is illustrated in Figure 7.11 which shows a point target moving away from the transducer, and the received ultrasound signal for consecutive ultrasound pulses. For each consecutive pulse the target moves further away from the transducer, and consequently, the echo is received at a later time from the start of the transmit pulse. As the echo pattern moves further away from the transducer with each consecutive pulse, so the amplitude of the signal at a specific depth changes, as shown in Figure 7.11. In PW Doppler systems the location of the Doppler gate defines the range of depths from which the Doppler signal arises. The Doppler signal is contained within the series of consecutive received echoes from the gate. The Doppler signal is then revealed by the subsequent signal processing.

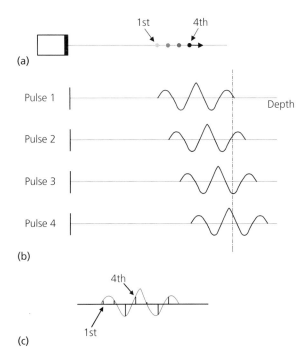

Fig. 7.11 Received echoes in PW Doppler. (a) A single target moves away from the transducer. Consecutive ultrasound pulses are emitted which strike the target at increasing depth. (b) The received echoes are displayed at increasing depth. A vertical dashed line is shown corresponding to a fixed depth. The amplitude of the echo changes as it crosses the dashed line for each consecutive pulse. It is from this change in amplitude of the received echoes with depth that contain the Doppler shift, which is extracted by demodulation. (c) Amplitude of consecutive echoes from the depth indicated by the dashed line in (b) shown as a function of time.

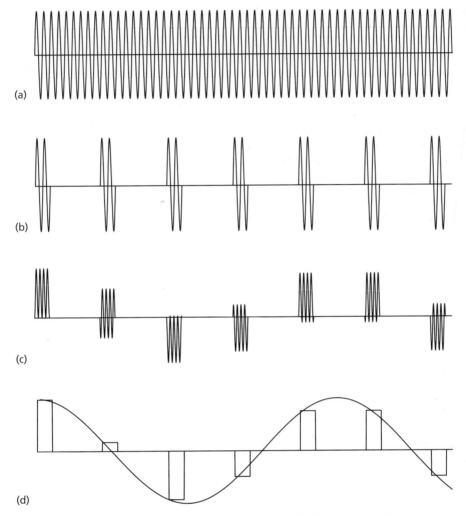

Fig. 7.12 Doppler demodulation for PW Doppler. (a) Reference signal of frequency f_t. (b) The received ultrasound signal consists of consecutive echoes which have passed through the electronic gate. (c) The reference signal is multiplied by the detected signal. (d) The high-frequency oscillations are removed by low-pass filtering. The end result is the Doppler frequency shift signal f_d (the example shown contains no clutter).

PW Doppler signal processor

In PW Doppler systems the basic steps of demodulation, high-pass filtering and frequency estimation are essentially the same as for CW Doppler. Figure 7.9 has shown how demodulation works for CW systems. Figure 7.12 shows the demodulator in action for PW Doppler. Although the reference signal (Figure 7.12a) is produced continuously, the received ultrasound signal (Figure 7.12b) from the Doppler gate is only produced once for every ultrasound pulse. The process of

"mixing" (Figure 7.12c) and low-pass filtering (Figure 7.12d) produces the Doppler signal. This signal has the same overall shape as the demodulator output from the CW Doppler system. This is the reason that the displayed Doppler signals from CW and PW Doppler appear to be very similar, often indistinguishable.

This process of Doppler frequency detection is usually referred to by physicists as the "phase-domain" method. PW Doppler systems which use it are referred to as "phase-domain systems". The term "phase" refers to the degree of correspondence between the received echo and the reference echo in the demodulation process. This can be explained by further consideration of the demodulation process. Figure 7.13 shows the received echoes from consecutive pulses with respect to the reference frequency. Figure 7.13 also shows the amplitude of the signal after the reference and received signals have been multiplied, and the amplitude of the detected Doppler signal. The peak positive amplitude of the detected Doppler signal arises when the reference and received signals are aligned or "in-phase". As the reference and received frequencies gradually become misaligned the detected Doppler signal amplitude gradually decreases. When the reference and received signals are completely misaligned or "out of phase" the demodulated amplitude reaches its peak negative value.

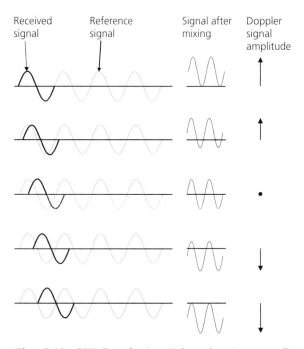

Fig. 7.13 PW Doppler is a "phase-domain process". The received ultrasound signal is shown in comparison to the reference signal for five consecutive ultrasound pulses. Also shown are the signal after the reference and received signal have been multiplied, and the final detected Doppler signal after low-pass filtering. The first ultrasound signal is in phase with the reference signal and the detected Doppler amplitude achieves its peak positive value. For consecutive echoes the received and reference signals become misaligned until, in the 5th pulse of this example, they are "out of phase" and the detected Doppler amplitude reaches its peak negative value.

For spectral Doppler estimation of the Doppler shift frequencies for the purpose of display is performed using the same FFT method as used for CW Doppler.

For colour flow an "autocorrelator" is used instead of the FFT method. In colour flow imaging, the estimator must calculate the mean (or average) Doppler shift frequency for each pixel of the 2D image. In order for colour images to be displayed at a suitable frame rate for real-time viewing, typically above 10 frames per second, the estimator must calculate this frequency value very quickly, usually in 1–2 ms. One possibility is to perform FFT, then calculate the mean frequency and colour code this value. This is not used in practice. The preferred option is to use a device called an "autocorrelator". This calculates the mean frequency directly, and is computationally more efficient (and hence faster) than the FFT approach.

Aliasing

The main difference between CW and PW Doppler, in terms of the display of blood velocities, is in the estimation of high velocity. Provided that there are a sufficient number of ultrasound pulses per wavelength it is possible to estimate the Doppler frequency shift accurately from the demodulated PW signal. If the prf is too low, the Doppler frequency shift cannot be estimated properly. This phenomenon is called "aliasing", and is a feature of pulsed Doppler systems, but not CW Doppler systems. This phenomenon can be explained with reference to Figure 7.14. The true Doppler signal is shown in Figure 7.14a. If the prf is high (Figure 7.14b) then there are a sufficient number of samples to enable the Doppler system to detect the frequency correctly. As the prf drops there comes a point at which the Doppler signal is only just sampled sufficiently. This is the case in Figure 7.14c where there are two samples per cycle. This is called the "Nyquist limit". This is equivalent to saying that the maximum Doppler frequency shift which can be detected is half of the prf, i.e. prf $= 2f_{d(max)}$. If the prf drops further (Figure 7.14d) the Doppler system can no longer calculate the correct frequency.

Do PW Doppler systems measure the Doppler effect?

There has been some debate in the literature about whether PW Doppler systems actually use the Doppler effect in their operation, and about whether PW Doppler systems have the right to be called "Doppler" systems. This is not an issue which impacts upon the clinical use of Doppler systems and these readers may wish to skip the remainder of this section.

The Doppler effect can be considered to be a dilation or expansion of the ultrasound wave. CW Doppler operates by directly measuring this dilation or expansion. For a PW Doppler system there will also be dilation or expansion of each individual echo arising as a result of the Doppler shift. However, PW Doppler systems do not measure this dilation or expansion, hence strictly speaking are not true Doppler shift detectors. However, the similarity in overall shape of the demodulator output for CW and PW systems is the reason that the equation describing the Doppler shift (Equation (7.1)) may be used for PW Doppler. In quantitative terms, these considerations are unimportant for the clinical use of CW or PW Doppler. The interested reader is referred to Section 4.2.2.5 in the textbook by Evans and McDicken (2000), and Example 4.2

in the textbook by Jensen (1996) for further explanations of this interesting phenomenon.

Time-domain systems

Another method for calculation of the velocity of a moving object such as blood, is to divide the distance the object travels by the time taken. This is the principle used in the time-domain Doppler system, which uses the PW approach. Figure 7.15 shows the position of a moving target and the corresponding echo for two consecutive ultrasound pulses. For the second ultrasound pulse the target and hence the echo are located further from the transducer. The estimation of the target velocity is performed by the following steps.

Estimate distance travelled by target

As described in Chapter 1, estimation of the depth from which echoes are received is performed automatically by the machine from the time between transmission and

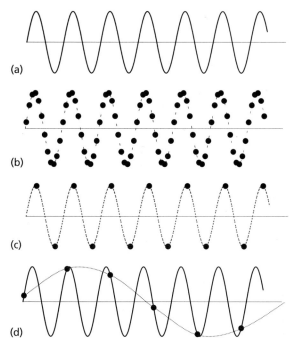

Fig. 7.14 Aliasing. (a) Doppler signal from CW system with a single frequency f_d. (b) PW Doppler, prf $> f_d/2$: there are many samples for each cycle of the Doppler signal, and as a consequence the Doppler frequency is correctly detected. (c) PW Doppler; prf $= f_d/2$: there are two samples per cycle and the Doppler frequency is estimated correctly. (d) PW Doppler, prf $< f_d/2$: there are less than two sample per cycle, and the detected frequency (dashed line) is less than the true Doppler frequency (solid line).

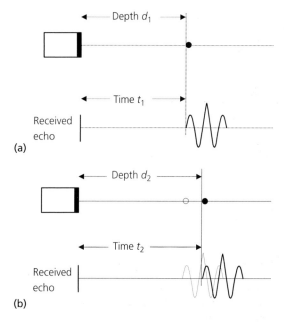

Fig. 7.15 Velocity estimated from time-domain method. A single target moves away from the transducer. The target position and echo are shown for two consecutive pulses: (a) first pulse (time t_1) and (b) second pulse (time t_2). The change in depth is calculated by estimating the depth the target has moved, and dividing this by the time interval between consecutive pulses.

reception of the echo, assuming that the speed of sound c is $1540\,m\,s^{-1}$. For the first and second pulses the depth of the moving target is estimated as

$$d_1 = \frac{ct_1}{2}, \quad d_2 = \frac{ct_2}{2}.$$

The factor of 2 above is to allow for the total distance travelled by the ultrasound, which is two times the depth of the target. The distance d_m moved between the two consecutive pulses is then estimated from the difference in estimated depths:

$$\begin{aligned} d_m &= d_2 - d_1 \\ &= \frac{c(t_2 - t_1)}{2}. \end{aligned} \quad (7.3)$$

The time-domain system estimates the difference in the time the echo is received between consecutive echoes using a process called "cross-correlation" which is described in more advanced text books.

Calculate time taken for target to move

The time taken for the target to move is simply the time between consecutive echoes, which is called the "pulse repetition interval" or pri. For Figure 7.15 the pri is the time between transmission of the first and second pulses, which is

$$\text{pri} = T_2 - T_1. \quad (7.4)$$

The pri is equal to the inverse of the prf:

$$\text{pri} = \frac{1}{\text{prf}}.$$

For example, if the prf is $1000\,Hz$, the pri is $1/1000\,s$, which is $0.001\,s$ or $1\,ms$.

Calculate velocity of target

The velocity of the target is calculated from the distance travelled and the time taken:

$$v = \frac{d_m}{\text{pri}}. \quad (7.5)$$

Using Equations (7.3) and (7.4) in combination with (7.5) gives Equation (7.6) in which the blood velocity is expressed in terms of the measured time difference between consecutive echoes:

$$v = (t_2 - t_1)\,c\,\frac{\text{prf}}{2}. \quad (7.6)$$

Commercial time-domain Doppler systems

Phase-domain systems use demodulated data, whereas time-domain systems require calculations to be performed on the RF data. The increase in computational power which the use of RF rather than demodulated data requires makes time-domain systems more expensive than phase-domain systems. This increase in cost is probably the main reason that, to date, there has only been one commercial system that has used the time-domain approach.

Other features

The basic steps of both spectral Doppler and colour flow systems are similar, as illustrated in Figure 7.8, so there will be a number of similar features. Below is a list of common features which are described in detail in the chapters on spectral and colour systems.

Feature	Description
Aliasing	The highest Doppler frequency shift that can be measured is equal to prf/2
Angle dependence	Estimated Doppler frequency is dependent on the cosine of the angle between the beam and the direction of motion
Doppler speckle	Variations in the received Doppler signal give rise to a "speckle" pattern seen in spectral and colour systems
Clutter breakthrough	Tissue motion giving rise to Doppler frequencies above the wall thump or clutter filter may be displayed on spectral Doppler or colour flow systems
Loss of low Doppler frequencies	Blood velocities which give rise to low Doppler frequencies (as a result of low velocity or angle near to 90°) will not be displayed if the value of the Doppler frequency is below the level of the wall thump or clutter filter

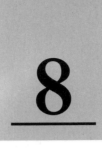

8

BLOOD FLOW

A Thrush

Introduction

The development of colour flow imaging has lead to an increase in the investigation of blood flow to aid diagnosis of both vascular and non-vascular disorders. An understanding of the physical properties of blood flow is essential when interpreting colour flow images and Doppler spectra. For example, the presence of reverse flow within a vessel as seen on a colour image may be due to the presence of disease or may be normal flow within the vessel. Changes in the velocity of the blood or the shape of the Doppler spectrum can help in locating and quantifying disease. A poor understanding of how blood flows in normal and diseased vessels may lead to misdiagnosis or to loss of useful clinical information. Blood flow is complex pulastile flow of a non-homogenous fluid in elastic tubes, however, some understanding can be obtained by considering the simple model of steady flow in a rigid tube (Caro et al., 1978; Nichols and O'Rourke, 1999).

Structure of the vessel walls

The structure of the arterial wall can change due to disease and these changes may be observed using ultrasound. Artery walls consist of a three-layer structure. The inner layer, the intima, is a thin layer of endothelium overlying an elastic membrane. The middle layer, media, consists of smooth muscle and elastic tissue. The outer layer, the adventia, is predominantly composed of connective tissue with collagen and elastic tissue. The intima–media layer is 0.5–1 mm thick in normal carotid arteries and can be visualised using ultrasound (Pignoli et al., 1986). Arterial disease will lead to changes in the vessel wall thickness that may eventually lead to a reduction of flow or act as a source of emboli. Vein walls have a similar structure to arteries but with a thinner media layer. Blood vessels not only act as a conduit to transport the blood around the body but are complex structures that respond to nervous and chemical stimulation to regulate the flow of blood.

Laminar, disturbed and turbulent flow

The flow in normal arteries at rest is laminar. This means that the blood moves in layers, with one layer sliding over the other. These layers are able to move at different velocities, with the blood cells remaining within their layers. However, if there is a significant increase in velocity, such as in the presence of a stenosis, laminar flow may breakdown and turbulent flow occurs (Taylor et al., 1995). In turbulent flow, the cells move randomly in all directions at variable speeds, but with an overall forward flow velocity. In the presence of turbulence, more energy is needed, i.e. a greater pressure drop is required if the flow rate is to be maintained. Turbulent flow may be seen distal to severe stenosis as shown in the spectral Doppler waveform in Figure 8.1. This demonstrates an increase in spectral broadening due to the range of velocities present within the turbulent flow and this may be used to indicate the presence of disease. The transition from laminar flow through disturbed flow and finally to turbulent flow is displayed diagramatically in Figure 8.2. The appearance of disturbed

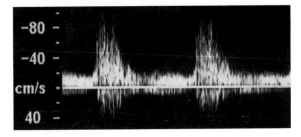

Fig. 8.1 Spectral Doppler display demonstrating turbulent flow.

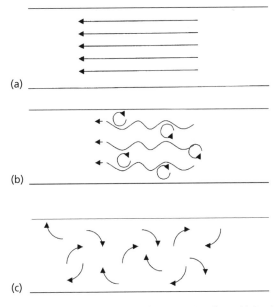

Fig. 8.2 Diagram showing the transition from (a) laminar flow to (b) disturbed flow and then (c) turbulent flow (after Taylor et al., 1995, with permission).

flow, such as the presence of vortices (spiral flow or eddies) or areas of flow reversal alone do not indicate the presence of disease but may be seen beyond a stenosis as well as in a normal bifurcation. For example, flow reversal in the carotid bifurcation (as seen in Figure 8.3) is considered to be a normal finding.

Velocity profiles

The blood within a vessel may not all be moving with the same velocity at any particular point in time. In fact, there is usually a variation in the blood velocity across the vessel, typically with faster flow seen in the centre of the vessel and slow moving blood near the vessel wall. This variation of blood velocity across the vessel is called the velocity profile. The shape of the velocity

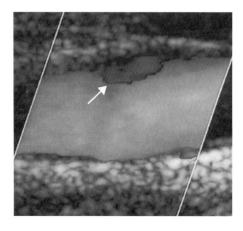

Fig. 8.3 Colour image showing flow reversal in the carotid bulb of a normal internal carotid artery.

profile will affect the appearance of both the colour flow image and the Doppler spectrum.

Considering a simple system of steady (i.e. non-pulsatile) flow of a homogeneous fluid entering a long rigid tube from a reservoir, the flow will develop from a blunt flow profile, with all the fluid moving at the same velocity, to parabolic flow (Caro *et al.*, 1978), as shown in Figure 8.4. This change of flow profile occurs due to the viscous drag exerted by the walls, causing the fluid at the wall to remain stationary. This generates a velocity gradient across the diameter of the vessel. The distance over which the flow profile develops from blunt to parabolic flow depends on the diameter of the tube and velocity of the fluid but is usually several times the tube diameter. Similar differences in velocity profile can be seen in different vessels within the body. For example, the flow profile in the ascending aorta is typically blunt but the flow seen in the normal mid-superficial femoral artery tends towards being parabolic. However, the shape of the velocity profile is further complicated by the fact that blood flow is pulsatile. The flow profile across a vessel may be visible on a colour flow image, as shown in Figure 8.5, with the slower moving blood seen near the vessel walls.

Velocity profiles in normal vessels

As the flow in arteries is in fact pulsatile, the velocity profile across an artery varies over time. The direction and velocity of the flow is dependent on the pressure drop along the length of the vessel. The pressure pulse, produced by the heart, travels down the arterial tree and is modified by the pressure wave that has been reflected back from the distal vessels. In the presence of high distal resistance to the flow, such as seen in the

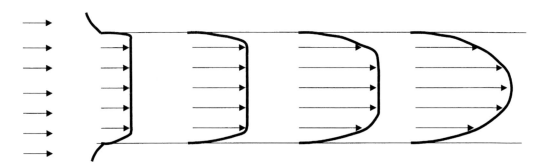

Fig. 8.4 The change in velocity profile, with distance along a rigid tube, from a blunt to a parabolic profile (after Caro *et al.*, 1978, with permission).

normal resting leg, this will lead to a reversal of flow during part of the diastolic phase of the cardiac cycle. This can be seen on the Doppler spectrum shown in Figure 8.6. This reversal of flow will affect the velocity profile seen in the vessel. Figure 8.7a and b shows

the predicted velocity profile at different points in the cardiac cycle for a normal common femoral artery and a common carotid artery, respectively (Evans and McDicken, 2000). This shows that reverse flow is not seen in a normal common carotid artery but flow reversal, during diastole, is demonstrated in the superficial femoral artery. Figure 8.7b also shows that it is possible for flow in the centre of the vessel to be travelling in a different direction from flow nearer the vessel wall. These changes in flow direction during the cardiac cycle can be observed, using colour flow imaging, as a change from red to blue or blue to red depending on the direction of flow relative to the transducer.

The shape of the velocity profile will also affect the degree of spectral broadening seen on the Doppler spectrum. If a parabolic profile is visualised with a large sample volume, both the low velocities near the vessel wall and the higher velocities in the centre of the vessel will be detected. This leads to a higher degree of spectral broadening in the Doppler spectrum than would be seen for a small sample volume placed in the centre of the vessel (see Chapter 9).

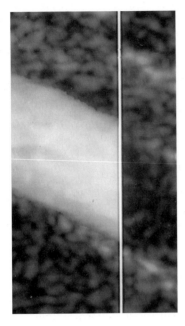

Fig. 8.5 Doppler image showing high velocities (paler) in the centre of a normal superficial femoral artery with lower velocities (darker) near the vessel wall.

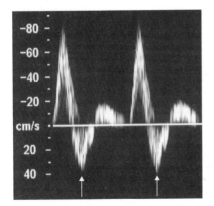

Fig. 8.6 Velocity waveform from a normal superficial femoral artery (arrows indicate reverse flow).

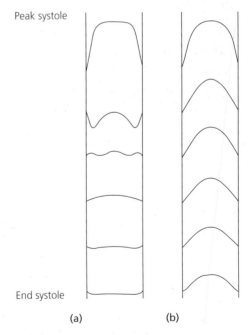

Fig. 8.7 Velocity profiles from (a) a common femoral artery and (b) a common carotid artery, calculated from the mean velocity waveforms (after Evans and McDickens *et al.*, 2000, with permission).

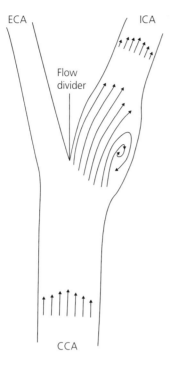

Fig. 8.8 Diagram of velocity patterns observed in the normal carotid bifurcation (from Reneman *et al.*, 1985, with permission).

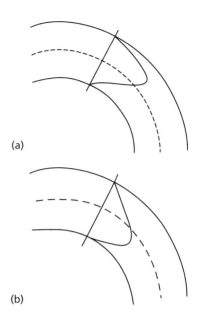

Fig. 8.9 Distortion of (a) parabolic flow and (b) blunt flow due to curvature of the tube (after Caro *et al.*, 1978, with permission).

Velocity profiles at branches and curves

The arterial tree branches many times along its length and this branching has an influence on the velocity profile. The velocity profiles found in the normal carotid bifurcation have been extensively studied and an example of this is given in the schematic diagram in Figure 8.8 (Reneman *et al.*, 1985). This shows an asymmetric flow profile in the proximal internal carotid artery with the high-velocity flow occurring towards the flow divider and the reverse flow occurring near the wall away from the origin of the external carotid artery. This profile results from pulsatile flow through a vessel of varying dimensions and will depend on the geometry of the bifurcation. An area of flow reversal is commonly seen on colour flow images of the normal carotid bifurcation (Figure 8.3).

Curvature of a tube will also influence the shape of the velocity profile. The peak velocity within the tube will be skewed off centre but whether this is to the inner or outer wall of the curve will depend on whether the underlying profile is blunt or parabolic. Figure 8.9

shows the effect of tube curvature on a flat and parabolic velocity profile.

Velocity profiles at stenoses

The velocity profile in the vessel can also be altered by the presence of arterial disease. If a vessel becomes narrowed, the velocity of the blood will increase as the blood passes through the stenosed section of the vessel. Beyond the narrowing, the vessel lumen will expand again and this may lead to flow reversal (Caro *et al.*, 1978) as shown in Figure 8.10. The combination of the velocity increase within the narrowing and an area of flow reversal beyond is often observed, with colour flow ultrasound, at the site of a significant stenosis (Figure 8.11). It is important to remember that the complex nature of both normal and abnormal blood flow is such that the flow is not necessarily parallel to the vessel walls.

Velocity changes within stenoses

The changes in the velocity of the blood that occur across a narrowing are used in spectral Doppler investigations both to identify the presence of a stenosis and to quantify the degree of narrowing. The relationship between the steady flow, Q, in a rigid tube of

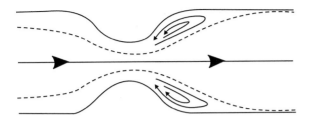

Fig. 8.10 Flow through a constriction followed by a rapid expansion downstream showing the region of flow reversal (from Caro *et al.*, 1978, with permission).

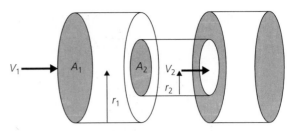

Fig. 8.12 For constant flow, Q, through a tube, the velocity of the fluid increases from V_1 to V_2 as the cross-sectional area decreases from A_1 to A_2 (r is radius).

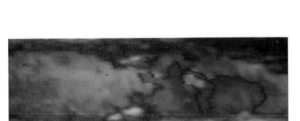

Fig. 8.11 Colour flow image showing the velocity increase as the blood flows through a stenosis, from left to right, followed by an area of flow reversal beyond the narrowing.

cross-sectional area, A, and the velocity of the fluid, V, is described by

$$Q = V \times A.$$

If the tube has no outlets or branches through which fluid can be lost, then the flow along the tube will remain constant. Therefore, the mean velocity at any point along the tube depends on the cross-sectional area of the tube. Figure 8.12 shows a tube of changing cross-sectional area (A_1, A_2) and, as the flow (Q) is constant, then:

$$Q = V_1 \times A_1 = V_2 \times A_2.$$

This can be rearranged to show that the change in the velocities is related to the change in the cross-sectional area as follows:

$$\frac{V_2}{V_1} = \frac{A_1}{A_2}.$$

This relationship actually describes steady flow in a rigid tube so cannot be directly applied to pulsatile blood flow in elastic arteries, however, it does give an indication as to how the velocity may change across a stenosis.

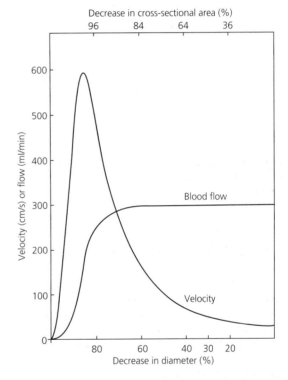

Fig. 8.13 Changes in flow and velocity as the degree of stenosis alters, predicted by a simple theoretical model of a smooth, symmetrical stenosis (after Spencer and Reid, 1979, with permission).

The graph in Figure 8.13 shows how the flow and velocity within an idealised stenosis varies with the degree of diameter reduction caused by the stenosis, based on the predictions from a simplified theoretical model (Spencer and Reid, 1979). This suggests that where the diameter reduction is less than 70–80%, the flow remains relatively unchanged; however, as the

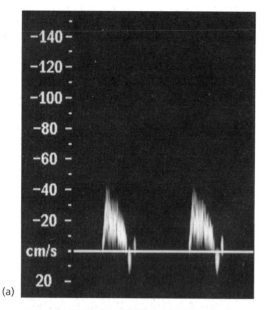

(a)

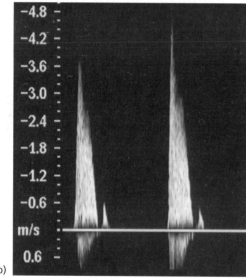

(b)

Fig 8.14 Doppler signal obtained (a) proximal to and (b) within a significant stenosis demonstrating a velocity increase.

diameter reduces further, the stenosis begins to limit the flow (known as a haemodynamically significant stenosis). The graph also shows that the velocity within the stenosis increases with diameter reduction and that these changes in velocity occur at much smaller diameter reductions than required to produce a flow reduction. For this reason, velocity changes are considered to

be a more sensitive method of detecting vessel lumen reductions than measurements of flow. Eventually, there becomes a point at which the flow drops to such an extent that the velocity begins to decrease and "trickle flow" is seen within the vessel. The relationships between vessel diameter reductions and velocity described above relate to simple steady flow models, and the velocity criteria used clinically to quantify the degree of narrowing are produced by comparing Doppler velocity measurements with arteriogram results. Figure 8.14 shows the velocity increase detected at the site of a superficial femoral artery stenosis.

Resistance to flow

The concept of resistance is used to describe how much force is needed to drive the blood through a particular vascular bed. Blood flows due to the pressure drop between different points along the vessel and also depend on the resistance to the flow. This relationship was described by Poiseuille as

$$pressure\ drop = flow \times resistance,$$

where the resistance to flow is given by

$$resistance = \frac{velocity \times length \times 8}{\pi \times radius^4}.$$

Therefore, in the presence of a given pressure drop, increased resistance would result in a reduction in flow. Again this equation describes non-pulsatile flow in a rigid tube and so cannot be directly related to arterial blood flow but indicates that flow not only depends on the pressure drop but is affected by the resistance to flow. It also shows how the resistance is highly dependent on the vessel diameter (r^4 term), with the resistance rapidly increasing as the diameter reduces. In the normal circulation, the greatest proportion of the resistance to flow is thought to occur at the level of the arterioles. The resistance to flow varies from one organ to another. For example, the normal brain, kidney and placenta are low resistance, compared to muscle at rest. Changes in the resistance to flow may occur during disease, either of the arteries or the arterioles. For example, abnormal development of the placenta may lead to the placenta being a high-resistance structure, making it difficult for blood to pass through the placenta, with the consequence that the foetus may obtain insufficient nutrition and oxygen and be small for its gestational age. Disease causing narrowing of the arteries, such as the superficial

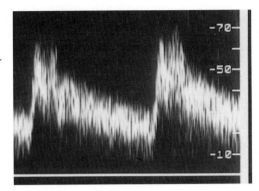

Fig. 8.15 Spectral Doppler obtained from a normal internal carotid artery.

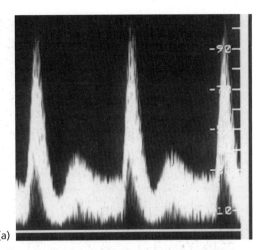

(a)

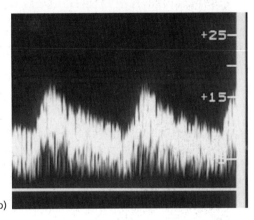

(b)

Fig. 8.16 (a) Doppler waveform obtained from an artery in the foot, in a normal leg following exercise, demonstrating monophasic hyperaemic flow. (b) Waveform demonstrating low-volume monophasic flow seen in the foot distal to an occlusion of the artery.

femoral artery, may lead to an increase in resistance to flow through the artery resulting in a reduction in blood flow, causing the patient to experience pain either when walking or at rest.

The waveform shape observed at different points in the body is dependent on the outflow resistance of the vessel, i.e. the vascular bed being supplied by the observed vessel. For example, the internal carotid artery supplies the brain which offers little resistance to flow and the Doppler waveform has continuous forward flow during diastole as shown in Figure 8.15. The renal arteries also supply a low-resistance vascular bed and, therefore, a similar waveform shape is observed. However, the peripheral circulation in the normal resting leg offers a higher resistance to flow and the typical waveform seen in the superficial femoral artery, supplying the leg, demonstrates a high-resistance waveform, with reverse flow seen during diastole (Figure 8.6).

Physiological and pathological changes that affect the arterial flow

Tissue perfusion is regulated by changes in the diameter of arterioles, thus altering peripheral resistance. For example, the increased demand by the leg muscles during exercise will lead to produce a reduction in the peripheral resistance, by dilation of the arterioles, leading to an increase in blood flow. This also leads to a change in the shape of the waveform, as seen in Figure 8.16a whereby the flow in diastole is now entirely in the forward direction (compared to Figure 8.6).

The presence of arterial disease can significantly alter the resistance to flow, with the reduction in vessel diameter having a major effect on the change in resistance. The Doppler waveform shape will be affected by an increase in the resistance distal to the site from which the waveform was obtained. This observed change in waveform shape may help indicate the presence of an occlusion distal to the vessel being observed. For example, the waveform in Figure 8.17 shows a Doppler spectrum obtained from a common carotid artery proximal to an internal carotid artery occlusion. This waveform demonstrates a short acceleration time but with an absence of any diastolic flow which is normally seen in the cerebral circulation (Figure 8.15).

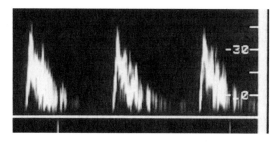

Fig. 8.17 Doppler waveform obtained from a common carotid artery proximal to an occluded internal carotid artery demonstrating a high-resistance waveform.

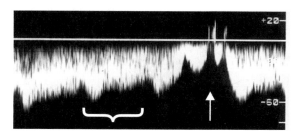

Fig. 8.18 Doppler waveform demonstrating the effect of respiration (indicated by the arrow) and the cardiac cycle (indicated by the bracket) on the blood flow in a subclavian vein.

Beyond an occlusion the spectrum may also appear abnormal. In the presence of severe disease in the superficial femoral artery, the arterioles may become maximally dilated to reduce the peripheral resistance to maximise the limited blood flow in an attempt to maintain tissue perfusion. A typical spectrum obtained distal to a superficial femoral artery occlusion is shown in Figure 8.16b with the characteristic damped waveform shape with longer systolic acceleration time and increased diastolic flow. The velocity of the flow seen in Figure 8.16b, distal to an occlusion, is lower than that seen in Figure 8.16a demonstrating hyperaemic flow in a normal leg. The presence of collateral flow, i.e. the blood finding an alternative route to bypass a stenosis or occlusion, will also influence both the waveform shape proximal and distal to the disease. Good collateral flow may alter the effect on the waveform shape expected for a given severity of disease, as the collateral pathway may affect the resistance to flow.

Venous flow

Veins transport blood back to the heart. To enable them to perform this function they have thin but strong bicuspid valves to prevent retrograde flow. There are typically a larger number of valves in the more distal veins. Venous flow back to the heart is enhanced by the influence of pressure changes generated by the cardiac cycle, respiration (Figure 8.18) and changes in posture as well as the action of the calf muscle pump. The flow and pressure in the central venous system is affected by changes in the volume of the right atrium which occur during the cardiac cycle. This pulsatile effect can be seen on Doppler spectra obtained from the proximal veins of the arm and neck due to their proximity to the chest. However, flow patterns in the lower limb veins

and peripheral arm veins are not significantly affected by the cardiac cycle due to the compliance of the veins, leading to a damping of the pressure changes. The presence of valves and changes in intra-abdominal pressure during respiration also mask the effect of the cardiac cycle on venous flow in the distal veins.

Changes in the volume of the thorax, due to movement of the diaphragm and ribs, also assists venous return. During inspiration, the thorax expands leading to an increase in the volume of the veins within the chest, resulting in an increase in flow into the chest. During expiration, a decrease in flow is seen. The reverse situation is seen in the abdomen because the diaphragm descends during inspiration, causing the abdominal pressure to increase encouraging flow into the thorax. When the diaphragm rises, the pressure drops encouraging flow from the upper leg veins into the abdomen. Respiration effects can be observed on the spectral Doppler display as phasic changes in flow in proximal deep peripheral vein, such as the common femoral vein. Augmentation of flow using breathing manoeuvres is often used in the investigation of venous disorders.

Changes in posture can lead to large changes in hydrostatic pressure in the venous system. When a person is lying supine, there is a relatively small pressure difference between the venous pressure at the ankle and right atrium. However, when standing there is a column of blood between the right atrium and veins at the ankle and this produces a significant pressure gradient which has to be overcome in order for blood to be returned to the heart. This can be achieved by the calf muscle pump mechanism assisted by the presence of the venous valves. The muscle compartments in the calf contain the deep veins and venous sinuses that act as blood reservoirs. When the deep muscles of the calf contract, thus causing compression of the veins, blood flow is forced out

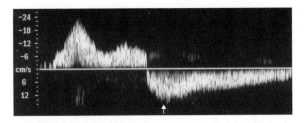

Fig 8.19 Sonogram demonstrating reversal of flow in the vein, reflux (shown by arrow), due to incompetent valves in the vein.

of the leg and prevented from returning by the venous valves. This also creates a pressure gradient between the superficial and deep veins in the calf causing blood to drain from the superficial to the deep venous system. If there is significant failure of the venous valves in either the superficial or deep venous system, reflux will occur leading to a less-effective muscle pump and a higher pressure than the normal in the veins following calf muscle contraction and relaxation. This may eventually lead to the development of venous ulcers.

Colour flow imaging and spectral Doppler can be used to identify venous incompetence seen as periods of retrograde flow, away from the heart, following compression of the calf (Figure 8.19). Venous outflow obstruction leads to a loss of the normal spontaneous phasic flow, detected by Doppler ultrasound, generated by respiration.

References

Caro CG, Pedley TJ, Schroter RC and Seed WA. *The Mechanics of the Circulation*. Oxford University Press. 1978.

Nichols WN and O'Rourke MF. *McDonald's Blood Flow in Arteries*, 2nd edition. Edward Arnold. 1999.

Pignoli P, Tremoli E, Poli A, Oreste P and Paoletti R. Intimal plus medial thickness of the arterial wall: a direct measurement with ultrasound imaging. *Circulation* 1986; **74**(6): 1399–1406.

Taylor KJW, Burns PN and Wells PNT. *Clinical Applications of Doppler Ultrasound*. Raven Press. 1995.

Evans DH and McDicken WN. *Doppler Ultrasound: Physics, Instrumentation, and Signal Processing*. Wiley. 2000.

Reneman RS, van Merode T, Hick P and Hoeks APG. Flow velocity patterns in and distensibility of the carotid artery bulb in subjects of various ages. *Circulation* 1985; **71**(3): 500–509.

Spencer MP and Reid JM. Quantitation of carotid stenosis with continuous-wave (C-W) Doppler ultrasound. *Stroke* 1979; **10**(3): 326–330.

Further reading

Oates C. *Cardiovascular Haemodynamics and Doppler Waveforms Explained*. Greenwich Medical Media Ltd. 2001.

9

SPECTRAL DOPPLER ULTRASOUND

A Thrush

Spectral display
Doppler ultrasound systems
Spectral analysis
Spectral Doppler controls and how they should
be optimised
Factors that affect the Doppler spectrum
Effect of pathology on the Doppler sonogram
Artefacts
Measurements and their potential sources of errors

Spectral display

A typical real-time spectral Doppler display is shown in Figure 9.1. This displays time along the horizontal axis and the Doppler frequency shift along the vertical axis. The brightness (or colour) of the display indicates the amplitude of each of the Doppler frequency components present, i.e. the relative proportion of the blood travelling with a particular velocity. The baseline indicated in Figure 9.1 corresponds to zero Doppler shift. The spectrum contains information about the speed and direction of the blood flow as well as the degree of pulsatility of the flow. Conventionally, it is arranged so that positive Doppler frequency shifts (blood flowing towards the transducer) are plotted above the baseline and negative Doppler shifts (blood flowing away from the probe) are plotted below the baseline, but the operator can invert this display as required. Both arterial and venous flow may be present within the beam and when, as is usually the case, the flow in these vessels is in opposite directions, the Doppler waveforms from the arterial and venous flow appear on opposite sides of the baseline as seen in Figure 9.1. The Doppler ultrasound signal from a blood vessel will contain a range of Doppler frequency shifts. These arise in part from the range of blood velocities present within the region of the vessel being investigated but also arise from a phenomenon called "intrinsic spectral broadening", which is described later in this chapter.

Doppler ultrasound systems

A spectral Doppler display is produced by performing spectral analysis of the Doppler signal. The Doppler signal can be obtained either from a stand alone continuous wave (CW) or pulsed wave (PW) system or from systems combing Doppler ultrasound with imaging, known as duplex systems. Some of the advantages and disadvantages of these systems are discussed below.

CW Doppler

The CW transducer consists of at least two elements: one to continually transmit and the other to continually receive ultrasound. The frequencies of Doppler signals generated by moving blood are conveniently in the audible range and so can be output to a loudspeaker after amplification and filtering to remove the signal generated by the slow-moving vessel wall. Early Doppler systems had only audio outputs, and this approach is still taken in the simple pocket Doppler devices used in peripheral vascular applications. However, useful information can be provided if spectral analysis of the Doppler signal is performed. The fact that the CW system is continually detecting the blood flow means that CW systems do not suffer from the artefact of aliasing (Figures 7.14 and 9.2). However, the large sensitive region (Figure 7.7) means it is difficult to identify the source of the Doppler signal.

Pulsed wave Doppler

Pulsed Doppler instrumentation has similarities to CW instrumentation. However, the transducer is excited with regular short pulses rather than continuously. In order to detect the signal from a specific depth in the

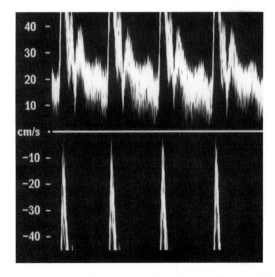

Fig. 9.2 Spectral Doppler display showing aliasing of the signal due to undersampling.

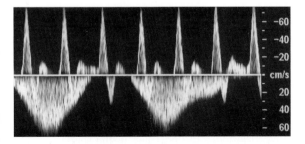

Fig. 9.1 Spectral Doppler display showing arterial flow towards the transducer displayed above the baseline and venous flow away from the transducer displayed below the baseline.

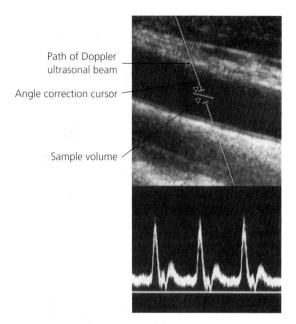

Path of Doppler ultrasonal beam

Angle correction cursor

Sample volume

Fig. 9.3 Ultrasound image of a vessel with the path of the spectral Doppler ultrasound beam, sample volume size and angle correction cursor displayed.

tissue, a "range gate" is used. This enables the system to only receive the returning signal at a given time after the pulse has been transmitted, and then for a limited period of time. The Doppler signal is, therefore, detected from a specific volume within the body, known as the sample volume, at an identified range (Figure 9.3). The length of time over which the range gate is open is often known as the gate length. The operator can control the depth and length of the sample volume, by varying the gate range and length. Thus, PW Doppler has the enormous advantage of allowing the operator to select the origin of the Doppler signal. However, PW Doppler does as a consequence, suffer from the artefact of aliasing if the blood flow is undersampled, as seen in Figure 9.2 (see Chapter 7).

Duplex systems

Initially, both the CW and PW Doppler were used without the aid of imaging and the vessels were located blindly, using only the detected Doppler signal to indicate the presence of the vessel. As imaging ultrasound developed, it become apparent that using Doppler ultrasound in conjunction with imaging, a combination known as duplex ultrasound, would enable better location of the relevant vessel. Duplex Doppler ultrasound

enables precise location of the Doppler sample volume, e.g. at the centre of a vessel, as shown in Figure 9.3. It is also possible to estimate the angle of insonation, between the beam and the vessel using the angle correction cursor, enabling the velocity of the blood to be calculated, using the Doppler equation.

Some early duplex systems used a separate CW or PW Doppler probe mounted by the side of the imaging transducer. The current approach is to use the same piezoelectric elements to produce the spectral Doppler waveform and the B-mode image. Modern duplex scanners use arrays of elements, as described in Chapter 3, to produce both the imaging and Doppler beam. These include curvilinear, linear and phased array transducers.

When combining B-mode imaging with Doppler ultrasound, there is a conflict in the optimal angle of insonation. Ideally, the vessel walls should be imaged with a beam that is at right angles to the vessel whereas the optimal Doppler measurements are made when the beam is parallel to the vessel. Therefore, a compromise has to be reached. Linear array transducers are able to steer the beam (using beam forming techniques) approximately 20° left or right of the path perpendicular to the transducer face (described later). This allows the Doppler beam to be set at an angle to the imaging beam enabling both the imaging and the Doppler recordings to be made in a vessel that runs parallel to the skin, such as vessels in the limbs and neck. Curvilinear and phased array transducers do not usually have the facility to steer the Doppler beam relative to the imaging beam so a suitable compromise for imaging and Doppler has to be obtained by angling the transducer.

Spectral analysis

The Doppler signal obtained by any of the systems described above can be analysed into its frequency components in the Doppler signal using a mathematical process known as the Fourier transform. The range of frequency components relates to the range of velocities present within the blood flow. Figure 9.4 shows how the sonogram is produced by displaying consecutive spectra, with frequency displayed along the vertical axis and time along the horizontal axis. A complete spectrum is produced every 5–40 ms and each of these spectra is used to produce the next line in the sonogram. The brightness of the display at each point indicates the relative amplitude of each of the component frequencies, which in turn is an indication of the backscattered power for each value of Doppler frequency shift. If the

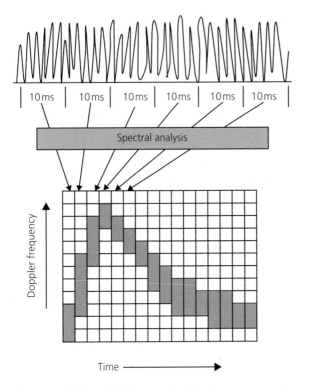

Fig. 9.4 Schematic diagram showing how consecutive spectra produced by the spectrum analysis of the Doppler signal are used to construct the spectral Doppler display.

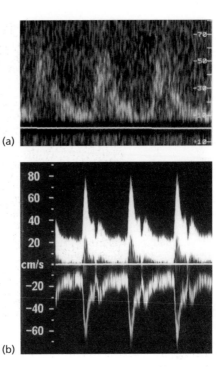

Fig. 9.5 (a) Doppler spectral displayed showing that when the amplitude of the Doppler signal and the background noise are similar, increasing the gain dose not help to improve the display. (b) Spectral Doppler display where the gain has been set to high causing signal to breakthrough on the reverse channel.

angle of insonation is known, the vertical frequency scale can be converted to a velocity scale.

Spectral Doppler controls and how they should be optimised

Transmit power

The ultrasound backscattered from blood is of much lower amplitude than the signals returning from the surrounding tissue. Increasing the output power will increase the amplitude of the transmitted ultrasound resulting in a higher-amplitude signal returning to the transducer. The output power of the transducer is altered by the scanner's transmit power control. On some ultrasound systems, the same control may be used to change the output power of all the three modalities: B-mode imaging, spectral and colour Doppler. However, increasing the output power will also increase the patients exposure to ultrasound. Therefore, the transmit power

should only be increased after other controls, such as the gain, have been optimised to obtain the best Doppler spectrum. On modern ultrasound systems, changes of the output power should be reflected in changes in the displayed mechanical index (MI) and thermal index (TI) (see Chapter 13).

Gain

As the received backscattered signal from blood is small it will need to be amplified before it can be analysed. Increasing the spectral Doppler gain increases the brightness of the spectrum on the screen. However, the gain control increases the amplitude of not only the Doppler signal but also the background electronic noise. If the Doppler signal is of similar amplitude to the background noise, then no matter how much the gain is increased, only a poor Doppler sonogram will be obtained, as shown in Figure 9.5a. In these situations, it may be necessary to use a lower transmit frequency (resulting in less attenuation) or a higher transmit power. If the gain is set too high, the Doppler system may become overloaded and may no longer be able to separate the forward and reverse flow accurately. This gives rise to an artefact whereby a mirror image of the true Doppler spectra appears in the reverse channel of the sonogram, as shown in Figure 9.5b. This is not true reverse flow but an artefact that can be eliminated by turning down the Doppler gain.

Transmit frequency

As high-frequency ultrasound is attenuated more than low-frequency ultrasound (see Chapter 2), the appropriate Doppler-transmit frequency needs to be selected to ensure adequate penetration of the ultrasound. The frequency required will, therefore, depend on the depth of the vessel to be investigated. The Doppler-transmit frequency is governed by the transducer that has been selected. Most modern ultrasound systems use broad-band transducer technology, which means it is possible to operate the transducer over a range of different frequencies without too much loss in efficiency. Therefore, for example, a transducer may use 5 MHz for imaging but use a lower frequency of 4 MHz for the Doppler measurements to ensure adequate returning backscattered signal from the blood. If the backscattered ultrasound signal from the blood is weak, it may be possible to improve the penetration of the beam by lowering the transmit frequency by 1 or 2 MHz. If this still does not provide sufficient penetration, it may be necessary to select a transducer that operates at a lower-frequency range.

Pulse repetition frequency (scale)

With pulsed Doppler ultrasound, the rate at which the pulses of ultrasound are transmitted is known as the pulse repetition frequency (PRF) and this can be controlled by the operator. The PRF can typically be set between 1.5 and 18 kHz, depending on the velocity of the blood that is to be detected. Not all systems display the PRF but may indicate this as a velocity scale. Most ultrasound scanners have application-specific pre-sets that, if selected, will set the controls, such as the PRF, to a suitable starting value. However, these values may need to be altered during the scan to obtain an optimal spectral display. If the PRF is set to low, aliasing may occur. This gives the appearance shown in Figure 9.2 where the high frequencies present are incorrectly displayed in the reverse channel. This can be overcome by increasing the PRF. There will be, however, an upper

limit to the PRF as the scanner will usually only allow one pulse to be "in-flight" at a time in order to prevent confusion as to where a returning signal has originated from. If PRF_{max} is the upper limit of the PRF, the maximum velocity, v_{max}, that can be measured will be given by the equation

$$\frac{PRF_{max}}{2} = \frac{2v_{max}f_t\cos\theta}{c}.$$

This can be re-written as

$$v_{max} = \frac{PRF_{max}c}{4f_t\cos\theta}.$$

For a depth of interest, d, and speed of sound, c,

$$PRF = \frac{c}{2d}.$$

The 2, in the equation above, arises from the fact that the pulse has to go to and return from the target. This gives

$$v_{max} = \frac{c^2}{8df_t\cos\theta}.$$

If too high a PRF is used to detect slower-moving blood, the scale of the spectral display will not be fully utilised and the ability to identify changes in the Doppler frequency will be reduced. It is, therefore, important to set the PRF such that the Doppler waveform almost fills the display, without any wrap around due to aliasing occurring.

When measuring very high blood flow velocities, as may occur in the presence of an aortic valve stenosis, some scanners will allow a "high PRF" mode to be selected. This allows more than one pulse to be "in-flight" at a given time. The higher PRF allows higher velocities to be measured, but also introduces range ambiguity, i.e. a loss of certainty as to the origin of the Doppler signal.

Baseline

The baseline represents zero Doppler shift and, therefore, demarcates the part of the display used for displaying forward flow from that used for reverse flow. The position of the baseline can be changed by the operator to allow optimum use of all the spectral display, depending on the relative size of the forward and reverse flow velocities present. For example, the position of the baseline may be lowered to prevent aliasing of a positive Doppler shift signal.

Invert

The invert control enables the operator to turn the Doppler display upside down, so that flow away from the transducer is displayed above the baseline and flow towards the transducer is displayed below. Typically, operators prefer to display arterial flow above the baseline.

Filter

The Doppler signal will contain not only the low-amplitude higher Doppler frequencies backscattered from the blood but also high-amplitude lower Doppler frequencies from the slow-moving tissue such as the vessel walls. These unwanted frequencies can be removed by a high-pass filter. As the name suggests, a high-pass filter removes the low-frequency signals while maintaining the high frequencies. There is, however, a compromise in the selection of the cut-off frequency to be used, as it is important not to remove the frequencies detected from the lower-velocity arterial or venous blood flow. Figure 9.6 shows the high-pass filter set at three different levels. The first (a) shows the filter is set too low and the wall thump, generated by the slow-moving vessel wall, and has not been removed. In the second situation (b), the filter has been correctly set to remove the wall thump and in the third situation (c), the filter has been set too high and the diastolic flow has been removed giving a false impression of the waveform shape, which could lead to a misdiagnosis.

Gate size and position

The size and position of the "range gate" or "sample volume" is selected by the operator and can typically be varied between 1 and 20 mm in length. The "gate size" or "sample volume length" may affect the appearance of the Doppler spectrum, as described below. It is important that care is taken to select the appropriate gate length, depending on whether the operator wishes to detect the velocities in the centre of the vessel only or velocities present across the whole vessel.

Beam steering angle

The angle of insonation can be altered by changing the orientation of the transducer in relation to the vessel, e.g. by tilting the transducer. Linear array transducers also have the facility to steer the Doppler beam 20° to the left or right of the centre. The ultrasound beam is electronically steered by introducing delays between the pulses used to excite consecutive active elements. This is similar to the method used to focus the beam, described in Chapter 3, but uses a different sequence of delays. Figure 9.7 shows how the delay between excitation pulses results in the wavelets produced by each element interfering in such a way that a wave front is no longer parallel to the front of the transducer. The path of the beam can be steered left or right of the centre depending on the delays introduced. Steering the beam in this way is necessary when using a linear array transducer it detects flow in a vessel that is parallel to the front face of the transducer. This enables a Doppler angle of insonation of 60° or less to be used while the imaging beam remains nearly perpendicular to the vessel wall, optimal for B-mode imaging. However, a steered Doppler beam has a lower sensitivity than a beam that

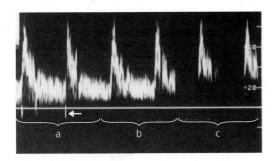

Fig. 9.6 Doppler spectral display showing how the appearance changes with different high-pass filters. (a) The filter is set to low allowing wall thump (shown by arrow) to be displayed. (b) The filter is set correctly. (c) The filter is set to high removing the diastolic flow component.

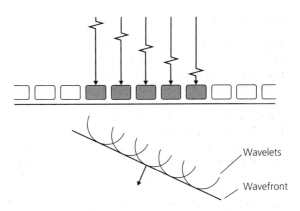

Fig. 9.7 The Doppler beam produced by linear array transducers may be steered by introducing delays between the pulses used to excite consecutive active elements in the array.

is perpendicular to the transducer face, which in combination with low-amplitude Doppler signal may result in a noisy or undetectable Doppler signal. The angle of insonation of the Doppler beam should be optimised to 60° or less to enable a good Doppler signal to be acquired and to minimise errors in velocity measurements (discussed later in the chapter).

Doppler angle cursor

In order to calculate the velocity of blood from the measured Doppler shift frequencies, the angle of insonation between the Doppler beam and the direction of flow must be known. Duplex scanners have the facility to allow the operator to line up an angle cursor with either the vessel wall, as seen on the B-mode image, or the direction of flow, as seen on the colour flow image. The scanner can then convert the Doppler shift frequencies to velocities and a velocity scale will be seen alongside the spectral display. Errors in the alignment of the angle correction cursor can lead to significant errors in velocity measurement (discussed later in the chapter).

Focal depth

In many systems the Doppler beam is focused. This may be fixed or adjustable, depending on the ultrasound system. In some systems the Doppler beam focal depth automatically follows the sample volume, when the operator moves it.

Grey-scale curve

The grey-scale curve governs the relative display brightness assigned to the different amplitude signals detected. The relative amplitude signal detected at each frequency relates to the relative proportion of red blood cells moving at each given velocity. The Doppler spectra may be displayed using different grey-scale curves or even colour scales. These are similar to the grey-scale curves used in B-mode image display (see Chapter 4).

Factors that affect the Doppler spectrum

Both the shape of the Doppler waveform and the velocity measurements made from it are used to diagnose the disease. However, the spectra may also be affected by factors other than disease. It is important for the operator to understand these effects in order to be able to correctly interpret the Doppler spectrum. Factors that may alter the Doppler spectrum are discussed below.

Blood flow profile

The velocity profile across a vessel, at a given point of time, may either be blunt, parabolic or part way in between (see Chapter 8). If the width of the Doppler beam and sample volume length is such that it covers the entire vessel, i.e. completely insonates the vessel cross section, then signals from flow across the full width of the vessel will be detected. With a blunt flow profile, all the blood is travelling at a similar velocity, therefore, the velocity spectrum would display a narrow spread of velocities as shown in Figure 9.8a. However, the spectral Doppler display for complete insonation of parabolic flow would demonstrate the wider range of velocities present in the vessel as seen in Figure 9.8b.

Non-uniform insonation

Modern linear array transducers typically have very narrow beams. When a linear array probe is aligned along the length of a section of vessel, it is the beam width in the elevation plane that is important. If a beam is narrow in this dimension, then the beam will not insonate the entire vessel and so the slower-moving blood on the lateral walls of the vessel will not be detected (as shown in Figure 9.9a). Therefore, the spectrum will no longer represent the true relative proportions of blood moving at the slower velocity in the presence of parabolic or near-parabolic flow.

Sample volume size

The sample volume size and position will also affect the proportion of the blood velocities within the vessel that will be detected. A large sample volume will enable the flow near the anterior and posterior walls to be detected, but, as discussed above, the narrow beam width in elevation may mean that the flow near the lateral walls will remain undetected. If only the fast flow in the centre of the vessel is to be measured, then a small sample volume should be selected (Figure 9.9b). It is also important to use a small sample volume when assessing the degree of spectral broadening, i.e. the width of the Doppler spectrum, as an indication of the presence of disturbed flow within a diseased vessel.

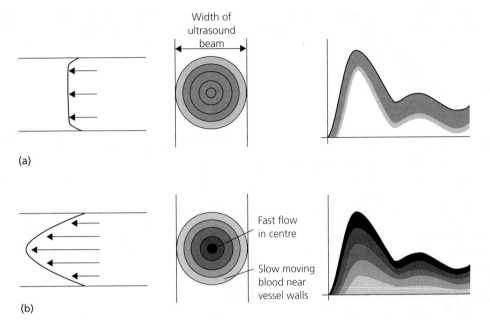

Width of
ultrasound
beam

(a)

Fast flow
in centre

Slow moving
blood near
vessel walls

(b)

Fig. 9.8 A schematic diagram showing how the velocities displayed in the Doppler spectrum will depend on the velocity profile within the vessel shown for idealised (a) blunt flow and (b) parabolic flow. (From Thrush and Hartshorne, 1999, with permission.)

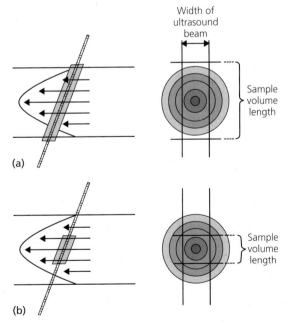

Width of
ultrasound
beam

Sample
volume
length

(a)

Sample
volume
length

(b)

Fig. 9.9 Effect of (a) incomplete insonation and (b) sample volume size on the detected Doppler signal. (From Thrush and Hartshorne, 1999, with permission.)

Intrinsic spectral broadening

The Doppler beam is produced by a sub-group of elements within the array (as shown in Figure 9.10), producing a Doppler aperture. This means that in reality, the Doppler beam insonates the blood with a range of different angles due to the shape of the beam. Linear array and curvilinear array transducers use a number of elements to form the Doppler beam and different elements will produce different angles of insonation. For example, in the diagram shown in Figure 9.10, the element on the far right of the sub-group will produce a smaller angle of insonation (θ_1) and will, therefore, detect a larger Doppler shift frequency than the element on the far left of the sub-group. This will lead to a spreading of the range of Doppler shift frequencies detected that is due to the beam shape rather than the blood flow. This effect is known as intrinsic spectral broadening (Thrush and Evans, 1995; Hoskins, 1996). It can be demonstrated by insonating a single moving target, such as a string driven by a motor at constant speed. The Doppler spectra produced using a 5 MHz linear array transducer and a moving string is shown in Figure 9.11. This demonstrates that, instead of Doppler spectra displaying a single velocity for the moving string, a spread of velocities is displayed. As the string (unlike blood) is moving at a

121

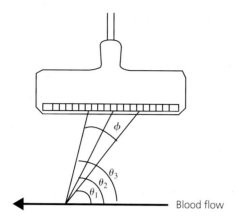

Fig. 9.10 A number of element of a linear array transducer are used to produce the Doppler beam leading to a range of angles of insonation (θ).

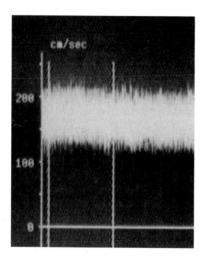

Fig. 9.11 Doppler spectrum obtained from a moving string test object showing a range of velocities despite the fact that the string can only move with a single velocity.

single velocity, the spreading of the detected velocities seen in the spectra is due to intrinsic spectral broadening. This spectral broadening effect can lead to errors when making velocity measurements, or estimating the range of Doppler frequencies relating to disturbed flow in the presence of arterial disease.

Pulse repetition frequency

If an inappropriately low PRF is used, this will result in aliasing of the signal. This will alter the appearance of

the waveform shape (Figure 9.2) and lead to an underestimate of the peak velocity.

High-pass filter

The high-pass filter is used to remove unwanted low-frequency signals arising from the slow-moving vessel walls. However, if the filter is set too high the waveform shape may be significantly altered (see Figure 9.6), e.g. the filter may remove the low frequencies detected during diastole which would alter the conclusions drawn from the scan.

Gain

If the gain is set too high, a mirror image of the spectrum will be seen (see Figure 9.4b). If the gain is set too low, all the detected signals may not be adequately displayed.

Effect of pathology on the Doppler sonogram

Changes in detected Doppler frequency shift

The velocity of blood increases as blood passes through a narrowing (as described in Chapter 8). For this reason, velocity measurements or velocity ratios are often used to quantify the degree of narrowing of a vessel. Velocity ratios compare the velocity in the normal vessel proximal to a stenosis with the highest velocity at or just beyond the stenosis. A significant stenosis or occlusion may lead to a reduction in flow and this will be indicated by the presence of untypically low velocities.

Changes in SB

The presence of disturbed or turbulent flow can lead to an increase in SB which may be used as an indicator of disease. However, SB should be interpreted cautiously as intrinsic spectral broadening can be introduced due to properties of the ultrasound scanner (as described earlier in this chapter).

Changes in spectrum shape

The shape of the Doppler spectrum will depend on which vessel is investigated. For example, the spectral shape detected in the carotid artery (Figure 8.15), which supplies blood flow to the brain, is very different from the spectral shape detected from the femoral arteries (Figure 8.6), which supply the leg. Significant disease either proximal or distal to the measurement site will also affect the spectral shape, and can, therefore, provide a useful indication of the presence and possible site of disease (Chapter 8).

Artefacts

Some of the artefacts that spectral Doppler suffers from are of the same origin as imaging ultrasound artefacts in that the ultrasound beam does not follow the expected path, or that the ultrasound has been attenuated. This leads to the following artefacts:

- *Shadowing:* This is due to highly reflecting or attenuating structures, such as bowel gas or calcified vessel wall, overlying the blood flow, leading to a loss of Doppler signal.

- *Multiple reflections:* In the presence of a strongly reflecting surface, e.g. bone–tissue or air–tissue interface, multiple reflections may occur, leading to the appearance that Doppler signals have been detected outside the vessel. This will affect both the spectral Doppler and the colour flow. An example of where this is often seen is when imaging the subclavian artery as it passes over the lung, leading to the appearance of a second vessel lying within the lung. This is known as a mirror image.

- *Refraction:* This occurs if an ultrasound beam passes a boundary between two media with different propagation speeds, at an angle of less than 90°. This can lead to misregistration of both the image and the Doppler sample volume.

Other artefacts seen in spectral Doppler relate to production of the Doppler spectrum. These artefacts include the following:

- *Aliasing:* This occurs due to undersampling of the blood flow (see Figure 9.2) and can be corrected by increasing the Doppler PRF.

- *Angle dependence:* The Doppler shift frequencies detected are dependent on the angle of insonation by the $\cos \theta$ term. The larger the angle of insonation the smaller the Doppler shift frequencies detected, possibly leading to a poorer-quality Doppler spectrum. As the angle of insonation approaches 90°, the Doppler signal may be very small and, therefore, will be removed by the high-pass filter.

- *Intrinsic spectral broadening:* This occurs due to geometry of the ultrasound beam and the vessel (see Figures 9.10 and 9.11).

- *Range ambiguity:* This occurs when more than one pulse is in-flight at a time, as may be the case when a high PRF is used, as the origin of the Doppler signal is no longer certain.

- *Inverted mirror image of the Doppler spectrum:* This can occur, if the gain is set to high (see Figure 9.5b).

Measurements and their potential sources of errors

Velocity

Measurements of blood velocities are often used to quantify disease. Duplex imaging allows an estimate of the angle of insonation (θ) between the Doppler ultrasound beam and the blood flow. The Doppler equation can be used to estimate the velocity of the blood (v) from the measured Doppler shift frequency (f_d), as the transmitted frequency of the Doppler beam (f_t) is known and the speed of sound in tissue (c) is assumed to be constant ($1540 \, \mathrm{m^{-1} s}$):

$$v = \frac{f_d c}{2 f_t \cos \theta}.$$

There is often a spread of velocities present within the Doppler sample volume. The effect of intrinsic spectral broadening will lead to a further spreading of the detected Doppler frequencies. Therefore, when measuring velocity, a choice has to be made whether to use the maximum or the mean Doppler frequency. The ultrasound system calculates the mean Doppler frequency by finding the average of all the frequencies in the spectrum at a given instant in time. The maximum velocity at peak systole is often used to quantify carotid artery disease and velocity ratios are used to quantify disease in peripheral arteries (Thrush and Hartshorne, 1999). The velocity ratio is given by the maximum peak systolic velocity within a stenosis, v_{sten}, and in the normal vessel proximal to the stenosis, v_{prox}, as follows:

$$\mathrm{Velocity} = \frac{v_{sten}}{v_{prox}}.$$

As well as spot measurements of velocity at given points in time, many ultrasound systems are also capable of providing velocity measurements averaged over time. One such measurement is the mean velocity averaged over a number of complete cardiac cycles, usually known as time-average velocity, TAV. This can be used to estimate blood flow as described later in the chapter.

Errors in velocity measurements due to the angle of insonation

An estimate of the angle of insonation is required to convert the detected Doppler shift frequency into a velocity measurement. Any inaccuracy in placing the angle correction cursor parallel to the direction of flow will lead to an error in the estimated angle of insonation. This, in turn, will lead to an error in the velocity measurement. As the velocity calculation depends on the $\cos\theta$ term, the error created will be greater for larger angles of insonation. Figure 9.12 shows the relationship between the percentage error in the velocity measurement as the angle of insonation increases where there is a 5° error in placement of the angle correction cursor. Ideally, the angle of insonation should be kept at or below 60° in order to minimise the effect of errors due to imperfectly positioning the angle correction cursor on an image. However, estimating the angle of insonation is not always straightforward, especially in the presence of disease. Some of the limitations are listed below.

DIRECTION OF FLOW RELATIVE TO THE VESSEL WALLS

The direction of the blood flow may not be parallel to the vessel wall, especially, in the presence of a stenosis. Therefore, lining the angle correction cursor to be parallel to the walls may lead to large errors in estimating the true angle of insonation, which, in turn, will lead to errors in the velocity estimation. If there is a clear image of the flow channel through a narrowing, it may be possible to line the angle cursor up with the flow channel. However, the maximum velocity may be situated just beyond the stenosis, and the direction of flow may be less obvious there.

LOCATION OF SITE OF MAXIMUM VELOCITY AND DIRECTION OF FLOW FROM COLOUR IMAGE

The advent of colour flow imaging has enabled better assessment of the direction of the blood flow, especially, if the B-mode image is unclear. The colour image may also be used to identify the site of maximum velocity, although this can be misleading since the colour image displays mean frequency, which is related to the blood motion in the direction of the beam, rather than the actual blood velocity. As the frequency measured is angle dependent, the point at which the highest frequency is displayed may not be the site of the highest velocity. Instead it may be the site at which the angle between the Doppler beam and the direction of the blood flow is small. If the direction of blood flow has changed relative to the Doppler beam, within the imaged area, there will be different angles of insonation at different sites in the image. Ideally, both the colour and the spectral Doppler assessment of velocity changes across a stenosis should be used to locate the site of the maximum velocity.

OUT OF PLANE ANGLE OF INSONATION

It is important to remember that the interception of the ultrasound beam with the blood flow occurs in a three-dimensional space and not just in the two-dimensional plane shown on the image. Therefore, the transducer should be aligned with a reasonable length of the vessel, as seen on the image, to ensure a minimal error (see Figure 9.3).

DOPPLER ULTRASOUND BEAM APERTURE CREATES A RANGE OF ANGLES

The wide aperture of the Doppler beam produced by multi-element transducers means that the beam contains more than one angle of insonation (Figure 9.10). Ideally, if the maximum velocity is to be measured, then the angle produced by the edge of the beam that gives the smallest angle (θ_1), should be used in the Doppler formula. However, the majority of modern scanners use the angle produced by the centre of the beam (θ_2), to covert from Doppler frequency to velocity. This can lead to an overestimate in the velocity. Because the velocity

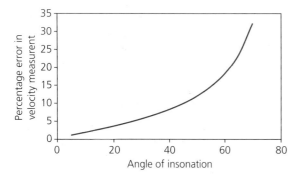

Fig. 9.12 Graph showing the relationship between the percentage error in the velocity measurement as the angle of insonation increases for a 5° error in the placement of the angle correction cursor.

measurement is dependent on the $\cos\theta$ term, this error is also angle dependent becoming greater with larger the angle of insonation. This again indicates that the angle of insonation should be kept to 60° or less when making velocity measurements. The error produced due to spectral broadening can vary with the changes in the active aperture that accompany changes in the sample volume depth. It also varies between manufactures.

Optimising the angle of insonation

There are many possible pitfalls when making velocity measurements and no single method of estimating the angle of insonation is completely reliable. The various possibilities and their advantages and disadvantages are discussed below.

VELOCITY RATIO MEASUREMENTS

Ideally, the angle of insonation used to make the velocity measurement proximal to and at the stenosis should be similar. This will result in the two velocities having similar errors that will cancel out when finding the ratio.

ABSOLUTE VELOCITY MEASUREMENTS

Firstly, the B-mode and the colour flow image are used to estimate the direction of flow in the area to be investigated so that the spectral Doppler beam can be steered appropriately. The angle of insonation is measured by lining up the angle correction cursor with the estimated direction of flow. There are two schools of thought about selecting the angle of insonation when making absolute velocity measurements:

1. *Always set the angle of insonation to 60°:* This ensures that any error in alignment of the angle correction cursor only leads to a moderate error in the velocity estimate (Figure 9.12) and that the errors caused by intrinsic spectral broadening are kept reasonably constant between measurements.

2. *Always select as small an angle of insonation as possible:* This ensures that any error in the alignment of the angle correction cursor produces as small an error in velocity estimation as possible. The error due to intrinsic spectral broadening will also be minimised. However, this error will be different for measurements made at different angles of insonation. This makes comparison between measurements made at different angles less reliable.

The blood velocity may need to be measured at a few points through and beyond stenosis to ensure the highest velocity has been obtained. Doppler criteria developed

over the years may not have been produced with a full understanding of all these possible sources of error. Different models of ultrasound systems may produce different results for the same blood flow. However, despite these sources of error, velocity measurements have been successfully used to quantify vascular disease for the past two decades. A greater understanding of the sources of error in velocity measurement may lead to improvements in accuracy.

Measurement of volume flow

Volume flow is a potentially useful physiological parameter that can be measured using duplex ultrasound. However such flow measurements are subject to many sources of error. Flow can be calculated by multiplying the TAV, obtained from the Doppler spectrum, by the cross-sectional area of the vessel, obtain from the B-mode image:

Flow = TAV × cross-sectional area of the vessel.

One method of estimating the cross-sectional area is to measure the diameter of the vessel, d, and calculate the area, A, as follows:

$$A = \frac{\pi d^2}{4}.$$

Some scanners allow the operator to trace around the vessel perimeter to calculate the area but this method relies on a steady hand and a good image of the lateral walls. Figure 9.13 shows how the vessel diameter has been obtained from the image and the velocity of the blood has been measured by placing the sample volume across the width of the vessel and estimating the angle of insonation from the image. Although the measurement of flow is relatively simple to perform there are many errors relating to both the measurement of the TAV and to the cross-sectional area (Evans and McDicken, 2000). These errors limit the value of one-off absolute flow measurements but serial measurements of flow may provide useful information on flow changes.

ERRORS IN DIAMETER MEASUREMENT

As the measurement of flow is dependent on the diameter squared, any error in the diameter will produce a fractional error in the flow measurement that is double the fractional error in the diameter measurement. The accuracy of the diameter measurement depends on the resolution of the image and the accuracy of the callipers. Calculation of the cross-sectional area from a diameter measurement assumes that the vessel

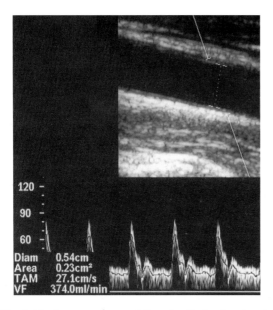

Fig. 9.13 Image and spectral Doppler display showing the technique used to measure time-averaged mean velocity (TAM) and volume flow (VF).

lumen is circular, which may not be the case in the presence of disease. Also the arterial diameter varies by approximately 10% during the cardiac cycle so, ideally, several diameter measurement should be made and the average found.

ERRORS IN TAV MEASUREMENT

Incomplete insonation of the vessel will lead to errors in the mean velocity measurements due to an under-estimation of the proportion of slower-moving blood near the vessel wall (Figure 9.9). This is the case even, if the sample volume is set to cover the near and far wall of the vessel as the out of imaging plane flow will not be sampled. Incomplete insonation of the vessel can lead to an overestimate in the measured value of TAV or flow of up to approximately 30%. The use of high-pass filters, if set to high (Figure 9.6), can also lead to an overestimate in the mean velocity since the low-velocity blood flow would be excluded. Aliasing would lead to underestimation of the mean velocity due to the incorrect estimation of the high frequencies present within the signal.

Waveform indices

The presence of significant disease can lead to alterations in the shape of the envelope of the spectrum

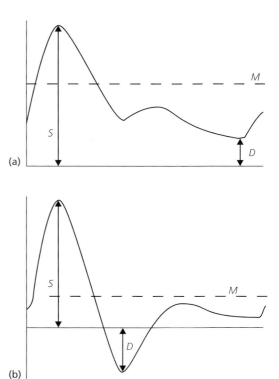

Fig. 9.14 Schematic diagram showing the indices (a) PI and (b) RI.

(waveform shape) and may indicate whether the disease is proximal or distal to the site at which the Doppler signal is obtained (Chapter 8). Over the years different methods of quantifying the waveform shape have been developed (Evans and McDicken, 2000) and modern scanners incorporate the facilities to calculate various indices to help identify changes in the wave-form shape.

PULSATILITY INDEX

The pulsatility index, PI can be used to quantify the degree of pulse wave damping at different measure-ments site. It is defined as the maximum, either fre-quency or velocity, of the waveform, S, minus the minimum, D (which may be negative) divided by the mean, M, as shown in Figure 9.14:

$$PI = \frac{(S - D)}{M}.$$

Damped flow, beyond significant disease, will have a lower PI value than a normal pulsatile waveform.

POURCELOT'S RESISTANCE INDEX

The resistance index, RI, is defined as (Figure 9.14(a))

$$RI = \frac{(S - D)}{S}.$$

SPECTRAL BROADENING

Over the years, there have been several definitions of spectral broadening to quantify the range of frequencies present within a spectrum (Evans) and one such definition is

$$SB = \frac{(f_{max} - f_{min})}{f_{mean}}.$$

When using these indices, it is important for the operator to understand how their ultrasound system calculates theses values. Increased spectral broadening indicates the presence of arterial disease but some broadening can also be introduced by the scanner itself, as discussed above.

Manual versus automated measurement

Most duplex systems enable the user to choose either to manually trace the maximum velocity over a cardiac cycle or to allow the system to automatically trace the maximum velocity. Manual tracing of the velocity can be both awkward and time consuming. Automatic measurements are usually quicker to implement but may be inaccurate in the presence of noise. Noise can include random background noise, electrical spikes or signals from other vessels, all of which may result in an incorrect estimation of the velocity. It is, therefore, preferable for the automated maximum trace to be displayed alongside the Doppler spectrum so that any large discrepancies can be seen. Automatic tracing of the maximum velocity also allows automated calculation of various indices. These can then also be displayed on the screen, sometimes in real time.

References

Evans DH and McDicken WN. Doppler Ultrasound: Physics, Instrumentation, and Signal Processing. Wiley. 2000.

Hoskins PR. Measurement of maximum velocity using duplex ultrasound systems. *Br. J. Radiol.* 1996; **69**: 172–177.

Thrush AJ and Evans DH. Intrinsic spectral broadening: a potential cause of misdiagnosis of carotid artery disease. *J. Vasc. Invest.* 1995; **1**(4): 187–192.

Thrush AJ and Hartshorne TC. *Peripheral Vascular Ultrasound: How, Why and When.* Churchill Livingstone. 1999.

10

COLOUR FLOW IMAGING

PR Hoskins and AL Criton

Introduction

Doppler ultrasound remained a minority-imaging methodology until the introduction of colour Doppler in 1982. In this technique, the motion of the blood is colour coded and superimposed on the B-mode image. This allows rapid visualisation of the flow patterns in vessels, allowing high-velocity jets in arteries and in cardiac chambers to be seen. It quickly became apparent that the ability to visualise flow patterns, such as the presence of intracardiac jets, was of great value. In addition, it considerably speeded up the placement of the Doppler sample volume in spectral Doppler investigation, hence reducing scanning time.

Prior to the introduction of commercial colour flow systems, several approaches were described to provide an image showing the pattern of blood flow. These often relied on manual scanning of the probe over the skin to build-up a two-dimensional (2D) image. These systems, which used electronic or mechanical sweeping of the beam, were not real time, having only a maximum of a few frames per second. These are reviewed in Evans and McDicken (2000) and in Wells (1994). In recent years, the technique of colour coding motion has extended from blood to tissue, giving rise to the technique commonly called Doppler tissue imaging (DTI) (see Chapter 14).

Terminology

In the development of any imaging modality, new terminology is introduced, usually by manufacturers. Unfortunately, this leads to a plethora of terms whose meaning may change with time. The term "colour flow" used to refer only to a system in which a 2D image of mean Doppler frequency from blood was displayed using colour coding; however, modern systems can display other quantities, such as the power of the signal. The terminology that will be used in this chapter is listed below:

- *Colour flow* – Imaging of blood flow. This is the generic term, which will be used in this chapter, and it encompasses the three modalities below.

- *Colour Doppler* – Image of the mean Doppler frequency from blood, displayed in colour superimposed on a B-mode image.

- *Power Doppler* – Image in which the power of the Doppler signal backscattered from blood is displayed in colour.

- *Directional power Doppler* – Image in which the power of the Doppler signal is displayed, including separate colour coding of blood velocities towards and away from the probe.

2D image production

Production of a 2D colour flow image includes elements of B-mode image formation and pulsed Doppler techniques. As in B-mode image formation, the image is built one line at a time, by transmitting ultrasonic pulses and processing the sequence of returned echoes. However, unlike B-mode image formation in which echo amplitude information is processed to form the image, the echoes are demodulated to produce a Doppler shift signal. In the pulsed wave spectral Doppler systems described in Chapter 9, Doppler information was obtained from only a single sample volume. In colour flow system, each line of the image is made up of multiple adjacent sample volumes.

As colour flow is a pulsed wave Doppler technique, the Doppler shift information for each line is obtained from several transmission pulses. Unlike spectral Doppler which relies on the fast Fourier transform (FFT) to extract the whole spectrum of frequencies that are present, colour flow imaging uses a technique known as "autocorrelation", which was introduced in Chapter 7. This calculates the mean frequency detected within each sample volume, which is then colour coded on the display. For the mean Doppler frequency to be detected, at least two pulses are required to be transmitted along each line. However, as a more accurate estimate of the detected mean frequency is obtained when more pulses are used, a typical colour scanner may use about 10 pulses. The requirement of several pulses per line to produce the colour image, compared with a minimum of one in the B-mode image, means that the frame rate for a comparable number of scan lines is much less in the colour image than it is in the B-mode image. For example, if 10 pulses were to be used for each colour line, and one pulse for each B-mode line, then the maximum frame rate for the colour image would be one tenth that of the B-mode image. There is, therefore, a compromise between the size of the colour image (number of scan lines), accuracy of the frequency estimate (number of pulses per line) and the rate at which the image is updated (frame rate). In order for a sonographer to appreciate the pulsatile nature of blood flow, it is preferable for the machine to maintain a frame rate above 10 frames per second. If the whole field of view were to be used, then the maximum achievable colour

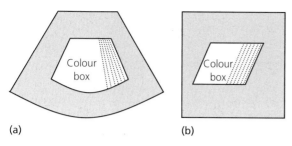

(a)   (b)

Fig. 10.1 Colour box shapes for (a) sector and (b) linear-array transducers. Within the colour box, the image is built-up as a series of colour lines. Each line consists of a series of adjacent sample volumes.

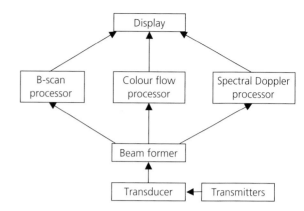

Fig. 10.2 Components of a colour system. For a colour flow system, three types of information are processed: B-mode, colour flow and spectral Doppler.

frame rate would be only a few frames per second. In order to improve the colour frame rate, the colour coded flow is only displayed in a limited region of interest called the "colour box" within the displayed B-mode image. The reduced depth and number of scan lines that this provides enables fewer ultrasound pulses to be sent per colour frame, and hence allows the use of higher colour frame rates. The width and depth of the colour box are under operator control, and the frame rate may be increased by narrowing the box, or by decreasing the box depth. In order to further increase frame rate, the line density may also be reduced on some systems. Typically, frame rates of 10–15 frames per second can be achieved in peripheral arterial applications, though this may fall to 5 frames per second or less in venous applications, where a large number of pulses are needed for each colour line in order to measure relatively low Doppler shifts. Low frame rates may also result for abdominal and obstetric applications, where the vessel depth is large. Typical colour box shapes and relative sizes are shown in Figure 10.1.

Phase and time domain techniques

The common theme of colour flow techniques is that the colour image is derived by consideration of the motion of the blood. There are two basic classes of instrument, dependent on whether they determine the presence of motion by analysis of the phase shift or the time shift as described in Chapter 7. Few commercial machines use the time domain approach, probably, as this is computationally more demanding, and hence more expensive to implement. Virtually, all modern commercial colour flow systems employ the phase shift approach using autocorrelation detection, and the sections immediately following will refer to this approach.

Colour flow system components

A colour flow system will independently process the received B-mode and colour flow echoes (Figure 10.2). In addition, a spectral Doppler display can be obtained from a single sample volume as selected by the operator. A small number of pulses, typically 2–20, is transmitted and received for each colour line that is produced. Each line is divided into a large number of sections each of which represents a different sample volume. The Doppler signal from all of the gates is processed simultaneously. This situation is different to pulsed wave spectral Doppler, where only one gate is considered. Figure 10.3 shows the essential components of the colour flow processor. The function of the components are described below.

Doppler transmitter

Colour flow imaging uses the pulse–echo technique. Modern colour flow systems do not use the same pulses that are used for the B-mode image, but instead use separate lower-frequency pulses as shown in Table 10.1.

Transducer

Any transducer used for B-mode imaging can, in principal, be used for colour flow. Commercial colour flow scanners typically use linear, curvilinear, or phased array transducers. The use of mechanically swept systems is possible, but is more problematic as the vibration that is produced can be picked up by the colour flow system, so that careful attention to design is needed in order to reduce false colour display.

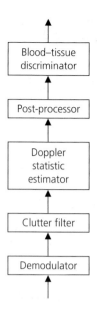

Fig. 10.3 Components of the colour flow processor.

Table 10.1 Typical B-mode and colour flow transmit frequencies.

Application	B-mode frequency (MHz)	Colour frequency (MHz)
Peripheral vascular	7–12	4–6
Abdominal/obstetrics	2–5	2–4
Transcranial	1.5–2.5	1–2

Beam former

This component of the system is the same as the B-mode beam former discussed in detail in Chapter 3. The beam former controls all aspects concerned with focussing and sweeping the beam through the tissue to produce a 2D colour image.

Demodulator

The demodulator extracts the Doppler shift frequencies as discussed in Chapter 7. This process is invisible to the user, with no relevant user controls.

Clutter filter

Clutter refers to signals from stationary and slowly moving tissue. It was noted in Chapter 7 that the signal from tissue is some 40 dB higher than the signal from blood. If

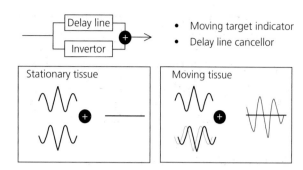

- Moving target indicator
- Delay line cancellor

Fig. 10.4 Simple clutter filter. The previous received echo is delayed and added to the current received echo. If the tissue is stationary, consecutive echoes will cancel out, whereas if there is blood or tissue motion, consecutive echoes will not cancel out. This simple method is also called a "delay line cancellor" or a "moving target indicator".

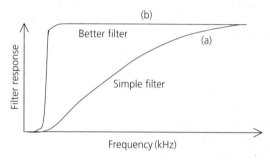

Fig. 10.5 Clutter filter response as a function of Doppler frequency. The ideal filter completely suppresses the clutter, and allows through the Doppler frequencies. (a) The simple delay line cancellor of Figure 10.4 causes suppression of high Doppler frequencies, which will prevent the display of low velocities; however, there is suppression of higher blood velocity signals also. (b) More complex clutter filter with better low-frequency behaviour.

it is moving blood that is of interest, then it is necessary to remove, as far as possible, the clutter signal, and so a clutter filter is present in colour flow systems. The clutter filter is analogous to the wall thump filter of spectral Doppler. Early colour flow systems used relatively unsophisticated clutter filters and were unable to detect low-velocity flow (Figure 10.4). The detection of low velocities by modern colour flow systems is linked to the use of a sophisticated clutter filter (Figure 10.5).

Mean-frequency estimator

The requirement for real-time scanning means that Doppler frequencies must be estimated in a much shorter time than is available for spectral Doppler; usually 0.2–2 ms for colour flow, as opposed to 5–40 ms for spectral Doppler. When colour flow systems were introduced in 1982, the processing capabilities available at that time meant that it was not possible to use an FFT approach. This would have meant calculating the full Doppler spectrum followed by extracting the mean frequency. The realisation by Namekawa *et al.* (1982) and Kasai *et al.* (1985) that a computationally simple algorithm termed 'autocorrelation' could be used to calculate mean frequency directly was the breakthrough that led to the introduction of real-time colour flow systems into commercial use. In addition to the short time that is available for calculation in colour flow, the number of pulses used for generation of each line is much less than in spectral Doppler; 2–20 in colour flow as opposed to 80–100 in spectral Doppler. The number of pulses used for generation of each colour line is called the "ensemble length".

The autocorrelator provides simultaneous estimates of three quantities:

- *Power* – Proportional to the square of the amplitude of the Doppler signal.

- *Mean-Doppler frequency* – The mean or average Doppler frequency.

- *Variance* – This is a quantity related to the variability of the Doppler signal. It is defined by the square of the standard deviation of the Doppler signal amplitude, estimated over the ensemble length.

Since the introduction of the autocorrelation technique, there have been many different techniques used to estimate the single quantity that can be displayed on a colour flow image. Some of these techniques have been alternative ways of estimating mean frequency. Other techniques have been for estimation of different quantities, such as maximum Doppler frequency. The descriptions of these techniques are beyond the scope of this book, and are reviewed in Evans and McDicken (2000). Most modern colour flow scanners use a technique called "2D autocorrelation" or variants of this. The 2D autocorrelation technique is described by Loupas *et al.* (1995a, b), and is an extension of the basic autocorrelation technique.

Post-processor

Even under conditions where the blood or tissue velocity is unchanging, the estimated mean-Doppler frequency will change to some extent in a random manner. On the colour flow image, this variation manifests itself as a speckle pattern called "colour speckle". The cause of this speckle is associated with the variation in echo amplitude received at the transducer arising from the variation in the detailed position of each of the red cells within the sample volume from one pulse to the next. This is the same reason that there is a speckle pattern on B-mode images and on spectral Doppler waveforms. This speckle pattern can mask changes in the displayed colour. However, it is possible to reduce the degree of noise by averaging over several frames. This is the same frame-averaging technique as used in B-mode imaging, and it gives rise to a persistence effect.

Blood–tissue discriminator

For each pixel of the image, it is possible to estimate the echo brightness level for the B-mode image and also the mean-Doppler frequency for the colour flow image. However, it is only possible to display one of these in the final composite image. The function of the blood–tissue discriminator is to ensure that colour is displayed only in regions of true blood flow and not in the presence of moving tissue. There are several methods by which discrimination between moving the signals from blood and moving tissue can be achieved. These include:

- *Doppler signal amplitude (noise) threshold* – In regions of tissue that are moving slowly with respect to the transducer, the Doppler frequency shifts from the tissue will be of high amplitude, but of low Doppler frequency. The clutter filter acts to eliminate these signals. After the clutter filter, the signal from blood is much stronger than the signal from tissue, and the use of a simple threshold set by the operator (the "colour gain" control) is sufficient to determine whether blood or tissue signals are displayed for a given pixel (Figure 10.6a and b).

- *Doppler signal amplitude (upper) threshold* – If the tissue moves sufficiently rapidly, then the clutter filter will not filter out the signal from the tissue. The Doppler signal amplitude from these regions is much higher than blood, by 40 dB, so the use of an upper threshold may be used to prevent colour display (Figure 10.6c).

- *Flash filter* – Rapid motion of either the tissue or of the transducer produces a Doppler shift, which may be displayed as region of colour; these are called "flash artefacts". The threshold method described above is often insufficient to remove such flashes, and manufacturers have developed more sophisticated removal methods, based on the detection of very rapid changes in the Doppler signal level, which could only be produced by motion of the transducer with respect to the patent.

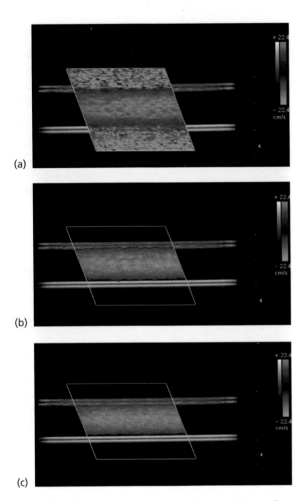

(a)

(b)

(c)

Fig. 10.6 Colour Doppler images acquired from a flow phantom with a blood mimic flowing through a tube. (a) No blood–tissue discriminator present – there is colour throughout the colour box consisting of a uniform colour in the region of flow, surrounded by random noise in the surrounding regions, (b) application of the noise threshold removes most of the colour from the region of no flow; however, there is some "bleeding" of the colour into the tube, (c) application of the upper amplitude threshold removes the bleeding.

Colour flow modes

The three outputs from the autocorrelator (mean frequency, variance and power) can be colour coded and displayed, either alone or in combination with each other. This produces a number of possible colour modes, which can be selected. In practice, only a few are sensible (Figure 10.7). These are considered below.

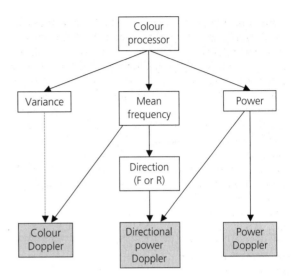

Fig. 10.7 Relationship between calculated quantities and colour flow display modes. The three quantities estimated by the colour flow system are the mean Doppler frequency, the Doppler power and the variance. The colour Doppler image is a display of the mean frequency in which the variance may be added, if required. The power Doppler image is a display of the Doppler power. For directional power Doppler, flow direction is obtained from mean frequency, and used to colour code the power Doppler image.

Colour Doppler

The earliest commercial colour flow systems concentrated on this mode, in which the mean frequency in each pixel is colour coded. Although in principle any colour scale could be used for the display, most manufacturers adopt a red-based scale for blood flowing in one direction, and a blue-based scale for blood flowing in the opposite direction (Figure 10.8).

Where variance is displayed alone, it is shown as a green colour, together with the red or blue representing the mean frequency, to produce a composite display. This option was widely available on early colour flow machines, where it was thought that variance was related to turbulence produced by narrowed arteries or cardiac valves. Figure 10.9 shows a cardiac jet, where the green colouration in the jet is seen. This mode is not used much outside cardiac applications.

Power Doppler

Display of the power of the Doppler signal had been a feature of early colour flow systems, however, the same

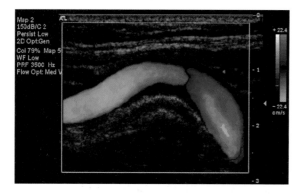

Fig. 10.8 Colour Doppler image of common carotid flow with a blue–red scale. This image shows very strong changes in colour, which are associated with changes in direction of flow.

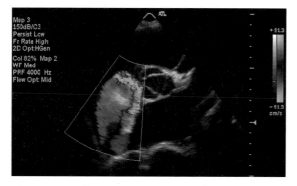

Fig. 10.9 Colour Doppler image of tricuspid regurgitation with variance admixed. Regions of green colouration associated with high variance are seen.

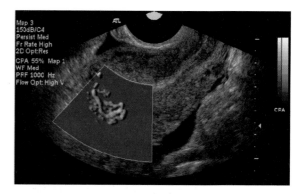

Fig. 10.10 Power Doppler image of arterio-venous fistulae, in which there is colour throughout the colour box.

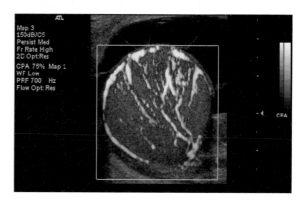

Fig. 10.11 Power Doppler image of testicular flow consisting of colour superimposed on the B-mode image.

instrument settings were used as for colour Doppler and, there was not much improvement over the colour Doppler image. It was only when the processing was optimised for power Doppler (Rubin *et al.*, 1994) that it became popular, largely due to improved sensitivity over colour Doppler. The first step in this optimisation is concerned with the display of noise. In colour Doppler, the noise is present on the image if the colour gain is set too high, and its appearance is a multi-coloured mosaic in which the true image from the vessel of interest may be difficult to observe. However, for power Doppler, the noise appears as a low-level uniform hue in which it is easily possible to observe the vessel of interest. Consequently, the first step in optimisation is to reduce the level of the lower threshold used to differentiate between the signal from blood and the signal from noise. The second step recognises that it

is not possible to follow the changes in blood flow with time using power Doppler, so it is not necessary to have good time resolution. Consequently, for power Doppler, the degree of averaging over successive acquired frames (persistence) is much higher than for colour Doppler. This averaging process acts to reduce the colour noise level, and hence make it easier to distinguish small vessels with low-signal levels. In order to make the best use of the increase in sensitivity, the first manufacturers to use Power Doppler displayed colour throughout the colour box. This is shown in Figure 10.10, where small vessels can be seen in yellow above the noise, which is shown in blue. The disadvantage of this mode is that the underlying tissue anatomy cannot be seen. Most manufacturers now prefer to display the power Doppler image superimposed on the B-mode image (Figure 10.11). A commonly used colour scale is a "heated body scale", in which the displayed colour changes through black, red, orange and yellow as the Doppler power increases.

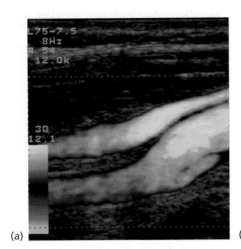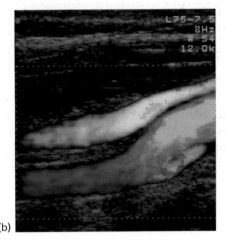

(a) (b)

Fig. 10.12 Images from the common carotid and jugular vein: (a) power Doppler image and (b) directional power Doppler image in which the direction is colour coded.

Directional power Doppler

In this mode, the directional information on blood flow is obtained from the mean-frequency data, and used to colour code the power Doppler data (Figure 10.12). This mode is supposed to combine the enhanced sensitivity of power Doppler with the directional capability of colour Doppler.

Colour controls

There are a large number of instrument settings, which affect the displayed colour image. Thankfully in most modern colour flow systems, the default value of the settings are pre-programmed by the manufacturer for particular clinical applications, which the operator can recall from the applications list. The operator must then adjust a small number of controls for individual patients. In the list below, the controls are classified according to four categories, controls which affect colour image acquisition, controls which affect Doppler signal extraction and frequency estimation, controls which affect the display of the colour flow signals. The section finishes with a description of the use of controls in clinical practice.

Controls affecting the acquisition of colour flow images

POWER

The amplitude of the ultrasound pulses used for generation of the colour flow images may usually be adjusted

over a wide range of values. The sensitivity of the instrument will improve as the power increases, however, in order to maintain patient exposure within safe limits, it is best if other controls, such as colour gain, are also used to obtain the desired image quality.

PULSE REPETITION FREQUENCY

The pulse repetition frequency (PRF) is the total number of pulses, which the transducer transmits per second. It is limited largely by the maximum depth of the field of view; the transmit–receive time is less for smaller depths and a higher PRF is then possible. The value of the PRF selected in the various system pre-sets, such as arterial or venous, will depend on the expected velocities present in the region of interest, but PRF may need to be altered by the operator, e.g. to prevent aliasing or to enable the detection of low flow. On modern systems, there is not a single control labelled "PRF". Instead, PRF is usually determined automatically from various controls including the colour box size and the velocity scale.

The total number of pulses transmitted is divided between the B-mode image, the colour flow image and spectral Doppler. Maximum PRF for the colour image is achieved when the spectral display is switched off, and the colour box depth and width are reduced as much as possible. This will result in a colour image with a high frame rate.

STEERING ANGLE

This control is applicable to linear-array systems, where it is possible to steer the colour beam in a variety of directions with respect to the B-mode scan lines. Most systems provide three angles (e.g. $-20°$, 0, $+20°$), though some provide a choice of five directions between this range. Steering the colour beams is desirable in colour flow imaging as many peripheral vessels run parallel to the skin surface, and an ultrasound beam perpendicular to the skin would provide zero Doppler signal. However, optimum B-mode imaging of the vessel is provided in this situation. By a combination of beam steering and probe angulation, it is usually possible to obtain a beam-vessel angle in the range 40–70°, which is sufficient for adequate colour flow image production, as well as good B-mode visualisation of vessel walls. The power Doppler image is much less dependent on the beam-vessel angle as explained below, and it is not necessary to steer the beam away from the $0°$ direction.

FOCAL DEPTH

Due to frame rate considerations, it is usual to only have one transmit focal depth for colour flow images. In some systems, the default is set automatically at the centre of the displayed field of view; in others, it is necessary to set this manually at the depth of interest.

BOX SIZE

The depth and width of the colour box are set by the user. The box depth directly influences the PRF, with higher PRF, and hence higher frame rates, being possible for box depths that are nearer to the surface. Higher frame rates may also be achieved by restriction of the width of the colour box as this reduces the number of Doppler lines required.

LINE DENSITY

It is not necessary for the line density (number of Doppler lines per centimetre across the image) of the colour image to be the same as the B-mode image. Reduction in line density increases frame rate; however, this is done at the expense of reduced lateral spatial resolution of the colour image.

GATE LENGTH

The gate length will determine the number of cycles in the transmitted pulse, and so alters the sample volume size. This improves sensitivity, but decreases axial resolution.

DEPTH OF FIELD

Reducing the image depth enables higher PRF to be used, and therefore, higher frame rates to be achieved.

Controls affecting the extraction and estimation of Doppler frequencies

FILTER CUT-OFF

It is common practice to set the filter cut-off frequency as a certain fraction of the total displayed frequency scale, rather than as an absolute value of say 200 Hz. This means that as the frequency scale increases, so does the level of the clutter filter. Observation of low blood velocities requires that the frequency scale is set to low values.

There are usually three or four clutter filter options to choose from. Selection of too low a filter level results in breakthrough of the clutter signal from slowly moving tissue.

ENSEMBLE LENGTH

The term "ensemble length" is used to refer to the number of pulses used to generate each colour line. Provided that flow is steady during the time spent measuring the Doppler shifts along one scan line, the variability of estimated mean frequency decreases as the ensemble length (number of pulses per estimate) increases. Low variability is required for accurate estimation of low velocities. In cardiology, it is higher blood velocities that are mainly of interest, whereas in radiology low venous blood velocity may be of more interest. Consequently, the ensemble length is partly determined by the selected application, with longer ensemble lengths used in radiology applications than in cardiology applications. Visualisation of low velocities is best achieved by adjustment of the velocity scale, so in many systems, the ensemble length is directly linked with the velocity scale. For example, a 10-pulse ensemble will take longer to complete when a low PRF is used than when a high PRF is selected. As the velocity scale is reduced to enable better visualisation of low velocities, the increased ensemble length will result in a reduction in frame rate.

BASELINE

If aliasing is a problem, then one method of dealing with this is to shift the baseline to enable higher positive velocities to be presented. This is identical to the technique used in spectral Doppler.

PERSISTENCE OR FRAME AVERAGING

Persistence refers to the averaging of Doppler shift estimates from current and previous frames. If flow is stable over the averaging period, then strong frame averaging will result in reduced colour noise, enabling better visualisation of the true flow pattern. If the degree of frame averaging is kept fixed through the cardiac cycle, then rapidly changing flow patterns will not be properly visualised. Some commercial systems attempt to overcome this by automatic adjustment of the level of frame averaging. For example, if the measured velocity is high, the persistence will be low, enabling visualisation of the high-velocity pulsatile flow patterns in arteries; when the velocity is low the persistence will be high, allowing the (usually) less pulsatile flow in veins to be observed.

Controls affecting the display of the colour flow signals

COLOUR GAIN

Colour is displayed if the amplitude of the signal after the clutter filter is above a threshold value set to exclude noise (Figure 10.13). The level of this threshold is set by the colour gain control. If the threshold is set to be too high, then no colour is displayed, whereas if this is set too low, then noise is displayed as a mosaic pattern throughout the image. This control is adjusted for each patient in a similar manner to spectral Doppler gain.

COLOUR-WRITE PRIORITY

The colour gain approach above, by itself, does not deal with high-amplitude signals from tissue, which have not been suppressed by the clutter filter. Colour is displayed, if the amplitude of the echo before the clutter filter is below a threshold value, which is set to exclude high-amplitude signals from moving tissue (Figure 10.14).

POWER THRESHOLD

This is a threshold on the calculated power value, with no display of colour, if the power is below the threshold.

FLASH FILTER

This is the process whereby the colour flashes from transducer or tissue motion are removed. Few details of these are available from manufacturers; however, one

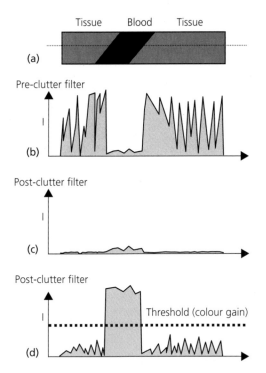

Fig. 10.13 Effect of the colour gain control. (a) A single echo through a region of tissue and flowing blood is shown; (b) the echo passes through the clutter filter, which removes the high-amplitude signals from the tissue; (c) there are residual signals in the region of the tissue due to noise; (d) imposition of a threshold enable the true flow to be identified as regions in which the signal amplitude is high.

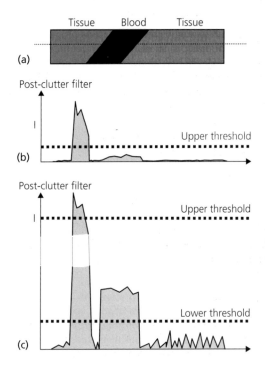

Fig. 10.14 Effect of an upper threshold. (a) Single echo through a region of tissue and flowing blood; (b) echo after it has passed through the clutter filter, with a high-amplitude spike from a region of moving tissue; (c) imposition of an upper threshold removes the spike.

139

possibility is that flash filters are based on the detection of very rapid changes in the Doppler signal level, which could only be produced by motion of the transducer with respect to the patent. The operator usually has the choice of turning the flash filter on or off.

Use of controls

The operator chooses the probe and the application from the pre-set menu. This provides default values relevant to the typical patient for the application selected. It is usual to start the examination using B-mode in order for the operator to familiarise themselves with the anatomy, then progress to colour flow. The operator adjusts the size of the colour box to cover the desired region. With a linear-array transducer, it is also possible for the operator to steer the colour box in order to optimise the colour Doppler angle of insonation. The mode is selected (Doppler or power), and the scale and baseline adjusted to enable display of the blood velocity range. The colour gain is adjusted, so that as much of the vessel as possible is filled with colour, but at the same time avoiding excess noise in the tissue. A further refinement for colour Doppler is to adjust the probe angulation and steering angle to ensure that a Doppler angle away from 90° is obtained. This avoids colour drop-out due to the action of the clutter filter on the low Doppler shifts obtained near to 90°. This limited sequence of control adjustments is often all that is needed in a colour flow or Doppler tissue examination, although the user can alter other controls, if necessary.

Features of colour flow

Penetration

The penetration depth is the maximum depth at which Doppler signals can be distinguished from noise. Improved penetration can simply be achieved by turning up the output power. High-output power is recognised as being hazardous to the patient as described in Chapter 13. For targets at the deepest depths, the returning ultrasonic signal and hence detected Doppler signal is of small amplitude due to the effect of attenuation within the tissue. The task of the Doppler system in this situation is to distinguish the true Doppler signal from noise, and good machine design uses low-noise components. A standard signal processing method to improve the detection of the signal is to combine a large number of measurements by some form of averaging. In this process, the signal size increases in comparison with the random noise that tends to cancel out, hence the signal

can be more easily detected from the noise. For Doppler systems, the averaging can involve the use of a larger ensemble length or frame averaging; however, both of these are done at the expense of a lower frame rate.

Display of low velocities

The most important component determining the visualisation of low velocities is the clutter filter, as noted above. Optimisation of machine settings in order to detect low velocities is achieved by increase in the ensemble length and by the use of persistence. This is performed automatically by selection of the clinical protocol and adjustment of the "velocity scale", but some may also be controlled directly by the operator in a hidden menu.

Display of flow in small vessels

The first requirement to display flow in small vessels is that the spatial resolution of the B-mode and colour flow images are adequate. It is the display of flow in small vessels where the superior characteristics of power Doppler over colour Doppler are demonstrated. It has been shown that power Doppler is superior in its ability to visualise small vessels. Figure 10.15 shows three pairs of colour and power Doppler images obtained with a simple flow test device consisting of a 1 mm diameter vessel embedded in tissue-mimicking material. For each pair, the same machine settings are used:

- *Drop-out* (Figure 10.15a) – In the first pair of images, there is no frame averaging, and the colour gain is set to just suppress noise in each case. The image of flow in the vessel should ideally be a contiguous line of colour. For colour Doppler, the image consists of several isolated colour spots whose position along the line varies randomly. This is associated with variations in the calculated mean frequency produced by the autocorrelator. Values of mean frequency that are low will trigger the blood–tissue discriminator, and colour will not be displayed. The calculated Doppler power is less variable than the calculated mean frequency, so the power Doppler image of the vessel demonstrates less drop-out.

- *Frame averaging* (Figure 10.15b) – In the second pair of images, persistence is used, and set to the same value for both power and colour Doppler. Both mean frequency and power demonstrate less variability, resulting in fewer values falling below the blood–tissue discriminator threshold. The colour line is contiguous in each case.

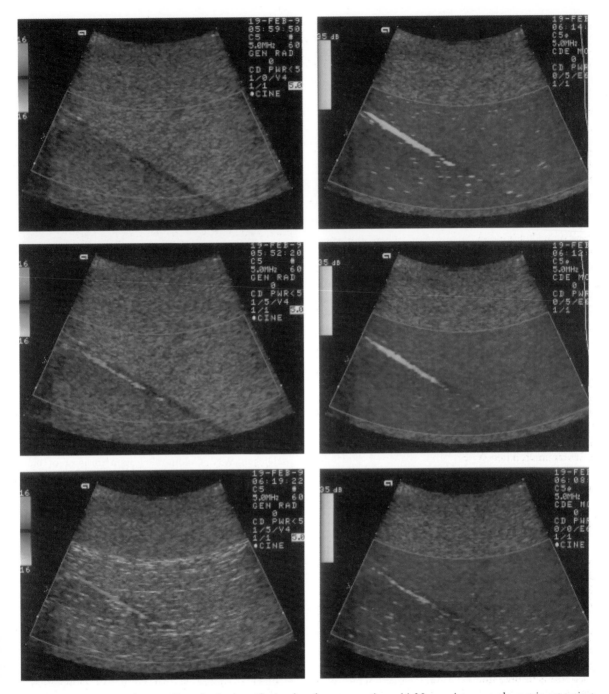

Fig. 10.15 Colour and power Doppler images obtained at the same settings. (a) No persistence, colour gain set to just suppress noise. Power Doppler shows a contiguous line of colour, but the colour Doppler shows considerable drop-out. (b) High persistence, same colour gain setting as for (a). There is now little drop-out on the colour Doppler image. (c) High persistence, high colour gain. The colour Doppler image shows substantial noise compared to the power Doppler image. Reproduced, with permission, from Hoskins PR and McDicken WN. Colour ultrasound imaging of blood flow and tissue motion. *Br. J. Radiol.* 1997; **70**: 878–890.

- *Display of colour noise* (Figure 10.15c) – Increase in colour gain will produce noise in regions of tissue. The colour image of the vessel must be distinguishable from the surrounding noise. Increase in the colour gain has a much more marked effect on the noise for the colour Doppler image than for the power Doppler image. For the power Doppler image, the noise values are of low amplitude, and in the example shown, the vessel can be clearly distinguished from the noise; however, for the colour Doppler image, the mean-frequency values of the noise change randomly, and are comparable with the displayed mean frequencies from the small vessel, making the vessel less clearly visible.

The above illustration shows that, when the same machine settings are used for power and colour Doppler, the penetration depth is similar for the two modalities. The improved detection of small vessels using power Doppler is due to the use of higher frame averaging, and also to the inherently less confusing nature of the power Doppler image, as there is no aliasing effect and only a limited angle dependence (Figure 10.16).

Display of complex flow patterns

The ideal colour Doppler display would provide images in which the displayed colour was related to the velocity of the blood in the scan plane. Similarly, the ideal power Doppler image would provide a display in which the colour was related to the presence or absence of moving blood. There are two phenomena that limit the ability of the technology to provide these ideal displays; angle dependence and aliasing.

The Doppler shift arises primarily from blood motion in the direction of the ultrasound beam; this leads to the cosine dependence on the angle between the beam and the direction of motion, when Doppler frequency is calculated (see Chapter 7). Consequently, colour Doppler demonstrates an angle dependence. In the colour shown in Figure 10.17a, the flow on the right side of the image is displayed towards the transducer, in red, and the flow on the left is displayed as away from the transducer, in blue. At first glance, the image gives the appearance that the flow is changing direction mid-way across the image; however, careful consideration of the changing angle of insonation allows the observer to establish that the flow is all in one direction. The flow in the centre of the image is not detected due to the poor Doppler angle resulting in small Doppler shift frequencies that are removed by the clutter filter. The

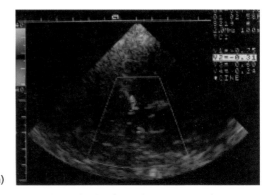

(a)

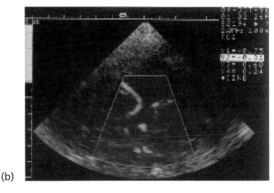

(b)

Fig. 10.16 Colour and power Doppler images from the circle of Willis. The power Doppler image shows the anatomy more clearly than the colour Doppler image. Reproduced, with permission, from Hoskins PR and McDicken WN. Colour ultrasound imaging of blood flow and tissue motion. *Br. J. Radiol.* 1997; **70**: 878–890.

power Doppler image maintains a uniform colour over a wide range of angles (Figure 10.17b); however, when the angle approaches 90°, the power signal may be lost. This may be understood with reference to Figure 10.18, which shows the received Doppler signal at different angles. As the angle increases the Doppler frequencies fall, but the total Doppler power, indicated by the area under the curve, remains constant. Near 90°, there is some loss of signal due to the clutter filter, and the power reduces. The angle dependence of directional power Doppler is similar to that for power Doppler, with the difference that flow towards and away from the transducer are coded with different colours. Display of tortuous vessels is often confusing using colour Doppler due to the angle dependence (Figure 10.19), whereas the corresponding power Doppler image has a uniform hue and is not confusing.

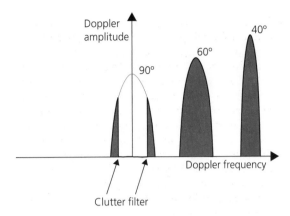

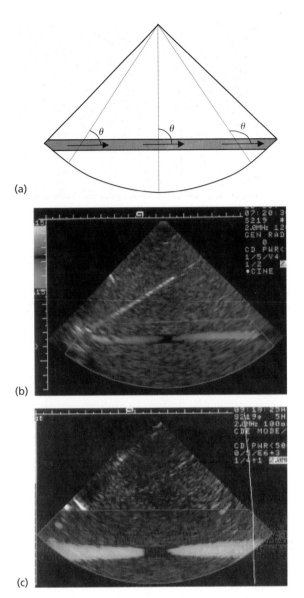

Fig. 10.17 Angle dependence of colour and power Doppler images. (a) A straight tube is shown in which the flow is identical at all points along the tube. For the sector scanner, the angle θ between the beam and direction of motion varies from the left to the right side of the image. (b) The colour Doppler image shows variation in the displayed colour throughout the length of the tube, with no colour shown at 90°. (c) The power Doppler image shows little variation of displayed colour, except for 90° when no colour is displayed. Reproduced, with permission, from Hoskins PR and McDicken WN. Colour ultrasound imaging of blood flow and tissue motion. *Br. J. Radiol.* 1997; **70**: 878–890.

Fig. 10.18 Effect of a change in angle on the Doppler spectrum, at constant blood velocity. As the angle decreases from 40° to 60°, the Doppler frequency shift decreases, but the power of the Doppler signal, represented by the area under the curve, remains approximately constant. However, at angles close to 90°, the Doppler frequencies are low and may be removed by the clutter filter, which causes a reduction in the Doppler power. In the figure, there is only partial removal of the Doppler signal at 90°.

Increase in blood velocity results in increase in Doppler frequency shift up to a maximum value set by the Nyquist limit (PRF/2). For frequency shifts above the Nyquist limit, there are two consequences of aliasing; the Doppler frequencies are inaccurately calculated, and the direction of flow is inaccurately predicted.

As the Doppler frequency is not estimated in power Doppler, aliasing will not affect the displayed image. An alternative way of understanding this is illustrated in Figure 10.20, which shows that the Doppler shift increases up to a critical velocity. Above this critical velocity aliasing occurs. However, in all cases the area under the curve, which represents the Doppler power, is the same. However, directional power Doppler does suffer from aliasing as directional information is calculated.

Both angle dependence and aliasing can occur in the same image. A flow model of a diseased artery may be used to illustrate these effects. In Figure 10.21a, the increase in mean Doppler frequency within the region of the stenosis is seen as a yellow-coloured area, and there is jet formation and recirculation in the post-stenotic region. Increase in flow rate (Figure 10.21b) leads to aliasing, where the previous yellow-coloured region is now coloured green. The corresponding power Doppler images are uniformly coloured (Figure 10.21c and d). At the low flow rate (Figure 10.21c), there is a gap in the region of recirculation, where the velocity is

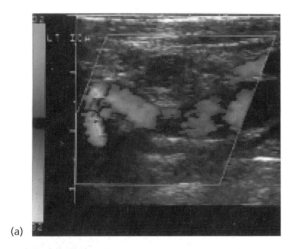

(a)

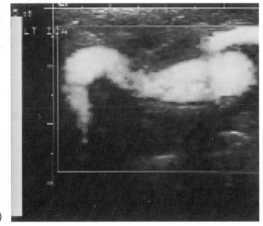

(b)

Fig. 10.19 Display of a tortuous carotid artery using colour Doppler and power Doppler. There are large changes in blood flow direction along the course of the carotid artery. This results in large changes in the displayed colour for the colour Doppler display (a), but only minor changes in colour for the power Doppler display (b). Reproduced, with permission, from Hoskins PR and McDicken WN. Colour ultrasound imaging of blood flow and tissue motion. *Br. J. Radiol.* 1997; **70**: 878–890.

low. The gap is filled when the higher flow rate is used (Figure 10.21d). The practical consequence of this last observation is that considerable care must be taken when using poor filling of the vessel in the power Doppler image as evidence of thrombus.

Display of rapidly changing flow patterns

The ability of the colour Doppler image to follow faithfully the changing flow pattern is determined by

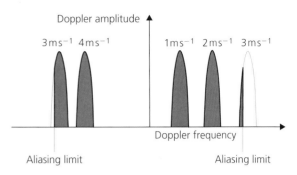

Fig. 10.20 Colour aliasing explanation. As velocity increases from 1 to $2 \, ms^{-1}$ the Doppler shift increases. However, when the aliasing limit (or Nyquist limit) is reached, at approximately to $3 \, ms^{-1}$, in the figure, the Doppler frequency is not estimated correctly. The Doppler signal for the velocity of $3 \, ms^{-1}$ consists of two components, one with a positive Doppler frequency and one with a negative Doppler frequency. The combined Doppler power, represented by the area under the curve of the combined signals, remains unchanged. Consequently, the power Doppler image is insensitive to aliasing.

frame rate and persistence. As noted above, the frame rate is maximised by the use of a small ensemble length, restriction of the colour box size and (in some systems) by the simultaneous acquisition of multiple beams. For display of lower velocities, a larger ensemble length is required, and the frame rate reduces accordingly. A degree of persistence is acceptable and also desirable as the effect of noise is reduced, and the visualisation of small vessels is improved. Although it is possible to observe changes in blood flow during the cardiac cycle using the colour flow image, this task is best performed using spectral Doppler.

In power Doppler, there is no information on the dynamic nature of blood flow, and persistence is set high to obtain maximum noise reduction.

Artefacts

Many of the features of B-mode images are applicable to colour flow images, as the propagation of the ultrasound pulse through the tissue will obey the same physics, whether it is used to produce a B-mode image or a colour flow image. Some of these artefacts have been described earlier in this chapter. The purpose of this section is to list all the major artefacts in one location.

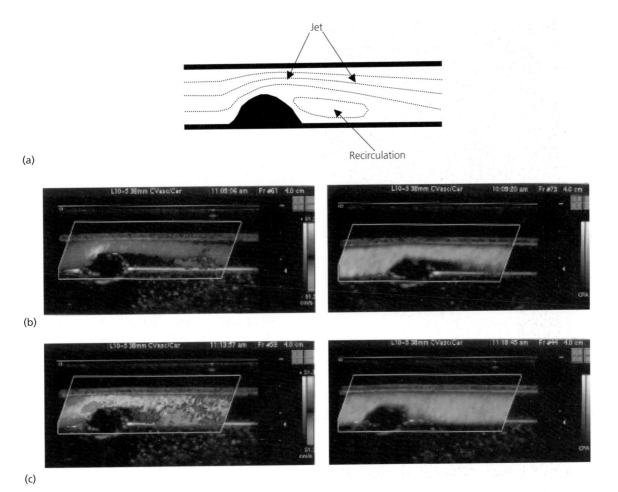

Fig. 10.21 Angle dependence and aliasing demonstrated in a stenosis flow model. (a) In the flow model, there is a localised narrowed region that mimics a stenosis. A blood-mimicking fluid is pumped from left to right through the tube. As the fluid passes through the stenosis, there is change in direction of the fluid, increase in velocity, with the formation of a jet and an adjacent region of recirculation in the post-stenotic region. (b) For the colour Doppler image, there is alteration of colour throughout the image; however, the power Doppler image is of a uniform colouration. The jet is clearly seen; however, the fluid in the region of recirculation has low velocity, and the Doppler shift frequencies are suppressed by the clutter filter, resulting in an absence of colour in this region. (c) The flow rate is doubled, resulting in a doubling of velocities. There is aliasing in the pre-stenotic region for colour Doppler. The power Doppler image is unaffected by aliasing and remains of a uniform colouration. The Doppler frequencies from the region of recirculation are now high enough to be not suppressed by the clutter filter, and both colour and power Doppler images no longer demonstrate a flow void. Reproduced, with permission, from Hoskins PR and McDicken WN. Colour ultrasound imaging of blood flow and tissue motion. *Br. J. Radiol.* 1997; **70**: 878–890.

Shadowing

There is reduction in the amplitude of the Doppler signal, whenever there is attenuation of the ultrasonic pulse. Hence, colour signal is lost when there is an intervening highly attenuation region or a region of high reflectivity, such as a calcified area or bowel gas.

This is similar to the production of shadows on a B-mode image.

Ghost mirror images

Ghost mirror images may be produced by partial reflection of the beam from a highly reflecting surface.

Angle dependence

The displayed colour is dependent on the angle between the beam and the direction of motion as illustrated in Figures 10.17 and 10.19:

- *Colour Doppler* – Displayed colour depends on the cosine of the angle.

- *Power Doppler* – Little angle dependence on angle except near 90°, where the Doppler frequencies fall below the clutter filter, if the velocity is too low.

- *Directional power Doppler* – Similar to power Doppler, except it is noted that flow towards and away from the transducer is coded in different colours.

Aliasing

As explained in Chapter 7, the maximum Doppler frequency shift that can be estimated is equal to PRF/2. Higher blood or tissue velocities will be displayed colour coded with opposite direction:

- *Colour Doppler and directional power Doppler* – Both suffer from aliasing.

- *Power Doppler* – Does not suffer from aliasing.

Drop-out

This is loss of colour due to the variable nature of the calculated mean frequency or power. If this is high, it is possible that the estimated mean frequency or power will fall below the threshold value used in the blood–tissue discriminator. When this happens, the system does not display colour. For colour flow, the effect is most marked at low velocities and in small vessels.

Noise

There are several types of noise present on the colour image:

- *Electronic noise* – This is produced within the colour flow system electronics. If the colour gain is set too high, the noise will be displayed as colour in regions of tissue in which there is no flow.

- *Flash artefacts* – These are false areas of colour on the colour flow image, which are produced when there is movement of the transducer with respect to the tissue. Some systems are able to remove these artefacts by use of a "flash filter".

- *Speckle* – The variation in the autocorrelator estimate of mean frequency and power gives rise to a noise superimposed on the underlying colour and power Doppler images; this noise is called "colour speckle". This speckle pattern may be reduced by the use of persistence.

Colour display at vessel–tissue boundaries

Ideally the power Doppler image would show a uniform colour up to the edge of the vessel. For colour Doppler, it is known that the blood velocities are low at the edge of the vessel, so that the displayed colour should show this. In practice, there are a number of effects that will lead to incorrect display of colour:

- *Partial volume effect* – At the edge of vessels, the colour sample volume is located partially within the vessel and partially in the tissue. This effect will lead to reduction in Doppler signal amplitude which will cause a change in displayed colour seen on power Doppler images. For colour Doppler, it is the mean frequency in that part of the sample volume that is located within the vessel which is displayed, so the displayed colour is not affected (Figure 10.22).

- *Image smoothing* – If there is any smoothing in the colour image, by averaging of adjacent pixels or by interpolation, this leads to false colours at the edge of vessels for both colour Doppler and power Doppler.

- *Clutter filter and blood–tissue discrimination* – Both of these will act to prevent the display of colour at the

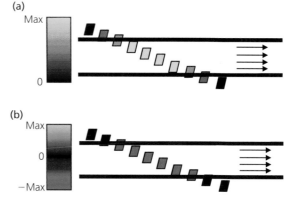

Fig. 10.22 Partial volume effect. In the vessel, it is assumed that all of the blood is moving at the same velocity. (a) Power Doppler – change in colour at the edge of a vessel. (b) Colour Doppler – no effect on the displayed colour.

edge of vessels as the velocities (and hence Doppler frequency shifts) are low, and the tissue signal strength is high.

Time domain colour flow systems

The essential features of this technique are described in Chapter 7, where it is noted that the change in target depth between consecutive echoes is estimated. Target velocity is then calculated by dividing the change in depth by the pulse repetition interval. The time domain approach was initially described by Bonnefous and Pesque (1986), and has been implemented by Philips Ultrasound, where it is called CVI (colour velocity imaging).

The time delay is calculated by comparing the echo pattern of consecutive transmission pulses by a mathematical technique called "cross correlation". This process is carried out by sliding one line of echoes past the other in a series of steps or time shifts, comparing the lines at each step. The time shift, which gives the closest correlation for each part of the line, gives a measure of how the corresponding target has moved between pulses. This method relies on the detailed echo pattern shifting as a whole, but not changing in its overall shape. However, as a region of tissue or blood moves, the echo pattern will change in overall shape, as it moves further away from its original site. This is associated with changes in the relative position of the scatterers as the blood or tissue moves, and also changes in the location of the red cells with respect to the transducer. The change in echo shape is called "decorrelation", and after a certain distance, the echo pattern has changed so much from the original echo pattern that the ultrasound machine cannot measure the time difference between the current and previous echo.

The time domain method has a number of features which lead to differences in performance to the phase domain method:

- *Aliasing* – As the time delay between pulses is measured, the technique does not suffer from aliasing. The upper limit of velocity detection is associated with the decorrelation described above.

- *Accuracy* – The time domain method calculates velocity more accurately than the autocorrelator, for the same ensemble length. Consequently, for the same accuracy, the time domain approach requires a smaller ensemble size, with gains to be made in either frame rate or line density. However, modern colour flow system use "2D autocorrelation", and

the accuracy for this technique is comparable with the time domain approach, so that this advantage is no longer present.

The time domain technique calculates the movement of blood cells along the beam. In other words, only the component of velocity in the direction of the beam is calculated. The time domain technique is, therefore, dependent on the angle between the beam and the direction of motion.

Measurements

This short section covers measurements, which are occasionally made from the colour flow image by clinical users, though it is noted that the vast majority of quantitative measurements are made using spectral Doppler. In research studies, quantitative analysis of the colour flow image using off-line computer analysis is widely performed; however, these techniques have yet to impact on clinical practice.

Single site velocity measurement

Some colour flow systems have the capability of showing the mean-frequency value at a specific location chosen by the operator. This can be converted to a velocity using the same angle correction techniques that are used in spectral Doppler. This information is occasionally useful in clinical research studies, e.g. estimation of the degree of arterial stenosis from peak velocity obtained from the colour Doppler image rather than the spectral Doppler waveform.

Quantitative analysis of flow patterns

Blood flow patterns are known to alter considerably in disease, as described in Chapter 5. However, there is little attempt to use the colour Doppler images to provide quantitative information on the colour flow patterns in disease, as there are not yet methods of quantification which have been shown to be clinically useful.

Volume flow

Calculation of volumetric flow requires estimation of the vessel cross-sectional area and the mean velocity. Ideally, the mean velocity and cross-sectional area should be estimated throughout the cardiac cycle to account for the expansion of the arteries, which occurs during the cardiac cycle. If colour flow images are obtained with the vessel imaged in the longitudinal plane, the velocity profile of the vessel can be obtained from the colour flow image, and the diameter obtained from the B-mode image. Estimation of the mean velocity requires an assumption that flow is symmetric within the vessel (i.e. all points at the same radius have the same velocity). Cross-sectional area is obtained from measured diameter assuming that the vessel has a circular cross section. Multiplication of the measured area and mean velocity give the volume flow.

This technique makes a number of assumptions, such as circular vessel, symmetric flow patterns, which limit its use to normal or relatively undiseased vessels. In practice, there is little call for volumetric flow measurement, and this method is not widely used.

References

Bonnefous O and Pesque P. Time domain formulation of pulse-Doppler ultrasound and blood velocity estimation by cross-correlation. *Ultrason. Imag.* 1986; **8**: 73–85.

Evans DH and McDicken WN. *Doppler Ultrasound: Physics, Instrumentation and Signal Processing.* Wiley, Chichester. 2000.

Kasai C, Namekawa K, Koyano A and Omoto R. Real time two-dimensional blood flow imaging using an autocorrelation technique. *IEEE Trans. Sonics. Ultrason.* 1985; **32**: 458–464.

Loupas T, Peterson RB and Gill RW. Experimental evaluation of velocity and power estimation for ultrasound blood flow imaging by means of a two-dimensional autocorrelation approach. *IEEE Trans. Ultrason. Ferroelec. Freq. Cont.* 1995a; **42**: 689–699.

Loupas T, Power JT and Gill RW. An axial velocity estimator for ultrasound blood flow imaging, based on a full evaluation of the Doppler equation, by means of a two-dimensional autocorrelation approach. *IEEE Trans. Ultrason. Ferroelec. Freq. Cont.* 1995b; **42**: 672–688.

Namekawa K, Kasai C, Tsukamoto M and Koyano A. Realtime bloodflow imaging system utilizing autocorrelation techniques. In: RA Lerski and P Morley (Eds) *Ultrasound '82.* Pergamon Press, New York. 1982, 203–208.

Rubin JM, Bude RO, Carson PL, Bree RL *et al.* Power Doppler US: a potentially useful alternative to mean frequency based color Doppler US. *Radiology* 1994; **190**: 853–856.

Wells PNT. Ultrasonic colour flow mapping. *Phys. Med. Biol.* 1994; **39**: 2113–2145.

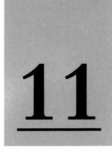

11

DISPLAY OUTPUT AND STORAGE

T Anderson

Displays for ultrasonic equipment
Printer technologies
Digital-imaging networks
Discussion

Unlike topics discussed in other chapters within this publication which have a significant physics content, the information presented here has a much more commercial bent and has been largely gleaned from sources of that type. These sources include the pages of manufacturers' publicity materials, data sheets, reference manuals, reputable sites on the World Wide Web and experience. While every effort has been made to ensure the accuracy of the material, it should nevertheless be used only for guidance, or as a basis for further investigation.

The selection of material included is based on treating the ultrasonic scanner simply as a source of image data made available as analogue or digital signals. The topics covered, therefore, include display, hardcopy, audio and video recorders and data storage devices. Because of this approach, it is also legitimate to include some discussion of digital-imaging networks in the form of patient archiving and communications systems (PACS), as well as associated topics such as networking and communication standards.

Developments in digital electronics, computers, signal processing and transducer design as well as a deeper understanding of the propagation of ultrasound in tissue, have lead to significant advances in the performance and range of imaging modalities available from current diagnostic ultrasound machines. Since an ultrasound system can be regarded as a collection of devices (scanner electronics, display, video recorder, printer, etc.), to gain maximum benefit from the system as a whole each component of the system must be optimised to complement the others. This is true whether all of the components of the system have been supplied by the manufacturer or additional devices, such as a video printer or recorder have been added by the user. The objectives of this chapter are twofold. Firstly, to provide the reader with a basic understanding of the operation of the various devices connected to an ultrasonic scanner. Just as a good understanding of the principles behind the operation of ultrasonic scanners is invaluable in their use, so to knowledge of the technology behind the peripherals is of value. Secondly, where appropriate, the chapter should also be of value to readers intending to expand the range of peripherals connected to their scanner, in helping them to select the most suitable device for their application.

Displays for ultrasonic equipment

In this section, the display devices required to transform the echoes collected by the ultrasonic scanner into a viewable image are discussed.

What qualities should a display for use in an ultrasound machine possess?

The type of display chosen by a manufacturer for a particular ultrasonic scanner depends on the intended application and resolution of the scanner. For most scanners, both general purpose and application specific, displays based on the cathode ray tube (CRT) are likely to be selected because of their general characteristics. If on the other hand, portability is a key feature then a liquid crystal display (LCD) may be chosen because of its flat rectangular shape and low weight. These same features also make the LCD an attractive proposition for image display where space is at a premium.

The characteristics of the CRT are summarised below:

- Greyscale or colour.
- High light output.
- Adequate range of brightness levels.
- Capable of resolution matching or exceeding that of the scanner.
- Moderate to high frame rates.
- Reasonable cost.

The size of a display is usually expressed in inches across the diagonal though increasingly sizes in centimetres are also given. Displays designed for medical applications currently range in size from a few inches up to 24 in. For an LCD display, the number given represents the true display area, however, for a CRT the actual display area is somewhat less due to the thickness of the glass used and the surrounding bezel. For a 17-in. monitor, the displayed image diagonal is reduced by these factors to approximately 16 in.

How does cathode ray tube work?

Though CRTs exist in many shapes and sizes those intended for image display, as opposed to those designed for use in electronic instruments such as oscilloscopes, come in two basic forms, black and white (greyscale) or colour. Although the principle of operation is the same, the construction of a black and white CRT is much simpler than that of a colour CRT.

MONOCHROME OR GREYSCALE (GS) MONITOR

In a monochrome or greyscale monitor (Figure 11.1), an electron beam produced by an "electron gun" is made to sweep over the phosphor coated inner surface

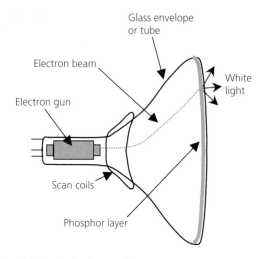

Fig. 11.1 Cathode ray tube.

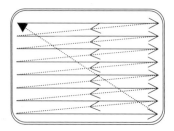

Fig. 11.2 Raster scan.

of the CRT screen in a raster pattern (Figure 11.2). The electron beam scans from left to right then rapidly "flies back" to the left-hand edge a little lower down ready to begin the next line. When the bottom right-hand corner is reached the beam is directed back to the top left to begin the next frame. As a result of the electron beam striking the phosphor and energising it, white light is produced. A greyscale image is formed on the screen by varying the intensity of the electron beam as it sweeps.

COLOUR MONITOR

To produce a colour image, three phosphors are required, representing the three primary colours from which all others can be formed. These red, green and blue phosphors are deposited on the inner surface of the screen as thousands of tiny dots arranged in groups of three, each group forming a single pixel (Figures 11.3 and 11.4). An electron gun is required for each of the three phosphors. The electron beams are made to sweep over the screen in the same way as in the monochrome display. To prevent the electron beam intended for one

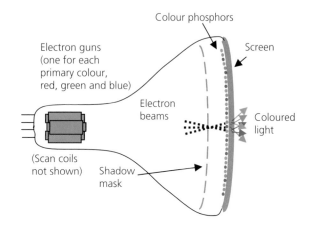

Fig. 11.3 Operation of colour CRT display. The electron guns produce varying intensity electron beams as required which scan across the phosphor dots on the inner surface of the screen. The shadow mask is designed and constructed such that the beams strike only their respective phosphors.

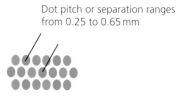

Fig. 11.4 Colour phosphor layout on inner surface of screen. The dot pitch indicates the resolution of the display.

phosphor striking the dots of another, a mask called a shadow mask is placed between the electron guns and phosphors. The shadow mask consists of a metal grid with a single hole for each pixel (group of three phosphor dots). The mask is positioned in front of the phosphors in such a way that as the electron beams sweep over the mask the beams pass through each hole and energise their respective phosphor dots. By varying the intensity of the electron beams independently, the combined light output, and hence the colour and brightness of each pixel can be controlled. If all three dots in a pixel are energised equally then a shade of grey is produced (Figure 11.5). If all three electron beams are turned off for a particular pixel, then that pixel appears black.

What is the resolution of a TV monitor?

As the name suggests TV monitors are designed to meet the standards developed for television. One of the main

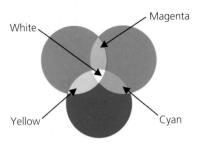

Fig. 11.5 Other colours are produced by mixing additive primary colours.

Table 11.1 Resolution of a TV monitor.

	Frame rate (Hz)	Vertical resolution (lines/ frame)	Horizontal resolution (TV lines)	Region
PAL	25	625	320	UK
NTSC	30	525	270	USA
SECAM	25	625	320	France

design objectives of these specifications was the production of an adequate image, while using a restricted bandwidth (to maximise the number of TV channels that could be transmitted). The standard that applies depends upon the region where the monitor is to be used. Without entering too deeply into the detail, these television standards define the horizontal and vertical resolution and the rate at which the image is updated, the frame rate. The basic information is summarised in Table 11.1.

Other regions use one or other of these standards or a variation, often dependent on political leanings or historical connections.[1]

Each TV frame is constructed from two interlaced raster scans or fields. Each field consists of half the total number of lines in a frame. When viewed from close range, as is the norm in ultrasonic scanning, interlaced fields often give rise to a flickering effect, which is most noticeable on display alpha–numerics.

Liquid crystal displays

LCDs, which first appeared as the display in watches and calculators, have now been developed to such an extent that they may be considered as a viable alternative to the colour CRT for image display. Where portability or space saving are key requirements then they are the display of choice despite their higher cost. Other flat panel display technologies under development may challenge this position in the future.

There are an increasing number of variations in the design and construction of LCDs but these mostly involve the method of control, with the objective of producing displays with a faster response (higher frame rate) and lower cost through reduced complexity of the drive and control electronics. The high cost of the LCD is a result of a rejection rate of around 40% on finished panels due to defects such as "missing" pixels rather than simply the cost of the materials used.

GREYSCALE LCD

Unlike a CRT, an LCD does not generate light, therefore, a light source of some kind, known as a "back light", is placed behind the display. Typically, an LCD is formed by sandwiching a thin layer of liquid crystal material between two polarised[2] glass plates where the polarisation is offset at 90°. Under normal circumstance, no light would pass through this arrangement as only say horizontally polarised light would enter the through the first plate but would be unable to pass through the following vertically polarised plate. Because of a twist in the structure of the liquid crystal layer, the polarisation of light passing through it is "rotated" 90°, thereby allowing it to pass through the second plate and be seen. However, when an electric field is applied by means of a matrix of transparent electrodes on the glass plates, the twist in the structure of the liquid crystal layer is straightened. The light now remains horizontally polarised and is, therefore, unable to exit through the vertically polarised second glass plate. The degree of twist and hence the amount of light able to pass through at each point or pixel, can be controlled by adjusting the strength of the electric field applied to the liquid crystal layer and a greyscale image formed as required (Figure 11.6).

COLOUR LCD DISPLAY

As in the CRT three sub-pixels coloured red, green and blue are required to form a single colour pixel. As the LCD does not generate light but only controls the light passing through, a colour filter layer must be included to produce these primary colours. The filters are arranged as strips running from top to bottom of the display as shown in Figure 11.7.

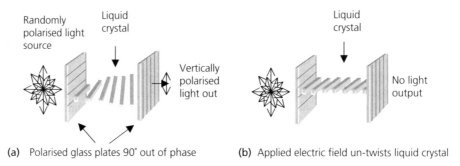

Randomly polarised light source

Liquid crystal

Vertically polarised light out

Liquid crystal

No light output

(a) Polarised glass plates 90° out of phase

(b) Applied electric field un-twists liquid crystal

Fig. 11.6 (a) The horizontally polarised light from the randomly polarised light source passes through the glass plate and into the liquid crystal. The twist in the structure of the liquid crystal "bends" the polarisation of the light through 90° enabling it to exit through the second plate. (b) When an electric field is applied across the liquid crystal, it straightens out and the light is no longer able to exit.

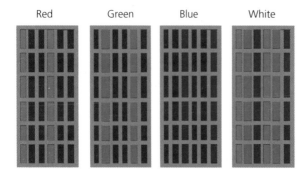

Red   Green   Blue   White

Fig. 11.7 Colours are produced through the use of RGB verical colour filter strips overlayed on top of an other wise greyscale LCD display.

What types of displays are used on the latest generation of high-performance scanners?

In the past, scanner displays were based on television monitors and associated standards. But for the latest generation of ultrasonic scanners with much improved image quality and also requirements for duplex display formats, these old standards are no longer adequate. There are two approaches which can be adopted to overcome the limitations of the standard TV monitor. One is to make use of monitors primarily developed for the computer industry. The second approach makes use of displays based on multi-standard monitors. The term "multi-standard monitor" is a vague term but any monitor claiming this title should be able to recognise the format of the signals supplied to it and perform the necessary signal processing to produce an image. This means that the multi-standard monitor is not limited to

a single national TV standard but is able to operate with virtually any TV standard without adjustment. More importantly, from the resolution standpoint, in addition to TV standards, they are also able to produce images using signal formats more commonly associated with high-resolution computer monitors. From a manufacture's point of view, both of these approaches allows the same monitor type to be fitted to every scanner no matter what the final destination of the machine might be.

Why do computer monitors have higher resolution than TV monitors?

As computer systems have developed so too has the resolution of their associated displays. These developments have been driven by the need for higher resolution displays for use with computer aided design, desktop publishing, graphic user interfaces and perhaps most significantly the mass market for computer games. As a result of this, mass market high-resolution colour graphic display systems are now typical on even the cheapest of personal computer. In addition, because of prolonged usage patterns, high frame rate low-flicker monitor technology has been developed to minimise operator fatigue. (In top of the range ultrasonic scanners, the monitor is usually the limiting factor as far as frame rate is concerned.)

From the performance viewpoint, higher frame rate monitors are especially suited to systems designed for echocardiology. Machines of this type often have a high ultrasonic frame rate capability, some over 200 per second. This has the potential to improve imaging of fast moving cardiac structures, such as heart valves and minimises time skew across the image. Where the scanner frame rate exceeds that of the display, at most 85 frames per second, ultrasonic frames must be dropped. However, the complete sequence of ultrasonic frames is available for review using the so-called video loop or video clip facility discussed below.

How can I record a video sequence?

In many situations, the ability to record sections of a patient exam can be very useful either for immediate review, without the distraction of scanning, for later review or for patient record purposes. Until recently, options were limited to the use of the video clip with possible storage to hard disk and to the video cassette recorder (VCR). A relatively new technique for recording video, at least to ultrasonic scanning, which overcomes the limitations of the video clip and VCR is "video streaming".

What is a video clip?

In all but the simplest of scanners, the last 10 s or so of exam images are stored in memory (RAM or random access memory) forming a "video clip". This facility is also referred as a cine loop, video loop or dynamic clip. When the "Freeze" button is pressed, the stored images may be reviewed, either singly by means of a tracker ball or on a continuous looping basis. The rate at which the images are displayed in video clip mode can often be varied as required. In some machines, the video clip images may be stored to disk and reloaded as required. On machines lacking these features or where a longer duration recording is required, a VCR represents the simplest means of recording a video sequence.

How good are video cassette recorders?

At the present moment, in the UK at least, virtually all video recording of ultrasonic images is performed using S-VHS recorders (S-VHS standing for super-video home system). The quality of reproduction approaches that of the original image but some degradation can be seen. This degradation takes the form of smudging, particularly of alpha-numerics, caused by the VCR's inability to respond to rapid changes in brightness (inadequate bandwidth). Also, slight variations in the start and end of scan lines caused by the mechanical nature of the device make vertical lines appear slightly uneven. Second generation copies show a significant reduction in quality, while third generation copies are unusable (Table 11.2). A further limitation is the difficulty in locating specific sections of interest.

Table 11.2 VCR resolution.

	Vertical resolution (lines/frame)	Horizontal resolution (TV lines)
VHS	625	240
S-VHS	625	400

Video recorders designed specifically for medical applications can be as much as 30 times more expensive than those intended for domestic use. The difference between the two forms may not always be obvious in terms of image quality but "medical" VCRs boast quick response industrial grade transport mechanisms, a control interface and digital frame freeze memory. Though the performance of VCRs intended for the domestic market may rival that of the medical grade VCR, they should never be used in the clinical setting, since they do not provide the same level of electrical safety particularly under fault conditions.

Some scanners provide auxiliary power outlets, which are supplied by an internal isolation transformer. Whenever possible, these auxiliary power outlets should be used instead of direct connection to the mains supply. However, even if an auxiliary power outlet is used, it advisable to have an electrical safety check carried out before using the modified system on patients.

How does a VCR work?

After a cassette has been inserted into a VCR and the play/record buttons pressed, the magnetic tape from the cassette is automatically threaded round read/write heads which read from the tape or record new images onto the tape. The read/write heads are contained in a rapidly rotating drum. The magnetic tape is partially wrapped round this drum in a spiral fashion as shown in Figure 11.8. The tape is moved slowly passed the rapidly rotating drum and the read/write heads read or write new information to or from the tape. This arrangement of rapidly spinning heads and moving tape causes TV frames to be written as diagonal tracks across the width of the tape. Also, because of this combined motion the tracks are slightly curved. In pause or still frame mode, tape movement is stopped. Unless a digital-image store is included as in some VCRs, the frozen image may appear to be "out of sync" or "torn" due to the inability of the heads to follow the curve track laid down during record.

Most of the limitations of the VCR can be overcome by a digital-recording technique called digital video streaming. This and other developments are likely to lead

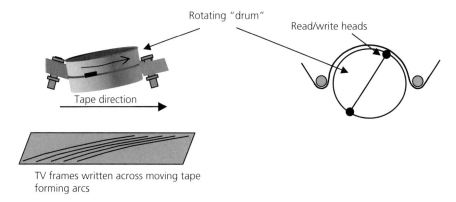

Rotating "drum"

Read/write heads

Tape direction

TV frames written across moving tape forming arcs

Fig. 11.8 VCR read/write heads.

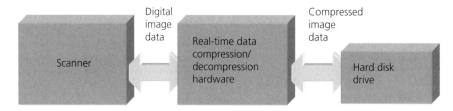

Digital image data

Compressed image data

Scanner

Real-time data compression/ decompression hardware

Hard disk drive

Fig. 11.9 Block diagram of digital video streaming hardware.

to the demise of the VCR with its analogue recording technique and highly complex mechanical construction.

What is "digital video streaming"?

Digital video streaming overcomes the short record length limitation of the video clip (limited by the amount of RAM available in the scanner for image storage) and the image degradation problems of the VCR. In this technique, the digital video or image data is compressed in real-time to reduce the data rate to manageable proportions prior to storage. It is then stored in real-time to hard disk. A block diagram is shown in Figure 11.9. The record period is specified prior to capture and multiple records can be stored dependent only on the size of the hard disk and the record period. During review, this process is reversed. The compression and decompression process is performed by specialised digital-signal processing hardware to achieve the necessary data flow rate.

What other video devices can be connected to a scanner?

Because video images are viewed, recorded, copied, edited, printed, etc. most video devices are equipped

with signal inputs and outputs to allow connection of multiply devices to one video source. The ultrasonic scanner manufacturer may also provide auxiliary audio and video signal outlets to enable users to connect additional audio/video devices as desired.

Before discussing, the details of connecting additional displays or hardcopy devices to a scanner, it is worth exploring the terminology used to describe the various video signals likely to be encountered. The three most widely used video signals on ultrasonic scanners are referred to as composite video, RGB and S–Video.

COMPOSITE VIDEO

Monochrome and colour TV monitors as well as many video-printers rely on a signal often simply referred to as the "video signal" but more correctly as the "composite video signal". In greyscale systems, this signal is composed of the horizontal and vertical synchronisation signals and the brightness signal, as illustrated in Figure 11.10. For colour displays, it also contains the colour or chrominace signal. Composite video is most commonly connected by means of a single core screened connector of the BNC type. For retention purposes, BNC connectors have a bayonet locking mechanism similar to that employed by many household electric light bulb fittings.

RGB

RGB (standing for red, green and blue) is a form of component video. That is, instead of all the necessary signals being encoded onto one conductor, each of the three-colour components of the image are made available on separate connectors, again the BNC type is the norm. The synchronisation or sync signal is encoded onto the green channel or may alternatively be linked by means of a fourth connector.

S-VIDEO

An improvement over composite video, the S-Video standard is utilised in S-VHS recorders. The improvement is achieved by separating the process path of the brightness signal (luminance) from the colour signal (chrominance). This modification achieves the horizontal equivalent of 400 lines of resolution. The synchronisation signals are encoded with the luminance signal. A multi-way cable with a special miniature four-way connector, "keyed" to prevent incorrect insertion, is used to link the signals between devices.

MAKING THE CONNECTION

Video devices, such as an additional display or printer, are connected together in a daisy chain fashion (Figure 11.11). With video systems, it is important to electrically terminate the final device in the chain. This avoids an electrical impedance mismatch which would otherwise cause a proportion of the signal to be reflected back down the cable. The result of this reflection is to produce a ghosting effect on the image. This appears, as a second usually fainter image overlaid on the first but slightly to one side. To facilitate proper termination, all video devices include a switch that connects or disconnects a "terminating" resistor. The switch is often labelled 75 Ω On/Off. Where only short cable runs are employed, as when an additional monitor is positioned next to the scanner to enable patients to see the image, a lack of a terminating resistor is unlikely to be noticed. However, on longer cable runs, say to an adjoining room, the effect may be very noticeable and takes the form of a "ghost" image. If two or more devices in a chain are inadvertently terminated, then the video signal amplitude is reduced, causing a reduction in display contrast.

With composite video and S-VHS-based devices, only a single cable need be connected from the "Video Out" connector of the scanner or other video device, to the "Video In" of the device being added. With RGB signals, the situation becomes a little more complicated. Instead of a single connecting video cable, three or possibly four cables are required. Alternatively, these cables may be combined in a single sheath, which splits to three or four separate connectors in combination with a single multi-way connector at the scanner end. The sockets for the individual connectors are labelled or coloured RGB, with possibly a fourth labelled Sync. Appropriate termination of each of the RGB signals is normally achieved by means of a single switch.

In the future, it is likely that external video equipment will be connected to scanners by optical means, thereby eliminating electrical connection and the possibility of compromising electrical safety (Table 11.3).

What type of hardcopy should I use?

The correct choice of hardcopy device depends largely on the task it must perform. The ideal printer for connection to a single scanner is unlikely to be the best choice, where a printer is required to service a number of machines. Similarly, the needs of different specialities are likely to require different hardcopy solutions. Factors

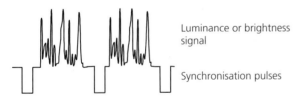

Luminance or brightness signal

Synchronisation pulses

Fig. 11.10   Composite video signal.

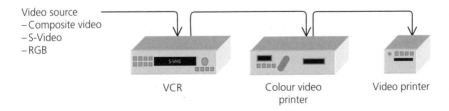

Video source
– Composite video
– S-Video
– RGB

VCR

Colour video printer

Video printer

Fig. 11.11   Video devices are connected in a daisy chain fashion.

Table 11.3   Typical display resolutions.

Type	Size	Frame rate	Horizontal	Vertical
GS TV monitor	All sizes	25	400	625
Colour TV monitor	All sizes	25	400	625
High resolution GS monitor	21″	70	2560	2048
Colour monitor	17″	50–120	1280	1024
LCD GS	18″	75	1280	1024
LCD colour	18″	75	1280	1024

which should be considered before even beginning the selection process are summarised below, though the order of their importance will depend on the nature of the application:

- Available budget

- Paper or film

- Light or heavy use

- Quality requirements

- Network connectivity

- Colour, greyscale or both

- Running costs

- Reliability

- Environmental factors, e.g. wet or dry, location

- Multiple scanner connection.

It may not be possible to satisfy every requirement with one printer. For example, if many greyscale prints are required each day from a mid-range ultrasound machine and the occasional colour image then a single printer able to produce both colour and greyscale might seem attractive. However, printers able to provide both greyscale and colour hardcopy are either very expensive to buy, or to run, or possibly both. A better solution might be a low-cost greyscale video printer satisfying the bulk of the hardcopy requirement and a low throughput colour printer for use when required. A second scenario might require a printer able to service the needs of a number of ultrasonic scanners and perhaps other imaging modalities as well. In this case, careful analysis of requirements must first be undertaken to select the most appropriate printer technology, one able to satisfy the imaging demands of all potential users. When considering printer sharing it should be borne in mind that this approach can add considerably to the final costs. Only after deciding on the most appropriate technology should the offerings of the various manufactures' be considered. Again, no single device may be able to fully satisfy requirements, though some printers combine two different print technologies in a single unit, effectively two printers in one.

GREYSCALE AND COLOUR IMAGE CONSTRUCTION

Before describing the various printer technologies available, it is worthwhile examining the methods used to produce hardcopy colour and greyscale images. In the section on colour displays three colours red, green and blue where described as primary colours from which all other colours can be produced. In a display system where light is emitted the desired colour is created by an additive process. However, in a colour photograph or printout, colours are observed by a subtractive process. When white light falls on the photograph or printout the colours that are seen are those that are reflected back from the picture. The base colours required to produce reflective colour images are the "subtractive" primary colours cyan, magenta and yellow. Black is sometimes included as a fourth "colour" to overcome the practical limitations of the coloured inks or dyes in producing pure black areas.

Images produced by continuously variable colour systems, such as photography, are referred to as contone images. Those in which the illusion of a full colour spectrum is simulated by laying down patterns of fixed or binary colours, in a process known as dithering, are referred to as halftone images. In some systems, even greyscale images are produced by changing the mix of black and white patterns (Figure 11.12). The illusion of a full range of grey shades is achieved by varying the size, shape and spacing of black dots or lines on a white background. Newspaper and magazine printing presses rely on halftone techniques for both greyscale and colour pictures. In newspaper pictures, the dots can often be seen with the "naked eye" while in magazines and books a magnifying glass is likely to be required. The resolution of printers is expressed in terms of dots per inch (dpi), the higher the number the better the resolution, at least in theory. However, increased resolution

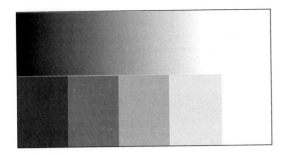

Fig. 11.12 The upper grey bar represents a continuous change from black to white, while in the lower grey bar the change is effected by a halftone technique.

can impact on the print rate, another important performance criterion. Print rate is expressed in pages per minute (ppm), with colour printouts usually taking much longer to produce than greyscale. Apart from photographic-based hardcopy systems, involving a single exposure, most other hardcopy production methods build up a complete image on the media as it is moved through the printer. Typically, the image is built up using some kind of scanning procedure, similar to the raster scanning process employed in a CRT or alternatively by printing a complete line at a time by means of a full width print head.

Printer technologies

For many years, the only practical way of producing hardcopies of images was by photographic means, such as the "Polaroid" print or onto X-ray film via a "multi-format camera" system. The options available today are much wider due to the development of new printing technologies[3] and media types.

Those discussed here include:

- laser printer types,
- dye sublimation printer,
- thermal wax transfer printer,
- video printer,
- ink jet printers.

Laser printer types

The term laser printer, not surprisingly, is applied to all printers which utilise a laser beam in their operation. However, there are two quite different types of printer which may be described by this term. The first is found almost universally in office situations where high-quality documents are required. This type of printer can produce images on plain paper or transparency film. A description of its operation is included here as it is being increasingly advertised for image hard copy applications. The second type which has until recently been restricted to larger radiology departments, due to both its size and high cost, is finding a wider market due to the arrival of alternative types of film media and handling methods which may or may not require further processing. These will be referred to as laser imagers.

LASER PRINTER

Available in "black and white" or colour versions this type of printer relies on halftone techniques for greyscale and colour image production. Charged areas are created on a rotating drum or belt by means of a scanning laser beam. These charged areas correspond to where ink, or more correctly toner, a very fine powder, is to be deposited on the media. As the charged areas on the drum pass the cartridge in which the toner is held, toner is attracted to the drum. As the drum continues to rotate with its toner load, it comes into close proximity with oppositely charged media to which the toner transfers. Before it emerges from the printer, the media is "baked" to fuse the toner on to the media preventing smudging of the printout. The media may be paper or special acetate film able to survive the heat of the baking process.

The colour laser printer is essentially four printers in one, since the process of toner deposition must be duplicated for all three primary colours in addition to black. In the colour laser printer, the number of parts which must be replaced after a specified period of usage approaches four times that of the black and white only version. For this reason, colour laser printers are both expensive to run and maintain, requiring a high level of staff competence compared to solid inkjet printers.

LASER IMAGER

The laser imager, depending on the media for which it has been designed, may utilise halftone or contone image formation techniques. In the laser imager, the laser beam scans the media directly as it passes through the imager (Figure 11.13). Again depending on the nature of media for which the imager has been designed to use, chemical processing of the output may or may not be required.

Dye sublimation printer

This type of printer is often regarded as the printer of choice for colour images because of its continuous tone

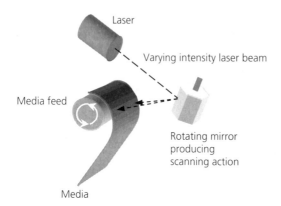

Fig. 11.13 In the laser imager the light or heat from the laser causes chemical changes in the media. In light sensitive media, chemical processing is required to "develop" the film. With heat sensitive (dry) systems no further processing of the media is required.

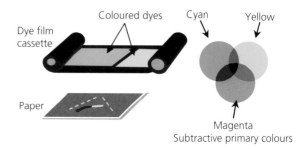

Fig. 11.14 In the dye sublimation printer a thermal print head transfers the coloured dyes to the media to form the image.

reproduction method. The dye used in the process is supplied on a roll of thin film (donor ribbon) stored in a cartridge, in successive panes of cyan, magenta and yellow; one set of three colours for each print. As the printing process proceeds, the film is wound from the source reel to a take up reel. The appropriate amount of each dye is successively transferred from the donor ribbon to the "acceptor media", either transparent film or white paper, by means of a full width thermal print head. As each layer of dye is deposited on the film or paper, the dyes flow together to form the intended colour at each pixel (Figure 11.14). Dye sublimation printers are able to reproduce up to 16.7 million colours inclusive of 256 shades of grey. The media may be as large as A4 with images arranged according to pre-set selectable patterns or formats.

Thermal wax transfer printer (solid ink jet)

Similar in operation to ink jet printers, thermal wax transfer printers use blocks of solid coloured wax instead of liquid ink cartridges. However, before a print session can begin the wax must first be melted. Discounting this daily warm up period, thermal wax printers can be significantly faster than colour laser printers. The quality of the printout is also high. Like the laser printer, colours other than the prime colours are produced by laying down primary colours in patterns to create the illusion of a full colour spectrum. The low cost of coloured waxes and relatively simple mechanisms, results in low maintenance costs and high reliability. The media may be paper or film. Thermal wax transfer printers may also

include a laminating option to protect the colour coating of the printout, making it much more durable by preventing scratching. Alternatively, the surface of the media may be coated to improve "ink" adhesion. Printers are available which combine dye sublimation printing, with its superior quality and thermal wax transfer printing, with its low cost, in one unit, with the aim of providing more flexible and hence economic printing options.

Video printer

The term "video" printer refers more to the method of capturing an image than the method of reproduction. These printers capture a video image using an internal "frame grabber". Available as colour or greyscale only, the input signals may be RGB, S-Video or composite greyscale video. The signals are digitised to 8-bit accuracy resulting in 256 levels of grey or for RGB, 16.7 million colours ($256 \times 256 \times 256$). Though both the colour and greyscale versions use a thermal print head, their method of operation is quite different. Colour versions use the dye sublimation approach described above, while the greyscale versions rely on heat sensitive paper. The print head consists of perhaps 256 elements. As the heat sensitive paper is drawn past the print head, the heat from each element is modulated causing the paper to change from white through grey to black as required for the image (Figure 11.15). This type of printer can be configured to suit a number of applications such as a low-cost printer commonly used for revenue generation in obstetrics departments to wide format versions for images and M-mode traces in cardiology applications.

Ink jet printers

Ink jet printers operate by projecting small droplets of ink onto paper or special transparent film as the print head or in some instances print heads sweep from side

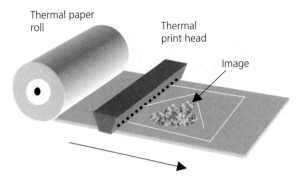

Thermal paper
roll

Thermal
print head

Image

Fig. 11.15 In the video printer, a thermal print head forms the image by changing the state of the heat sensitive paper from white to grey or black.

to side, while the paper is advanced. As yet not widely used for medical imaging directly, in large format type, they are used for the production of quality posters for exhibition use. Available with black and coloured inks with as many as 2400 dpi, they are capable of producing very high-resolution printouts, particularly when used with special high-quality papers. As the ink remains "soluble" in water, printouts are easily damaged and are, therefore, best laminated (sandwiched between two layers of clear plastic film) where durability is required.

Making the final choice

Choosing a printer for a particular application can be a daunting exercise, but one which can be made easier with a basic understanding of the technologies involved. Each technology has its own strengths and weaknesses which have to be taken into consideration, however, the application and its requirements often dictate which type to use. Once the type of printer has been selected, but before committing to a particular manufacturer or model, sample hardcopy should be viewed. If possible, a selection of printers should be tried on an evaluation basis. Where this is not possible the views of others providing a similar service could prove valuable.

Digital-imaging networks

The developments in computing and data storage technology over the last 10 years or so are such that it is now possible to collect, store and manage all of the medical images produced within even the largest of hospitals by digital means. These multi-modality image collection and storage systems referred to as PACS. The components, which form a PACS, are the main theme of this

section. The objective of this brief discussion is again one of familiarisation with the basics of the technology.

Why PACS?

A properly designed and implemented PACS can overcome many of the difficulties and limitations associated with a hardcopy- and paper-based method of recording the results of patient scans, X-rays, reports, etc. and provide benefits such as

- ready access to previous examination images,
- make acquired images immediately available to all authorised users,
- guarantee legibility of reports,
- reduce demographic information entry,
- greatly reduce hardcopy storage space requirements,
- eliminate repeat examinations and procedure cancellation through non-availability of images,
- eliminate time lost searching for patient records,
- enable higher patient throughput.

A PACS is able to deliver these benefits, since it provides for the total management of acquisition, distribution, reporting, storage, retrieval and display of images acquired by digital means or converted to digital form.

A sophisticated PACS might include CT, MRI, DR and Ultrasound and provide centralised image storage, reporting, distribution and shared hardcopy facilities. A PACS is not limited to a single floor or building but may link imaging devices across a site and even remote medical facilities. Importantly, it must be linked to the hospital information system (HIS) if all of its potential benefits are to be fully realised.

Apart from imaging devices, what other systems are required to form a PACS?

To form a PACS, systems other than imaging devices are required. These include the cable to form the network, ports or connection points, workstations for image reporting and review, short- and long-term storage systems for current and archived records and hard copy devices.

THE NETWORK INFRASTRUCTURE

A PACS is essentially a "local area network" (LAN) which has been designed for a particular application. The type and grade of cable used to form the network determines the maximum rate at which information (images) can be transferred. The choice also has a bearing on the overall reliability of the network. The fastest networks are based on fibre optic cables. These are typically used to provide a high-speed "backbone" to which other network components are connected. This optical fibre "backbone" plays a similar roll to a motorway in a road system. Fibre optic cables currently have transfer rates up to 40 Gbps (40,000 million bits per second), roughly the equivalent of the contents of seven data CDs transferred in 1 s.

A communications network requires more than the physical connection of computer systems. To enable the transfer of information across a network a common set of rules or protocols must be followed. The most widely used set of protocols in PACS is the Transmission Control Protocol/Internet Protocol (TCP/IP).[4] This provides for the low-level process of transferring information. But to allow the utilisation of the services provided by one device on the network, e.g. a printer, by another device, e.g. a scanner, a standard method of communicating is required. This is provided by a standard known as DICOM and is discussed later.

WORKSTATIONS

Acquired images can be transferred to workstations for reporting or review. Workstations are simply computer systems configured for image display and management. Two levels of workstation are commonly available on a PACS. One able to display images at very high resolution, comparable with film, using one or more large format high-resolution greyscale monitors. The other, usually intended for review rather than reporting, using a lower resolution and, therefore, lower cost monitor. Colour and possibly sound may also be included in the configuration. The operation of the workstation and the reporting facilities offered are determined by its physical configuration and by the software installed. Common facilities offered include:

- Icon-based user interface with drag and drop features.
- Work list management.
- Dual monitors for image comparison.
- Windowed display capable of showing multiple images.

Image storage

Images of any type require large amounts of disk storage space, particularly, when compared to the space required to store a single page of text. Ultrasound images, for example, require approximately 0.5 MB of storage for greyscale and 1.5 MB for colour images. If a number of images and possible a cine loop are required, then the per patient storage space requirement could easily exceed 100 MB. Storage requirements for other modalities can be higher.

Image storage within a PACS can occur at a number of locations depending on how the system is organised. Images may initially be stored within or locally to the imaging device and only deleted, when they have been successfully transferred to other storage locations within the PACS. The ability to store images within the modality or associated computers ensures that the modality will be able to function normally even if the network should fail temporarily. After capture, images may be transferred or copied across the network to a pre-selected workstation for reporting or may be sent to a rapid access short-term storage. The images may also be made available, instantly, over the network to all interested parties prior to reporting.

Up to three levels of information storage are implemented in a PACS, short term, long term or short term, medium term and long term. The longer the images are stored at any one location, the larger the storage capacity must be. The actual storage strategy employed depends to a degree on the vendors preferred approach to storage and to the storage technologies employed. A wide range of high-capacity storage devices is available to choose from based on electromagnetic and optical techniques.[5]

SHORT-TERM STORAGE

Recently, acquired or active images are liable to be copied to a variety of users for reporting, second opinions, etc. To ensure that this can be done quickly these active images are stored in a fast retrieval system which is able to located and copy the images to other locations in a matter of seconds. This type of fast retrieval storage is provided by hard disks drives, the same or similar to those found in most PC systems. Since hard disk drives are not 100% reliable short-term storage is implemented using an array of disk drives or RAID system (redundant array of inexpensive drives). By using multiple drives and including redundancy in the form of duplication or a checksum to enable errors to be detected and corrected, a much higher level of reliability is achieved than would otherwise be the case with a single drive. Using these techniques, RAID storage systems are "fault tolerant" in that they are able to continue to operate normally despite the failure of

Table 11.4 Storage technology, media capacity and cost.

Drive type	Media	Use	Capacity	Mb/£ (approximately)
Hard Disk	Fixed	Read/write	60 Gb	1000
MO Disk	Removable	Read/write	5.6 Gb	54
CD-R	Removable	Write once	640 Mb	900
CD-R/RW	Removable	Read/write	640 Mb	640
WORM	Removable	Write once	14 Gb	74
DVD-Ram	Removable	Read/write	5.2 Gb	288
DLT	Removable	Read/write	40 Gb	450

one of the drives in the array. When the faulty drive is replaced, usually without even switching the system off, the information that had been stored on the failed drive is restored to the replacement drive.

LONG-TERM STORAGE

After a predetermined period, perhaps 30 days, images, which have been reported on, are moved from the rapid access short-term storage to long-term storage. This level of storage can be based on optical drives of one form or another or magnetic tape. Three types of optical drive are available, all featuring high-reliability media. These are magneto optical (MO), recordable CD (CD-R) or read/write CD (CD-RW) and "write once read many" (WORM) optical drive. All of these provide random access to stored information at medium to high-transfer rates. The cost of storage per megabyte or number of megabytes per currency unit (pound/dollar, etc.) over the range of storage systems varies dramatically (see Table 11.4). An alternative to optical disk based systems is magnetic tape storage. The most commonly used magnetic tape storage in PACS is known as DLT (digital linear tape). DLT provides the highest storage density, tens of gigabytes per cartridge, and reliability similar to optical disks due to built in error checking and correction. Storage systems in the terabyte (million megabyte) range can be constructed in cabinet sized enclosures using robotic systems to automatically locate and insert the required tape cartridge into a drive.

What is DICOM?

Initially, PACS was essentially a proprietary technology whereby a single manufacturer would supply the complete system. Linking equipment from another supplier required the use of interface units to make the physical connections and interpret data formats. In 1983, the American College of Radiology (ACR) and the National Electrical Manufacturers Association (NEMA) formed the Digital Imaging and Communication Standards Committee. The objective of this committee was to develop an open communications standard enabling imaging equipment to link to devices, such as computers and printers independent of manufacturer.[6] As well as specifications for hardware the Committee were charged with developing the necessary data structures required for image display and evaluation. The standard has developed with each implementation to the current level, DICOM 3.

DICOM provides the means to negotiate a mutually acceptable level of interaction between say an imaging device and a printer much in the same way a FAX machine negotiates the highest possible resolution and speed of transfer with another FAX machine of an unknown type.

To be DICOM Compliant, a device must be able to support minimum communication syntax. Unlike earlier versions, DICOM 3 has been designed to be an evolving standard, able to accommodate the needs of an ever-increasing list of imaging modalities.

In principle, the use of this standard allows information to be passed between equipment supplied by different manufacturers since it specifies the details of the physical link between equipment, data communication protocols, and a command structure for controlling the interoperation of equipment. Every piece of equipment for which DICOM compatibility is claimed must have a corresponding DICOM conformance statement. This conformance statement is intended to provide sufficient information so a user or potential user can determine what services a device will be able to provide. Most suppliers make the conformance statements for their equipment available over the World Wide Web.

Discussion

In this chapter, displays, hardcopy, digital-imaging networks and storage devices have been discussed at an introductory level. These are areas that continue to be subject to very rapid developments. In the case of displays, improvements in resolution are brought about not only as a result of refinements to existing technologies but also as a result of completely new technologies and materials being developed. This is, particularly, true for flat panel displays. Hardcopy devices have progressed rapidly too in recent years, with the arrival of dry film systems and thermal wax transfer technologies. Computing and storage devices also continue to drive forward the capabilities of imaging networks as a result of the doubling of computing power available in a given space every 12–18 months.[7] All of these forces combine to make the task of specifying and selecting the types of device and systems discussed here more difficult. As in many fields, independent advice as to which product is best for a particular application can be hard to come by. Therefore, where practical, on site evaluation remains the best strategy before the final decision to purchase is made.

Notes

1. www.ee.surrey.ac.uk/Contrib/WorldTV/compare.html

2. www.physicsclassroom.com/Class/light/U12L1e.html

3. www.kodak.com/US/en/digital/dlc/book2/chapter2/index.shtml

4. www.webopedia.com/TERM/T/TCP_IP.html

5. www.sel.sony.com/SEL/rmeg/mediatech/overview.html

6. //medical.nema.org/dicom/geninfo/dicomstrategyv105/dicomstrategyv105.htm

7. www.webopedia.com/TERM/M/Moores_Law.html

12

QUALITY ASSURANCE

AJ Evans and PR Hoskins

Introduction

The term "Quality Assurance" is normally associated with schemes for the assessment of the quality of a process or activity. Such an assessment might be used to demonstrate that the outcomes of the process meet a required standard or specification.

The use of ultrasound in diagnostic processes and services leads hopefully to clinically useful outcomes, such as measurements of anatomical features or identification of abnormalities. Such outcomes would be affected by process elements, such as machine technical performance, operator competence and reporting procedures and would be assessed within schemes under the heading of clinical audit.

Quality assurance, as described in this chapter, relates specifically to the assessment of the performance of diagnostic ultrasound systems, and might be described more correctly as performance testing or performance assessment. However, the term quality assurance is used commonly in this context and will be used here.

Clinical and technical assessment

Two approaches to quality assurance of diagnostic ultrasound systems are in common use. Clinical users of ultrasound equipment often assess performance using diagnostic criteria in images of real patients. These might involve evaluating how well a system images challenging anatomical detail or differentiates subtle changes in tissue. Technical assessments of system performance make use of inanimate test objects. These are constructed from materials designed to mimic the ultrasonic properties of human tissue and contain a range of targets designed to test specific system parameters, which are related to imaging performance.

Clinical assessments, it is often argued, are useful because they are made on images of real patients. However, they yield only qualitative assessments of performance, which are affected by operator skill and judgement, and by wide biological variations in patients. Technical assessments are more quantitative and repeatable as they use standard test objects, but still involve some subjective judgement and may not mimic performance in real tissues very closely. This chapter describes test objects and methods for carrying out technical assessments of performance.

Applications of quality assurance

Purchase evaluation

In purchase evaluation, the objective is first to specify what is required of the imaging system in terms of functions and performance, and then evaluate available models against the specification. As for any medical equipment, the evaluation criteria should be relevant to the intended purpose. For example, a system intended for use only for dating in pregnancy, will not need the same range of functions and imaging performance, as one intended for in-depth abdominal and vascular investigations in a radiology department. However, it will be important to ensure that any growth charts included in the measurement functions are relevant to the population to be studied (see Chapter 6). For first trimester investigations, it may be relevant to specify an upper limit on worst case thermal and mechanical acoustical indices (see Chapter 13).

In principle, imaging performance can be specified and evaluated against *absolute* criteria using technical assessments with standard test objects or alternative measurement equipment. In practice, the best that can be achieved is to *compare* performances on standard test objects, as there are no widely agreed absolute criteria for different applications. The advantage of standard test objects is that they are relatively stable in terms of their properties and dimensions, and performance tests are fairly repeatable, when carried out by a suitably qualified and experienced operator.

Although it is difficult to make clinical assessments against absolute criteria due to patient variability and operator judgement, evaluation should include clinical assessments in the intended area of application. Comparisons of clinical performance of two or more systems side by side on the same subject can be useful. More limited comparisons might be carried out on different days in the same subject by storing images of carefully chosen anatomy in digital form or as hard copies. Clinical comparisons, which are not on the same subject, are likely to be of limited use.

Acceptance testing

Quality assurance tests may be carried out on new equipment, before it is accepted into clinical service. Such acceptance tests also may be against absolute criteria, where they are used to ensure that the new system performs as specified by the manufacturer or as specified in the purchase contract. Acceptance tests also provide baseline measurements of performance against which to evaluate performance in the future. Technical assessments are most useful in acceptance tests, due to the requirement for absolute measures of performance. Clinical assessments should be made to ensure that the system functions adequately in the intended area of application. Acceptance testing of ultrasound equipment should include inspection and testing of electrical, mechanical and acoustical safety. These tests will require the involvement of the local Medical Physics Department. Acceptance tests should include rigorous testing of measurement functions (Chapter 6).

Continuing performance assessment

Regular assessments of ultrasound systems are made to demonstrate that the system performance has not deteriorated from that measured in acceptance tests. Technical assessments are most useful in this application, but to be valuable, need to be reproducible and sensitive to change in performance. Clinical assessments are unlikely to be useful in monitoring performance over long periods (e.g. several years), as the subject is likely to change over this time scale.

Standards and guidelines

All medical devices sold in the European Community (EC) must meet the "Essential Requirements" of the Medical Devices Directive (93/42/EEC) for safety and performance. Manufacturers can demonstrate compliance with requirements for electrical and mechanical safety by referring to internationally agreed standards published by the International Standards Organisation (ISO) or the IEC (International Electrotechnical Commission), which have been adopted by the EC. There are as yet no standards for acoustical safety, which have been adopted by the EC. As described in Chapter 13, the American FDA regulations are the *de facto* standard for most manufacturers.

At present, it is not possible for manufacturers of ultrasound-imaging systems to demonstrate that they meet requirements for performance, as there are no agreed standards to work to. Some international standards have been published, which describe standard methods for measuring the performance of ultrasound pulse–echo-imaging equipment (BS 5724 Section 3.26; IEC 61390), but there are no standards, which specify how well a system should perform in a particular application.

Guidelines on methods for performance testing of ultrasound-imaging equipment have been published by the American Association of Physics in Medicine (Goodsitt *et al.*, 1998) and the Institute of Physical Sciences in Medicine (Price, 1995). These do not have the status of international standards, but have been agreed by panels of each organisation's experts and give practical guidance on how to perform technical assessments and when to test particular parameters. These also offer little guidance on absolute performance criteria.

Test objects for B-mode imaging

Measurement parameters

Test objects are designed to allow measurement of parameters, which relate to imaging performance. As described in Chapter 5, the performance of ultrasound-imaging systems may be described in terms of spatial, amplitude and temporal properties. Spatial properties determine the smallest target or target separation that can be imaged, amplitude properties the lowest echo amplitude or smallest change in amplitude, and temporal properties the most rapidly moving target. For many targets, these properties are interrelated. Standard-imaging test objects have fixed targets designed only to assess spatial and amplitude properties. Specifically, the most common test object targets are those designed to assess:

- spatial resolution (axial, lateral and slice thickness);
- maximum penetration (weakest echo/noise);
- the smallest and the largest echo amplitudes (dynamic range); and
- measurement accuracy.

Test object design

A wide range of test objects is available commercially. The most common form is a closed container filled with a medium, whose acoustic properties are similar to those of tissue. Within the medium, there are a number of targets designed to facilitate testing of the parameters listed above. The shape and size of the test object created in this way is determined by the type of systems it is designed to evaluate. Thus, if low-frequency (2–5 MHz) equipment is to be tested, the test object will need to be relatively large. Typically, this will be $150 \times 150 \times 50$ mm. For higher-frequency transducers, the targets and their separation will typically be smaller and the overall dimensions reduced. Targets intended for the measurement of spatial resolution and measurement accuracy usually consist of thin (0.1–0.5 mm) nylon filaments or wires, which are imaged in cross section. Targets for measurement of dynamic range, typically, consist of cylinders of the medium, which scatter more or less strongly than the medium in the bulk of the test object. More detailed descriptions of specific test object designs are given later in this chapter.

Test object media

There are three main categories of medium used to fill test objects. These are liquids, aqueous gels and polyurethane rubbers. Liquid media are useful in test objects designed specifically to test measurement functions of imaging systems. Figure 12.1 shows an example of an "open-topped" test object. The test object targets consist of a matrix of 0.5 mm diameter steel pins mounted 25.0 mm apart between two plates of Perspex. The test object is used in an open container of liquid whose speed of sound is 1540 m s^{-1}. The most widely used liquid is a mixture of ethanol (9.5% by volume) and distilled water, which gives a speed of sound of 1540 m s^{-1} at 20°C. The temperature of the mixture must be maintained within a few degrees of 20°C, as the speed of sound is temperature dependent (Martin and Spinks, 2001).

The open-topped test object is useful for testing measurement accuracy, because the speed of sound in the liquid is known accurately and good acoustic contact is made, even to curved transducers, by immersing the transducer face in the liquid. Open-test objects are not

available commercially, but are usually manufactured within hospital Medical Physics Departments.

Most commercially available enclosed test objects are filled with an aqueous gel material loaded with graphite particles designed to scatter ultrasound and produce an image with a speckle pattern similar to that produced by human tissue (e.g. liver). The typical characteristics of such "tissue-mimicking" materials are

- speed of sound = 1540 ± 10 m s^{-1} at 22°C,
- attenuation = 0.5–0.8 dB cm^{-1} MHz^{-1},
- scattering characteristics similar to tissue (produces similar speckle pattern).

In practice, such gels tend to dry out after a few years, potentially changing the relative positions of the targets and the speed of sound and attenuation. Also, the attenuation may not change with frequency as it does in real tissue, and the speed of sound may change with temperature. These properties should be specified in the user manual supplied with the device, and care should be taken to use the test object under the conditions advised by the manufacturer.

Polyurethane rubber materials have been used in some more recent commercial test objects. These materials are very stable and robust and do not need to be totally enclosed to reduce drying out. They can be made to have scattering properties similar to those of tissue, but have the significant disadvantage that the speed of sound is typically 6–7% lower than that in tissue. Manufacturers have attempted to correct for this discrepancy by reducing the vertical separation of targets within the test object by the same percentage, so that distance measurements in the vertical direction give the expected reading. Care must be taken in making measurements of the horizontal separation of targets, however, as it is not possible to make corrections that work for all scan formats (linear, sector and curvilinear) (Goldstein, 2000). Also focusing of the ultrasound beam is less effective leading to an apparent reduction in spatial resolution.

Performance testing of B-mode systems – How to do it?

Setting up

Measurement of the parameters listed above will be affected to some extent by the way that the imaging system and its display are set up. To obtain optimum and reproducible results, it is important to take a rational and consistent approach to system and monitor settings.

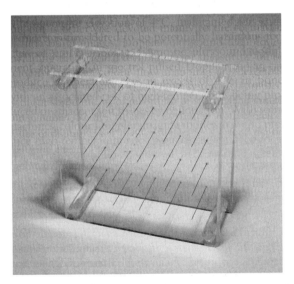

Fig. 12.1 An open-topped test object. The matrix of 0.5 mm diameter steel pins is mounted between two perspex plates using 25.0 mm spacing between pins.

The display monitor has two controls, which affect the grey-scale image, i.e. contrast and brightness (see Chapter 11). Contrast is effectively a gain control, which can be used to expand or reduce the range of grey levels in the displayed image. A low-contrast setting results' in a washed-out image, where there is little difference in displayed grey level between the brightest and darkest parts of the image. A high-contrast setting may result in saturation and loss of detail in the brightest part of the image, and the darkest parts being too dark to see. The brightness control is used to lift the overall brightness level up or down without affecting the range of levels used.

The range of grey levels visible on the display monitor is affected by the room lighting, which reflects from the screen. In bright room lighting, it is necessary to use a high monitor brightness setting to see the darkest parts of the image above the glare from the screen. This effectively reduces the range of grey levels that the observer can see. Subdued room lighting allows lower brightness settings to be used, extending the usable range of display brightness.

When testing a new imaging system or working in a new room, it is worth spending a little time optimising the room lighting conditions and display monitor settings. This should be done for a grey-scale image, which contains regions of low-level and high-level echoes. The aim is to adjust the controls, so that the darkest shades in the image are just discernible above the display background and the brightest levels appear almost at the peak white level of the display. The settings can then be recorded and used again when tests are repeated.

MACHINE SETTINGS

Ultrasound-imaging systems make internal adjustments to many system parameters, when a different application (e.g. abdominal, small parts) is selected. These changes may have a significant effect on imaging performance as measured with a tissue-mimicking test object. Also, transducers are often optimised for particular applications.

Hence, it is sensible to test abdominal transducers on a large test object with the system set to abdominal mode. Small parts test objects are available to test small parts transducers in small parts mode. The same combinations should be used, when the test is repeated as in consistency checks. Gain, time–gain compensation (TGC) and focusing may need to be optimised for individual tests, but in general are set to produce uniform mid-grey speckle throughout the image from a tissue-mimicking

test object. Again, reuse of the same conditions is necessary for consistency checks.

Resolution

The spatial resolution of an ultrasound-imaging system is defined most commonly in terms of its ability to display closely spaced targets as separate images (Chapter 5). Spatial resolution can be estimated in the scan plane using this approach for targets separated by a small distance along the beam axis (axial resolution) or at 90° to the beam axis (lateral resolution).

AXIAL RESOLUTION

Most commercial tissue-mimicking test objects contain sets of targets designed for the assessment of axial resolution. The most common arrangement is a set of five or six filaments, whose vertical separation reduces with depth from approximately 5 mm down to 1 mm as illustrated in Figure 12.2a. Note that the filaments do not form a vertical column, but each target is also offset in the lateral direction from the one above to avoid being shadowed by it.

With the scanning plane carefully aligned at 90° to the filaments and the system gain set to ensure that their images are not saturated, i.e. not at peak white, an image of the targets is obtained on the largest possible scale. The observer then decides which pair of targets is just resolved separately in the image and records their separation as the axial resolution. This method has the disadvantage that only a small range of discrete values of resolution can be reported.

An alternative approach to estimating axial resolution is to obtain an image of a single filament target and estimate its axial extent using the system callipers (Figure 12.2b). This is essentially a measurement of pulse length, but is closely related to the measurement from the first technique. This approach has the advantage that a continuous range of values can be reported. However, the measurements may be subject to poor repeatability, due to the difficulty in making a visual estimate of the extent of the image and the effects of image pixelation and minimum calliper increment (see Chapter 6). To minimise this variability, it is important to use the largest scale possible, when acquiring the image. Measurement accuracy can be improved further by viewing the stored image in zoom mode.

The length of an ultrasound pulse does not change significantly as it propagates into the tissue. However, some imaging systems may use the lower frequencies in the

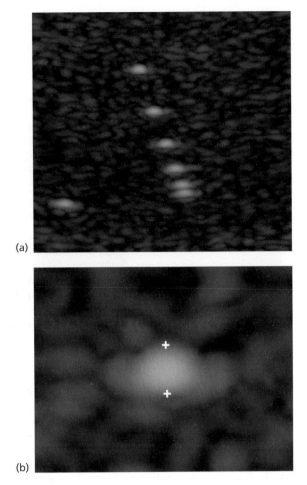

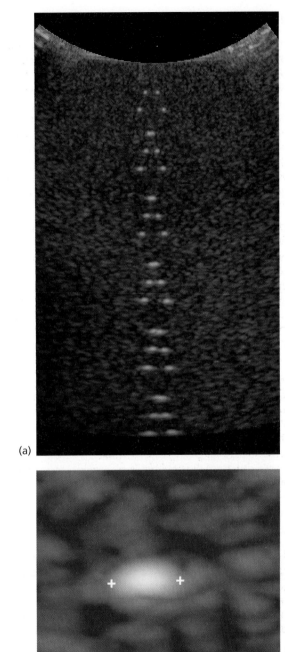

Fig. 12.2 (a) An image of axial resolution targets. The spacing of the filaments reduces from 5.0 to 1.0 mm and each is offset from that above to avoid shadowing. (b) Measurement of axial resolution. A single filament is imaged using a large-scale setting to minimise errors, when its axial extent is measured.

pulse or separate, lower-frequency pulses to image the deeper parts of the image, resulting in longer pulse lengths and poorer axial resolution in these areas. Hence, it may be useful to measure axial resolution at several depths.

LATERAL RESOLUTION

Lateral resolution may be estimated also by imaging groups of filament targets set at different spacings in the lateral direction or by measuring the lateral extent of the image of a single filament. Figure 12.3a shows an image using a particular test object (the Cardiff Resolution Test Object), where pairs of filaments are arranged in

Fig. 12.3 Measurement of lateral resolution using target pairs. (a) Pairs of targets are spaced at 1.25, 2.5 and 5 mm in each group. The smallest resolvable spacing is a measure of lateral resolution at the depth of each group. (b) The lateral extent of the target is measured using a large display scale to minimise errors.

groups with lateral spacings of 1.25, 2.5 and 5 mm. The pattern is repeated to allow estimation of lateral resolution at different depths. The image is inspected and a judgement made on whether two targets are separately resolved, i.e. whether there is a gap between them. If a pair separated by 2.5 mm is resolved, but a nearby pair with 1.25 mm spacing is not, then the resolution is quoted as being between 1.25 and 2.5 mm at that depth. The measurement using this test object is rapid but, as for axial resolution, suffers from the disadvantage that only a small number of discrete values of resolution can be reported.

The alternative approach of measuring the extent of the image of a single wire using the system callipers may be applied also in the lateral direction (Figure 12.3b) to give a continuous range of values. All the above methods for estimating resolution suffer from variability, due to the effects of image speckle.

In most imaging systems, lateral resolution changes significantly with depth due to the beam shape (Chapter 5), and is strongly affected by the setting of the focus control. A fixed focal depth, as may be used in a routine clinical examination, will not give the best available lateral resolution at all depths. It is suggested here that lateral resolution is measured at each available target depth with the focal setting, which gives the most optimistic answer at that depth. This approach is more likely to show any deterioration in performance on subsequent checks than a fixed focal setting for all depths.

SLICE THICKNESS

Several methods have been described for estimating slice thickness based on the assumption that targets set in a plane at 45° to the imaging plane will appear in the image with an axial or lateral extent, which is equal to the slice thickness. The most readily available method is that described by Skolnick (1991), which makes use of a vertical column of parallel filament targets as found in many test objects for assessing in-plane resolution and linear measurement accuracy. For in-plane resolution measurement, such line targets are aligned at 90° to the scan plane (Figure 12.4a). For slice thickness measurements, the scan plane is set at 45° to the line targets. Echoes are registered in the image for each beam pos-ition, where the sample volume overlaps part of the line target (Figure 12.4b). If the lateral extent of the sample volume in the scan plane is much less than its extent in the slice thickness direction, the lateral extent of the image is approximately the slice thickness. This method can be used to estimate slice thickness

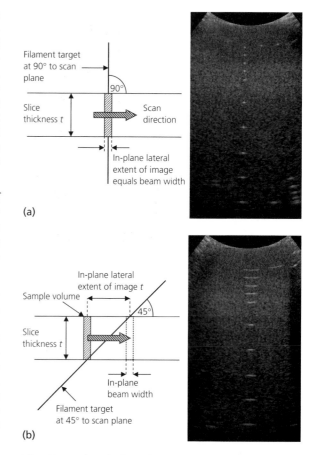

(a)

(b)

Fig. 12.4 Slice thickness by the Skolnick method. (a) The lateral extent of the filament targets indicates the in-plane beam width, when the scan plane is at 90° to the filament targets. (b) The lateral extent of the filament targets indicates the slice thickness, when the scan plane is rotated to 45° to the filaments. The slice thickness is small only in the out-of-plane focal region.

over a range of depths, but requires that the best available in-plane focusing be used at each depth. Figure 12.4b shows that the slice thickness is quite large near this transducer and reaches a focus at a distance of about 5 cm. This transducer would be poor at imaging small lesions, such as cysts within 3 cm of its surface.

An alternative method is available in the Cardiff Resolution Test Object, where groups of filament targets are set at known separations in planes at 45° to the vertical at different depths (Figure 12.5). The scan plane is aligned parallel to the filaments and the number of targets from each group, which appear simultaneously

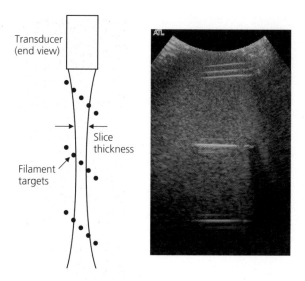

Fig. 12.5 The Cardiff scheme for estimation of slice thickness. The number of filaments imaged simultaneously in each group indicates the slice thickness at that depth.

in the image gives an indication of the slice thickness at that depth.

Penetration

As discussed in Chapter 4, echoes received from targets deep within the tissue are relatively small in amplitude, due to attenuation of the transmitted pulse and the returning echoes. TGC is applied to the echo signal to allow echoes from similar targets to be displayed with similar image brightness regardless of their depth. With increasing depth, however, the echo signal from typical scattering targets is reduced eventually to the level of electronic noise in the signal-processing circuits. Further amplification results in the display of random noise in these deeper parts of the image and no useful echo information. The maximum depth at which real ultrasonic echo information from small scattering targets can be identified in the image is referred to as the penetration depth. This depth is effectively an indication of the noise level in the system. A well-designed system with low noise will be able to display weaker echoes from greater depths. Penetration depth is affected strongly by system parameters, such as output power, transmit frequency and focal depth. Measurement of penetration depth is useful as a consistency check and a loss of penetration depth may indicate a fault in the transducer, transmit or receive beam formers or increased noise in the signal-processing circuits.

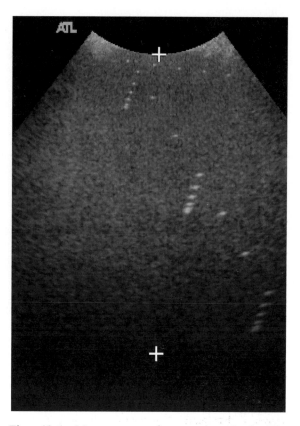

Fig. 12.6 Measurement of penetration depth. The observer judges the maximum depth at which ultrasonic information can be detected, as indicated by the caliper marker.

Penetration depth is normally measured by imaging the tissue-mimicking material within a test object and judging the maximum depth at which real echo information can be detected (Figure 12.6). This should be done on a real-time image rather than a frozen image to make it easy to distinguish the relatively constant ultrasonic speckle pattern from the constantly changing random electronic noise. The measurement is made normally with the system settings, which give the maximum value of penetration depth for a given transducer and frequency. This would normally include maximum transmit power and a deep focus setting. It is essential also to ensure effective acoustic coupling of the transducer to the test object by using lots of coupling gel or other coupling fluid. If ultrasonic speckle is identified to the bottom of the test object, a deeper test object should be used, if available or the output power may be reduced until a limit is achieved.

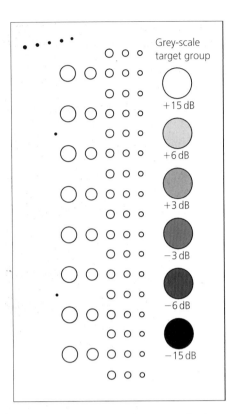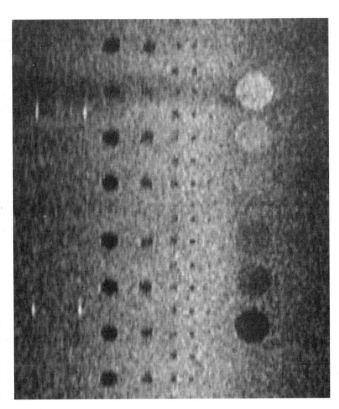

Fig. 12.7 A test object with regions of enhanced and reduced scattering strength. Dynamic range is estimated from the difference between the brightest and darkest regions, which can be imaged simultaneously. (By courtesy of ATS Laboratories Inc, Bridgeport, CT, USA.)

Dynamic range

The dynamic range of a system is the ratio of the largest signal, which can be processed to the smallest (usually the noise level). The ratio is usually expressed in decibels (see Appendix A). Within an ultrasonic image, these two levels are determined by the echo levels at the transducer, which result in peak white in the display and that which is just discernible above background noise or black level for particular settings of system controls. Dynamic range should be large enough to image echoes from strongly reflecting interfaces of interest without image saturation at the same time as echoes from weakly scattering tissues of interest (Chapter 4). The way in which the dynamic range of echoes at the transducer is related to the dynamic range of brightness levels on the display is controlled by system settings, such as dynamic range and compression controls and grey-scale curves used to enhance the image for different clinical applications.

The dynamic range of displayed echoes may be estimated using a tissue-mimicking test object, which includes regions with increased and reduced scattering strength in relation to the main body of tissue-mimicking material. Figure 12.7 shows an example of such a test object containing cylinders of material with scattering strengths ranging from −15 to +15 dB with respect to the background material. Dynamic range is estimated from the difference in scattering strengths in decibels between the area that just reaches saturation in the displayed image and that which is just detectable above background black level or noise. The values for scattering strength of the cylindrical inserts are valid only within the frequency range specified by the test object manufacturer.

Measurement accuracy

The most common measurements in ultrasound diagnosis are linear distance measurements, such as organ

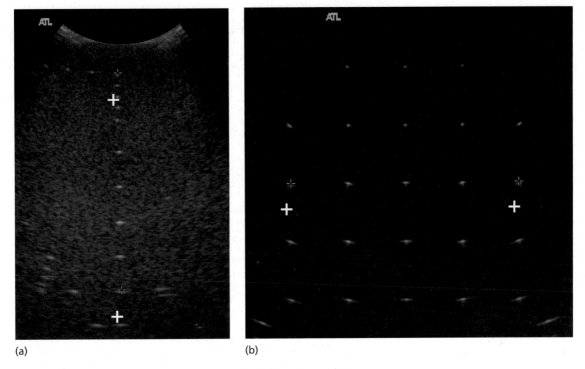

(a) (b)

Fig. 12.8 (a) Calibration of axial distance measurements. Target spacing is measured over a large axial distance to minimise positioning errors. (b) Calibration of lateral distance measurements using an open-topped test object. Caliper markers are placed at the centres of the target images. The focus is set to the depth of the measurement to minimise target width.

length or diameter. Perimeter and cross-sectional area measurements are also common in obstetric applications. Ultrasonic measurement systems are unlikely to change with normal use. However, careful checks of measurement accuracy are advised on new systems or following upgrades, particularly, for area and perimeter measurements, where accuracy may be affected by the choice of internal calculation method (Chapter 6). Regular checks of measurement accuracy ensure that where ultrasound measurements directly affect patient management, a loss of accuracy will affect a limited number of patients and may allow corrective action to be taken.

LINEAR DISTANCE MEASUREMENTS

It is usual to carry out accuracy checks of linear distance measurements in the axial direction and the lateral direction, even though most clinical measurements are not made along these axes. Axial measurement accuracy is determined by timing and scaling factors within the measurement system including the assumed speed of sound, whereas lateral measurement accuracy is affected by other geometrical factors. Hence, axial and lateral

checks may reveal different sources of error. Accuracy checks are carried out almost exclusively by imaging a set of targets of known separation within a test object containing a medium of known speed of sound. This is most commonly designed to be $1540 \, \mathrm{m \, s^{-1}}$, the value assumed by the ultrasound system. Measurements of target separation using on-screen callipers should agree with the specified separation of the targets.

AXIAL DISTANCE

To check the accuracy of measurements in the axial direction, a vertical column of filament targets of known separation is imaged. For sector and curvilinear probes, the column is aligned with the central beam and the scan plane aligned at 90° to the filaments to avoid any geometric errors. Checks are made on the frozen image by aligning the on-screen callipers with the leading edges of the most superficial and deepest targets available (Figure 12.8a). Use of the leading edge avoids ambiguity in target position due to reverberation within the target, and mimics the way that callipers should be used in clinical practice.

Using the most distant targets available ensures that any errors in placing the marker on the image are minimised in relation to the distance measured. Agreement to within 1% is expected normally. Errors which exceed 2% should be investigated.

LATERAL DISTANCE

Lateral (horizontal) calliper checks require targets positioned with known separation at the same depth. The callipers in this orientation are aligned with the centres of the displayed echo (Figure 12.8b). This is facilitated by selecting the focal zone, which minimises the lateral extent of the images of the filament targets. As for axial measurements, alignment of the scan plane at 90° to the line targets and selection of the largest target separation helps to minimise errors. Measurement values within 2% of the expected values can normally be achieved. Discrepancies greater than 4% should be investigated.

PERIMETER AND AREA

Test objects designed specifically for checking accuracy of perimeter and area measurements are not widely available from commercial sources. Limited checks on these measurements can be made using test objects designed for axial and lateral measurements by drawing around a 2 dimensional shape formed from targets in the axial and lateral directions. More accurate assessments require specially designed arrays of targets as described in more detail in Chapter 6.

Testing of spectral Doppler and colour flow systems

Virtually, all testing of ultrasound systems performed in hospitals covers only B-mode imaging. In clinical use, Doppler ultrasound is also important yet, at the time of writing, this aspect of machine performance is not usually tested in hospitals. This section describes relevant guidance and standards, the design of test objects for Doppler ultrasound, and some quantities, which can be measured. A review of Doppler testing is given in Hoskins and Ramnarine (2000).

Standards and guidance

Both the IPEM and AIUM have produced documents, which describe in detail the design and use of test objects (Hoskins *et al.*, 1994; AIUM, 1993). IEC standards have been produced for fetal Doppler (IEC 61266) and for CW Doppler (61206); however, both are out of date and currently being revised.

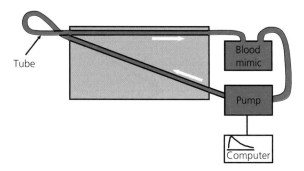

Fig. 12.9 Components of a flow phantom. These are the tissue mimic, tube and blood mimics. The pump may be controlled using a computer to obtain physiological flow waveforms.

Test objects for Doppler ultrasound

The design of test objects suitable for Doppler is more difficult than for B-mode imaging as the Doppler test object must include a moving target to simulate the moving blood. There are two types of moving-target test object, which are available commercially; the string phantom and the flow phantom.

FLOW PHANTOM

This device simulates flow of blood within a vessel. The components of the flow phantom are illustrated in Figure 12.9. The main design criterion is that the acoustic properties of the tissue mimic, the blood mimic and the vessel must be matched to those of human tissue. The tissue mimic is usually a gel-based material, as described above. The blood mimic must have the correct viscosity, as well as correct acoustic properties. A suitable blood mimic has been described by Ramnarine *et al.* (1998), which is based on the use of nylon particles suspended in a solution of glycerol and dextran. Matching the acoustic properties of the artery is much more difficult. Rubber-based materials, such as latex, have the correct acoustic velocity, but the attenuation is high. This mismatch of acoustic properties results in distortions in the shape of the Doppler spectrum obtained from flow within the tube. This is mainly important when flow phantoms are used for calibration of quantities involving the mean frequency, such as volumetric flow. In this case, the mean frequency in the flow phantom is overestimated as a result of the spectral distortion. Unfortunately, all commercial-based flow test objects are based on the use of tubes of latex or similar material, and the calibration of volumetric flow using these devices is, therefore, unreliable. A "wall-less" approach in which the

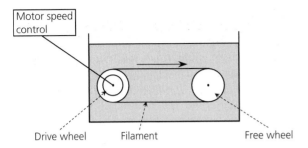

Fig. 12.10 Components of a string phantom. The string is driven in a circuit by a drive wheel. The speed of the drive wheel may be controlled using an external computer to produce waveforms with a physiological appearance.

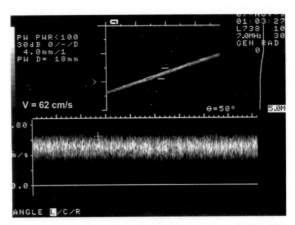

Fig. 12.11 Ultrasound imaging of a string phantom for checking of Doppler velocity estimation. The angle cursor is aligned with the string. The maximum velocity is measured using the manual cursor.

tissue mimic is in direct contact with the blood mimic is the ideal arrangement. The most stable of wall-less test objects uses polyurethane as the tissue mimic; however, this approach is unreliable as the acoustic velocity is not correctly matched to tissue as noted above. In research laboratories, flow phantoms can be designed, which are correctly matched to human tissue (Hoskins and Ramnarine, 2000; Ramnarine, 2001).

STRING PHANTOM

In this device, the moving string simulates moving blood. The components of the string phantom are illustrated in Figure 12.10. Choice of the string is important as the scattering characteristics of blood need to be matched. Filaments, such as cotton and silk, are spiral-wound, with a repeat pattern at distances that are comparable with the wavelength of ultrasound. This repeat pattern gives rise to high-amplitude scattering along certain directions, which distorts the Doppler spectrum making this type of filament unsuitable Cathignol, 1994). The use of commercial systems based on the use of spiral-wound filaments is not advised. A suitable filament is O-ring rubber, as this scatters ultrasound in all directions in a similar manner to blood (Hoskins, 1994). The most important feature of the string phantom is that the velocity can be accurately measured. The true string velocity may be calculated from the speed of rotation of the drive wheel. This makes this device especially suited to the checking of velocity estimates made using Doppler.

Quantities of interest

There are three main classes of quantity that are of interest: velocity, sensitivity and resolution. The use of test objects to measure these quantities is described below.

VELOCITY

The estimation and display of blood velocity is the key task of Doppler systems; hence, it is appropriate to test the accuracy of this quantity. Maximum velocity is used clinically in estimation of the degree of stenosis in arterial disease. Velocity measurements may be checked using a string phantom (Figure 12.11). The string is set at a constant velocity. The spectral Doppler sample volume is positioned at the level of the moving string using the B-mode image to guide placement. Spectral Doppler data is acquired, and maximum velocity estimated using the manual measurement cursor. The string velocity is then compared to that estimated using spectral Doppler. In general, modern commercial systems overestimate maximum velocity, as explained in Chapter 9.

SENSITIVITY

The acquisition of noise-free Doppler signals from vessels which are deep, or which are small, is a key task determining Doppler performance. This task is dependent on the strength of the Doppler signal from blood, compared to the clutter signal from the tissue and the strength of the electronic noise. The flow phantom is a suitable test object to assess penetration depth. The flow phantom design should include a vessel, which is angled at 30–45° with respect to the surface. The penetration depth is the maximum depth from which spectral Doppler or colour flow signals can be obtained (Figure 12.12).

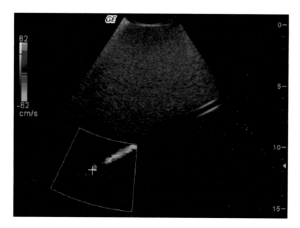

Fig. 12.12 Penetration depth measurement. The depth is measured at which the colour flow can no longer be distinguished.

RESOLUTION

The measurement of both spatial and temporal resolution is relevant for Doppler systems. Spatial resolution in the context of colour flow refers to the ability of the system to distinguish adjacent regions of blood moving at different velocities or in different directions. Temporal resolution refers to the ability of the system to distinguish rapidly changing flow patterns at a single location. These are important aspects of performance; however, procedures for measuring these quantities have not been adequately developed at the time of writing.

References

AIUM. *Performance Criteria and Measurements for Doppler Ultrasound Devices.* Laurel, MD, American Institute of Ultrasound in Medicine. 1993.

BS 5724 Section 3.26. *Method for Declaring Parameters for Ultrasonic Diagnostic Equipment Using Test Objects.*

IEC 61390. *Ultrasonics. Real-Time Pulse–Echo Systems. Guide for Test Procedures to Determine Performance Specifications.* 1996.

IEC 61206. *Ultrasonics – Continuous-Wave Doppler Systems – Test Procedures.* 1993.

IEC 61266. *Ultrasonics – Hand-Held Probe Doppler Foetal Heartbeat Detectors – Performance Requirements and Methods of Measurement and Reporting.* 1995.

Cathignol D, Dickerson K, Newhouse VL, Faure P and Chaperon JY. On the spectral properties of Doppler thread phantoms. *Ultrasound Med. Biol.* 1994; **20**: 601–610.

Goldstein A. The effect of acoustic velocity on phantom measurements. *Ultrasound Med. Biol.* 2000; **26**: 1133–1143.

Goodsitt *et al.* Real-time B-mode ultrasound quality control test procedures. Report of AAPM Ultrasound Task Group No.1. *Med. Phys.* 1998; **25**: 1385–1406.

Hoskins PR. Choice of moving target for a string phantom. I. Backscattered power characteristics. *Ultrasound Med. Biol.* 1994; **20**: 773–780.

Hoskins PR and Ramnarine KV. Doppler test devices. In: DH Evans and WN McDicken (Eds) *Doppler Ultrasound*, 2nd edition. Wiley. 2000, 382–404.

Hoskins PR, Sherriff SB and Evans JA (Ed). *Testing of Doppler Ultrasound Equipment.* Institute of Physical Sciences in Medicine. 1994.

Martin K and Spinks D. Measurement of the speed of sound in ethanol/water mixtures. *Ultrasound Med. Biol.* 2001; **27**: 289–291.

Medical Devices Directive, 93/42/EEC. *Official Journal EC.* 1993; **36**: L169.

Price R (Ed.). *Routine Quality Assurance of Ultrasound Imaging Systems.* Institute of Physical Sciences in Medicine. 1995.

Ramnarine KV, Nassiri DK, Hoskins PR and Lubbers J. Validation of a new blood mimicking fluid for use in Doppler flow test objects. *Ultrasound Med. Biol.* 1998; **24**: 24, 451–459.

Ramnarine KV, Anderson T and Hoskins PR. Construction and geometric stability of physiological flow rate wall-less stenosis phantoms. *Ultrasound Med. Biol.* 2001; **32**: 245–250.

Skolnick ML. Estimation of ultrasound beam width in the elevation (section thickness) plane. *Radiology* 1991; **180**: 286–288.

13

SAFETY OF DIAGNOSTIC ULTRASOUND

FA Duck and A Shaw

Introduction: risk and hazard

What does ultrasound exposure mean?

What happens to tissue exposed to ultrasound, and does it matter?

How is safety managed?

Safety for specific uses of diagnostic ultrasound

Summary and conclusions

Introduction: risk and hazard

The words "risk" and "hazard" are emotive terms when used commonly. They are sometimes used to imply that an action should be avoided so as to ensure that there are no risks involved. Strictly, hazard describes the nature of the threat (e.g. burning, falling) while the associated risk takes into account the potential consequences of the hazard (e.g. death, injury) and the probability of occurrence. Ultrasound scanning is potentially hazardous, but the real questions are

1. is there any risk for the patient and

2. if so, what is the correct way to manage this risk?

The purpose of this chapter is to explain the scientific basis informing the responses to these safety questions, and to describe the ways by which the enviable safety record of diagnostic ultrasound may be maintained.

Whenever an ultrasound scan is carried out, some part of the patient is exposed to an external influence – the ultrasound beam. As it travels through the body, the ultrasound beam interacts with the tissue in ways giving a lasting biological effect, if the exposure is sustained and of sufficient strength. For instance, it is well known that elevated temperature affects normal cell function and that the risk associated with this particular hazard is dependent on the degree of elevation, the duration for which the elevation is maintained and the nature of the exposed tissue. During every scan with every transducer, some of the ultrasound energy is converted to heat and causes temperature elevation; the ultrasound is, therefore, a source of thermal hazard. The degree of elevation (i.e. the severity of the hazard) will vary throughout the region of the scan and will depend on many properties of the ultrasound field and the exposed tissues. If the maximum temperature increase within the exposed region lies within the range normally occurring in tissue, the hazard may be considered to be small, and so may the risk to the patient. If the maximum temperature increase is outside of the normal range, factors such as the duration of the elevation and the sensitivity of the tissue to damage must be borne in mind when assessing risk.

A second hazard arises from the presence of gas within soft tissues. Gas may occur naturally, for instance air in the alveoli of lungs or gas in the intestines. Alternatively, gas bubbles may be introduced deliberately in the form of gas-contrast agents. When such "gas bodies" are exposed to ultrasound they can give rise to a variety of local mechanical effects which can cause damage to cells or tissue structures. The oscillation of the gas surface, which causes the mechanical effects, is termed "acoustic cavitation" for a free bubble, or "gas-body activation" for the more general case. In these cases, the hazard, a bubble which is caused to oscillate by the ultrasonic wave, gives a risk of tissue damage which will vary depending on the size of the oscillation, where the bubble is, and what cellular changes result.

The prudent sonographer, therefore, should consider the safety aspects of each examination, and undertake it only if the benefits to the patient from the expected diagnostic information outweigh the risks. This chapter aims to provide the sonographer with the information needed to assess the risks associated with ultrasound examinations. It first reviews how ultrasound output and exposure are related to hazard and risk. Thermal and mechanical processes and effects are then reviewed, leading to a discussion of the safety indices now presented on scanners to assist users in making risk–benefit judgements. A brief review of epidemiological evidence is given. The partnership between manufacturers and users in managing safety is reviewed, including an overview of standards and regulations. Finally, situations giving rise to specific safety issues are discussed.

Those wishing to gain further background knowledge or explore the topics in greater depth are recommended to refer to other recent texts on ultrasound safety (Barnett and Kossoff, 1998; ter Haar and Duck, 2000). Succinct tutorials on a number of safety topics have also been prepared by the European Committee for Medical Ultrasound Safety (ECMUS) on behalf of the European Federation for Societies of Ultrasound in Medicine and Biology (EFSUMB), and are freely available on the EFSUMB web site (www.efsumb.org/ecmus.htm).

What does ultrasound exposure mean?

During an ultrasound scan, the imaged tissues are exposed to ultrasound beams and pulses (the ultrasound field) used to acquire the image or Doppler waveform. To measure the ultrasound exposure of the tissue, it is necessary to characterise the ultrasound field in terms of a number of standard parameters. We have seen in Chapter 2 that the ultrasound is a longitudinal pressure wave and so, as the ultrasound wave passes a particular point, the pressure at that point will increase and decrease in a cyclic manner. Figure 13.1 shows a representation of the acoustic pressure variation with time for a typical pulsed Doppler ultrasound pulse near to the focus. The very rapid change from negative to positive pressure and the larger positive than negative pressure is normal for these pulses. There are many different properties that can be measured. The main parameters used to describe output and how they are measured are described in Appendix 13C.

From a safety perspective, we want to know what is happening inside the exposed tissue. Obviously, this is not an easy thing to do, so, instead of using tissue, measurements are made in a substitute medium, which is well characterised and reproducible; and the medium, which is currently chosen, is water.

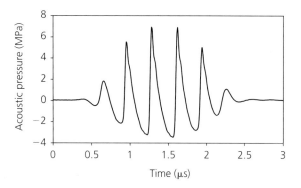

Fig. 13.1 Variation of acoustic pressure with time in a pulsed Doppler ultrasound pulse near the focus.

Seventy per cent of most soft tissues is water and, in many ways, ultrasound travels through water in a similar way to how it travels through soft tissue. The main difference is that water absorbs very little ultrasound compared to tissue and so the measured values in water are higher than would be expected in tissue. Measurements made in water are called acoustic output measurements (or, more correctly, "free-field acoustic output measurements"). Using this term allows the concept of "exposure measurements" and "exposure parameters" to be reserved for what happens in tissue rather than what happens in a tank of water.

Very often this important distinction is not properly made when values are reported. Whatever names are attached to them, it is almost certain that any values for acoustic output and exposure parameters you see have come from measurements made in water. Estimates of exposure levels in tissue made from these, usually referred to as "estimated *in situ* values", are usually approximations derived from very simple models of tissue properties and structure.

The relationship between risk, hazard, exposure and acoustic output is outlined in Figure 13.2. It can be seen that as we move from actual measurements of acoustic output parameters in water to estimates of exposure, hazard and risk, our assessments become less and less certain.

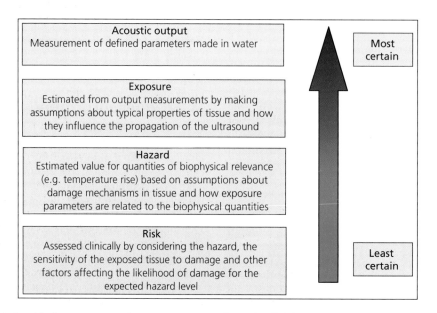

Fig. 13.2 Relationship between acoustic output, exposure, hazard and risk.

What happens to tissue exposed to ultrasound, and does it matter?

Thermal effects

When an ultrasound pulse travels through tissue, some of the energy in the pulse is absorbed by the tissue and is converted to heat, which in turn produces a temperature rise. In most soft tissues, the rate at which energy is absorbed per unit volume, q_v, depends on the amplitude absorption coefficient, α_0, of the tissue, the acoustic frequency, f, of the pulse and the intensity, I:

$$q_v = 2\alpha_0 f I. \qquad (13.1)$$

The factor 2 arises because the intensity absorption coefficient is twice the amplitude absorption coefficient. Since the intensity varies throughout the field, the rate of energy absorption and the temperature rise also vary. To discuss the effects on tissue temperature in more detail, it is easiest to consider a fixed beam mode, such as a pulsed Doppler beam interacting with soft tissue, in which the temperature is initially uniform. When the field is first applied, energy will be absorbed at a rate proportional to the local intensity, which means that the temperature will increase fastest at the focus. As time goes on, the temperature will continue to increase as more energy is absorbed, but the regions where the increase has been greatest (e.g. at the focus), will start to lose some of their heat by conduction to neighbouring cooler regions, and so the rate of increase will begin to slow. Commonly, the rate of heat loss by conduction will nearly cancel out the rate of energy absorption after approximately 30 s and so the temperature at the focus approaches its equilibrium value very rapidly. In wider regions of the beam, where the initial temperature increase was more uniform, such as near the transducer, very little heat will be lost by conduction and so the temperature will continue to increase at its initial rate. A second effect also becomes significant: as it generates ultrasound, the transducer itself begins to heat up. This heat conducts into the tissue enhancing the temperature rise near the transducer. In many cases, after several minutes of exposure, the temperature near the transducer may significantly exceed the focal temperature. Where the beam is broader, conductive losses will be smaller and perfusion becomes more important, particularly close to large blood vessels.

The presence of bone in the field will increase the temperature rise. Bone strongly absorbs ultrasound at all frequencies and so the ultrasound energy is almost completely absorbed in a very small volume and the temperature increases rapidly. Because the absorption takes place in a small region, the temperature gradients and also the conductive heat losses will become large. This means that the temperature will quickly approach its final value. The large conductive heat losses also dominate the perfusion losses so the presence of blood flow is unlikely to significantly reduce the temperature.

It is, sometimes, argued that you would have to hold the transducer stationary for hours to get any significant temperature rise and that, anyway, blood flow takes all the heat away. This argument is misleading. Most of the temperature increase occurs within the first minute and it is certainly not safe to assume that blood flow will limit the temperature rise to levels which pose no risk.

TEMPERATURE PREDICTIONS

In principle, it is possible to predict the temperature distribution using theoretical models, if enough is known about the *in situ* intensity distribution and the properties of the tissue. In practice, accurate predictions are difficult since the *in situ* intensity can only be approximated from acoustic output measurements and because of lack of knowledge about the properties of living tissue. Values reported in the literature show large variations. This means that all estimates of temperature rise in tissue are uncertain. Consequently, alternative approaches have been developed such as the use of tissue-mimicking phantoms to make measurements of temperature rise and simplified, approximate methods of estimating the maximum temperature increase, e.g. thermal indices (TIs).

TEMPERATURE MEASUREMENT

Ideally, of course, it would be possible to measure the temperature rise in the patient during the ultrasound examination. Unfortunately, with current technology, this is not yet possible. However, it is possible to measure the temperature rise in a tissue-mimicking phantom, also called a Thermal Test Object or TTO (Shaw *et al.*, 1999). Figure 13.3 shows a schematic diagram of one of these TTOs. This is a much more direct way of evaluating the heating potential of ultrasound scanners which automatically caters for most of the complexities which are ignored by other methods. Although still at the experimental stage, studies using TTOs have provided important results (e.g. Shaw *et al.*, 1998; which is discussed later) and it is likely that direct measurement of temperature rise in phantom materials will become more widespread over the next few years. This will

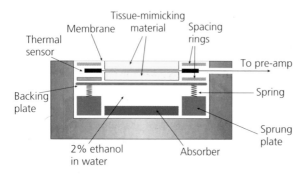

Fig. 13.3 Schematic diagram of a TTO. The temperature rise in the middle tissue-mimicking material is measured with a small thermocouple of less than 0.5 mm in diameter.

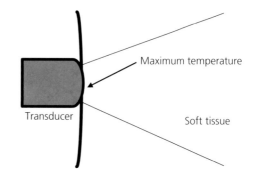

Fig. 13.4 Diagram showing conditions for TIS for scanning (these conditions are also assumed to apply for the calculation of TIB for scanning).

undoubtedly allow the relationship between ultrasound exposure and biological hazard to be put on a much firmer foundation than it is currently.

THERMAL INDICES

Since it is impossible for the user to know how much temperature increase is occurring in the body, the idea of the TI was developed to provide some guidance. A TI is a rough estimate of the increase in temperature that occurs in the region of the ultrasound scan. A TI of 2.0 means that you can expect a temperature rise of about 2°C. TI values can provide extra information to help weigh-up the risks and benefits to an "average" patient as the examination progresses. They are not supposed to apply to any particular patient and other factors such as the physical state of the patient must be considered when making a risk assessment.

The TI itself has a very simple definition. It is the ratio between two powers. The first is the power exposing the tissue during use, W. The second is the power, W_{deg} required to cause a maximum temperature increase of 1°C anywhere in the beam, with identical scanner operating conditions. This temperature is that reached with the beam held stationary under "reasonable worst-case conditions" allowing thermal equilibrium to be achieved, and is intended to be a temperature which could be approached but never exceeded *in vivo*.

The difficulty with calculating the TI lies mostly in the estimation of W_{deg}, the power giving a worst-case 1°C rise. In order to simplify the problem, three tissue models have been chosen to distinguish three applications. They give rise to three TIs: the Soft-tissue Thermal Index (TIS); the Bone-at-focus Thermal Index (TIB); and the Cranial (or Bone-at-Surface) Thermal Index

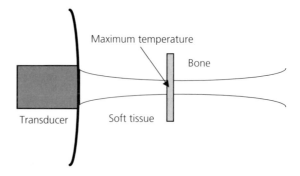

Fig. 13.5 Diagram showing the conditions for TIB.

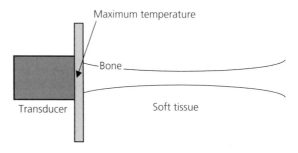

Fig. 13.6 Diagram showing the conditions for the TIC.

(TIC). Figures 13.4–13.6 show these three conditions. The tissue models are based on simple assumptions about the acoustic and thermal properties of tissue, including the assumption that the tissue attenuation coefficient is uniformly $0.3\,\text{dB}\,\text{cm}^{-1}\,\text{MHz}^{-1}$. For bone, a fixed proportion of the incident power is assumed to be absorbed in the bone layer. Clearly, from the basic definition of TI, all the three TI values depend linearly on the acoustic power emitted by the transducer. If the machine controls are altered in such a way as to double the power output, the TI displayed will increase by a factor of 2.

In addition to the dependence on power, one of the TIs, that for soft tissue (TIS) also depends on the frequency of operation of the transducer. This is because the absorption coefficient of soft tissue depends on frequency, and hence so does the heating (see Equation (13.1)).

A practical feature of the models is the prediction of where the greatest heating occurs. For a stationary beam (such as in pulsed Doppler or M-mode) the greatest heating for bone (TIB) is at the focus (see Figure 13.5). On the other hand, for scanned transducers it is predicted that the greatest heating will always be at the surface (see Figure 13.4), and the calculation is for this and not the temperature which may be found elsewhere within the imaged organ.

Until better methods are developed, these TI values are more helpful than any other information you are likely to see and you should take note of the values when you can. However, do not be misled by the apparent precision of the value on the screen. The methods for calculating TI ignore several important complications, such as transducer self-heating and the simplicity of the models, and the true temperature rise may be a factor of two (or sometimes more), higher or lower than the number indicated.

On current generation equipment, TI values can usually be found around the edge of the scanner screen – often in the top right corner – indicated by the letters TIS, TIB or TIC followed by a number which changes when the scanner controls are altered. The mechanical index (MI) is displayed similarly (see below). If the scanner was bought before about 1996, it will probably not display the index values (unless the firmware has been upgraded more recently). If they are not visible, it may be necessary to turn on the display of these values. Check the manual or ask your supplier how to do this. Smaller, portable or low-output equipment will often not display TI or MI. The same applies to older equipment. Again, check the manual or ask your supplier if you are not sure.

Although they do provide useful information to the user, the regulatory reason behind displaying TI (and MI) values is so that the manufacturer can meet certain requirements imposed by the Food and Drugs Administration (FDA) for selling in the USA. Following this route allows

the manufacturer to generate higher-output levels than was allowed previously for most types of examination, including obstetric.

DOES TEMPERATURE RISE MATTER?

What are the risks or benefits associated with an increased temperature? According to Miller and Ziskin (1989), the range of "normal" core temperatures is approximately 36–38°C in man, and a temperature of 42°C is "largely incompatible with life". To maintain life requires the careful balance of many chemical processes. Changing cellular temperature not only changes the rate at which these reactions take place, it also affects the equilibrium position between the competing reactions. A further complication is the denaturing of enzymes and other large molecules: this becomes particularly important above 45°C.

Clearly it is undesirable to elevate the whole body above its natural temperature, but during an ultrasound examination only a small volume of tissue is exposed. Does it matter if this is affected? Generally, the human body is quite capable of recovering from such an event. There are, however, several regions that would not tolerate it so well, namely the reproductive cells, the unborn fetus and the central nervous system (brain and spinal cord). In view of the large number of obstetric examinations carried out, damage to the fetus is, particularly, a sensitive issue.

There is growing evidence that clinical ultrasound scanners operating towards the top end of their power range are capable of producing temperature rises above the World Federation for Ultrasound in Medicine and Biology (WFUMB) recommendations. One study carried out at the National Physical Laboratory for the UK Department of Health (Shaw *et al.*, 1998) measured, amongst other things, the temperature rise produced in tissue-mimicking phantoms by a range of clinical pulsed Doppler ultrasound systems. The front panel controls of the systems were adjusted to produce the maximum spatial-peak temporal-average intensity and the temperature rise produced in these phantoms was then measured at different positions in the ultrasound field.

From the 21 Doppler and two other fields studied, it appeared unlikely that a temperature rise above 1.5°C would occur in soft tissue in the absence of bone or other strongly absorbing material. The exceptions might be for exposure of the first-trimester fetus through the full bladder, when a temperature rise up to 3°C was considered possible, or the use of intra-cavity probes, where prolonged exposure may result in higher temperature rises within 1 cm of the transducer face. However, when the ultrasound beam impinges on bone or other strongly absorbing material (even if that material is not the subject of the examination), the temperature rise may be much higher. Seventy-five per cent of the systems studied produced a temperature rise in a bone mimic of between 1.5°C and 4°C with even higher temperatures considered possible, if these same fields were used for examinations through the full bladder, for instance for the third-trimester fetus. Although it is important to remember that the exact study conditions are unlikely to be replicated in most examinations, under the modelled conditions 50% of the systems gave temperature rises in excess of 4°C and 15% in excess of 8°C.

Non-thermal mechanisms and effects

Ultrasound is a mechanical vibration. It follows that biological responses may arise directly from mechanical disturbances of the tissue structure, rather than indirectly from heating as described above. In past discussions, two main categories of non-thermal effects have been identified which have been referred to as "cavitation effects" and "non-thermal, non-cavitation effects". While this general division remains valuable, it will be seen from the following that a clearer division is between those effects which are mediated by the presence of gas in the tissue and those which arise in the absence of gas. The first includes a number of effects which should not strictly be called "cavitation" and have been referred to as "gas-body activation".

CAVITATION AND OTHER GAS-BODY MECHANISMS

Acoustic cavitation refers to the response of gas bubbles in a liquid under the influence of an acoustic (ultrasonic) wave. It is a phenomenon of considerable complexity (Leighton, 1994; 1998), and for this reason it is common to simplify its description into two categories. Stable, or non-inertial cavitation refers to a pulsating or "breathing" motion of a bubble whose diameter follows the pressure variation in the ultrasonic wave. During the compression in the wave the bubble contracts in size, expanding again as the rarefaction phase in the wave passes. Over time, the bubble may grow by a process of "rectified diffusion", or it may contract and dissolve back into the liquid. Cavitation only occurs if there exist suitable cavitation nuclei which serve to seed the cavitation process. These nuclei are typically micro-bubbles or solid particles in suspension or bubbles trapped in crevices at a solid surface. For safety discussions, the most important sources of cavitation nuclei are those introduced *in vivo*

in the form of contrast materials, and these are discussed below.

Bubbles have a resonant frequency, f_r, depending on their radius, R_0, which, for a spherical air bubble in water, is given by:

$$f_r R_0 \approx 3\,\text{Hz}\,\text{m}. \qquad (13.2)$$

This expression is a reasonable approximation for bubble radii greater than $10\,\mu\text{m}$, but also suggests that typical diagnostic frequencies cause resonance in bubbles with radii of the order of $1\,\mu\text{m}$.

Of course the existence of an oscillating bubble (i.e. a hazard) does not automatically result in a risk. It is necessary to relate its behaviour with something which could be potentially damaging. When a suspension of cells is exposed to ultrasound, stable cavitation occurs and shear stresses can rupture the cell membranes. Shear is a tearing force, and many biological structures are much more easily damaged by tearing than by compression or tension. Destruction of blood cells in suspension by ultrasound may occur in this way, and this has been shown *in vitro* for erythrocytes, leucocytes and platelets. In addition, the existence of a second effect, not causing cell destruction, may occur. Gaps can open transiently in the cell membrane during ultrasound exposure, an effect known as sonoporation, allowing the passage of larger biomolecules such as DNA.

The second class of cavitation activity has been termed inertial cavitation. It is more violent and potentially more destructive than stable cavitation, occurs at higher pressures, and can be generated by short ultrasound pulses. The bubble undergoes very large size variations, and may violently collapse under the inertia of the surrounding liquid (hence the term "inertial cavitation"). As with stable cavitation, local shear stresses are generated which may cause lysis of adjacent cells. Acoustic shocks are generated which can propagate stress waves outwards. In addition, enormously high, localised pressures and temperatures are predicted to occur, and the energy densities are sufficient to cause free-radical (H• and OH•) generation local to the collapsing bubble.

While bubbles may undergo stable (and non-harmful) oscillations in ultrasound beams at very low pressures, the onset of inertial cavitation only occurs above a threshold for acoustic pressure. An analysis by Apfel and Holland (1991) quantified this threshold, assuming that a full range of bubble sizes were present to provide nucleation centres. This resulted in the formulation of a mechanical index (MI), which was intended to quantify the likelihood of onset of inertial cavitation:

$$MI = \frac{p_r}{\sqrt{f}}, \qquad (13.3)$$

where p_r is the peak rarefaction pressure *in situ* (see Appendix 13C), and f is the ultrasound frequency. For $MI < 0.7$, the physical conditions probably cannot exist to support bubble growth and collapse. Exceeding this threshold does not, however, mean there will automatically be a mechanical bioeffect caused by cavitation.

The destructive outcome of cavitation on cells in culture is well documented. *In vivo*, there is evidence for acoustic cavitation when using extracorporeal lithotripsy. However, there is no evidence at present that diagnostic pulses generally cause cavitation within soft tissues. There are only two specific conditions when the presence of gas *in vivo* can alter this. These are with the use of contrast materials and for the exposure of soft tissues in the presence of gas bodies, such as in the lung and in the intestine.

Contrast materials

Much of the previous discussion would appear to be of direct relevance to the use of contrast materials. When injected into the bloodstream, ultrasound-contrast agents introduce a plentiful supply of cavitation nuclei, which in principle could result in the generation of free radicals, cell lysis, or sonoporation as described above. Extrapolation from studies carried out *in vitro* to what may happen *in vivo* is, however, notoriously difficult. For example, free-radical scavengers in blood strongly limit the lifetime of any radicals generated in vivo, and hence the potential for damage. Most contrast agents break up when they are exposed to ultrasound. Nevertheless, there is good evidence that bubble fragments continue to circulate for a considerable time after the initial disintegration. For this reason, it is considered unwise to use contrast materials during lithotripsy and at any time during the preceeding day in order to minimise the chance of the contrast fragments acting as cavitation nuclei in the lithotripsy field. More seriously, recent evidence suggests that micro-vascular damage may often result from exposure of gas-filled contrast agents *in vivo* to pulsed ultrasound at *in situ* rarefaction pressures of less than 1 MPa, well within the diagnostic range (Skyba *et al.*, 1998). The establishment of safety criteria for the use of contrast agents is becoming a high priority in international safety discussions.

Lung capillary haemorrhage

Exposure of the pleural surface of lungs to diagnostic levels of ultrasound has been consistently shown to cause alveolar capillary bleeding. This has been observed in experiments on a variety of small mammals. Pressure thresholds for damage in small animals are about 1 MPa, which is well within the diagnostic range. Exactly the mechanism responsible is unclear. Similar small haemorrhages (petechiae) have also been observed in the exposed intestines of small animals, and related to the presence of intestinal gas. Whatever the cause, diagnostic pulse amplitudes can cause damage when fragile tissue structures are exposed to pulsed ultrasound while being adjacent to gas bodies.

Lung and intestinal haemorrhage from ultrasound exposure has never been observed in humans. It has been suggested that the lungs of smaller animals are more susceptible to this form of damage than those of larger mammals where the pleural layers and perhaps the alveolar membranes are thicker and stronger. If so, the relevance of these animal studies to clinical scanning may be restricted to studies in neonates, particularly cardiac examinations. Even so such alveolar haemorrhages would, generally, be almost without clinical importance, provided they were limited in extent.

Epidemiological evidence for hazard

Epidemiology is concerned with the patterns of occurrence of disease in human populations and of the factors influencing these patterns. Epidemiological methods have also been used to search for risks associated with any external agents, such as diagnostic ultrasound, and to look for associations between exposure and unwanted outcome. There have been a number of studies to investigate the possible association between exposure to ultrasound *in utero*, and childhood maldevelopment.

This section summarises briefly the outcome of the more important epidemiological studies into ultrasound exposure *in utero*. Fuller reviews may be found elsewhere (Ziskin and Petitti, 1988; EFSUMB, 1996), in which the details of the literature may be found.

Birth weight

The outcome of a review of available data on birth weight suggests that on average, those children exposed to ultrasound imaging were heavier than those not exposed. Conversely, a non-significant reduction in birth weight was noticed within a large randomised controlled trial using CW Doppler examinations. Subsequent studies have been unable to demonstrate an association between exposure and birth weight or subsequent growth. In view of the conflicting evidence presented by these studies, it is presently concluded that there is no evidence to suggest an association between exposure to ultrasound and birth weight.

CHILDHOOD MALIGNANCIES

There have been three well-managed case–control studies into ultrasound and childhood malignancies, all of which were of sufficient size to have statistical validity. No association with childhood malignancy was found in any study.

NEUROLOGICAL DEVELOPMENT

A range of neurological functions has been examined and no association between ultrasound exposure *in utero* and subsequent hearing, visual acuity, cognitive function or behaviour has been found. An association with dyslexia reported earlier was not found in later larger studies. Further studies have suggested a possible association between ultrasound exposure and handedness, with a gender-biased tendency towards left handedness. The effects were small and remain to be confirmed by others.

SPEECH DEVELOPMENT

Reports of altered speech development associated with ultrasound exposure are confusing, showing in one case delayed speech development and in another a lower level of referral to speech therapist in the exposed group. There is no clear evidence associating ultrasound with altered speech development.

In summary, there is no independently verified evidence to suggest that ultrasound exposure *in utero* has caused an alteration in the development and growth of the fetus. All studies have either proved to be negative, or, when positive findings have appeared they have not been verified, or have been shown to result from poorly designed studies. New studies will be difficult to structure, because of the difficulty of finding an unexposed control group, because of the widespread use of ultrasound during pregnancy throughout the world. It is necessary to sound a note of caution, however. Details of ultrasound exposure are missing in many of the studies, which commonly record neither exposure intensities nor dwell time. There are no studies which have explored outcomes following exposure to pulsed Doppler or Doppler imaging, where intensities and powers are known to be higher than in pulse–echo imaging. While the results of epidemiological studies so far are comforting, they cannot be used to support an argument that it is safe to extend exposure *in utero* to include the higher

levels associated with Doppler ultrasound. Further epidemiological studies focused, specifically, on Doppler exposure would be needed before such confidence can be claimed.

How is safety managed?

The successful management of safety for medical ultrasound involves everyone: manufacturers, users and other experts. Manufacturers must comply with standards intended to make the equipment safe. Users must make sure that they use the equipment in an appropriate and safe manner. Both groups, together with other experts such as embryologists, biochemists and physicists, must contribute to the development of national and international standards to keep ultrasound safe without unduly restricting its use and benefits.

The manufacturers' responsibility

The Medical Devices Directive (MDD) in Europe, and the Food and Drug Administration (FDA) in the USA both make demands of manufacturers regarding safety of their scanners and provision of information to purchasers and users. The standards supporting these directives are generated by the International Electrotechnical Commission (IEC) and by the American Institute of Ultrasound in Medicine and the National Electrical Manufacturers Association (AIUM/NEMA) in the USA. AIUM/NEMA have defined TI and MI, and these were discussed earlier. They are intended to give some safety-related indication to sonographers; these indices are now available on most current ultrasound scanners. The IEC has published a number of measurement and performance standards.

US FOOD AND DRUGS ADMINISTRATION

Any equipment sold in the USA must meet the US FDA Regulations requiring that manufacturers supply information on acoustic output and ensure that certain derated acoustic parameters do not exceed allowable levels. Most commonly, manufacturers follow what is known as "Track 3". The exposure limits are set out in Table 13.1.

In order to comply, manufacturers must also however, provide on-screen indication of TI and MI according to the methods set out in the Output Display Standard (ODS). Track 3 has the potential benefit of improved imaging through removing lower-output restrictions which had been used previously. Removing these restrictions also means that the potential risk to the patient

Table 13.1 The upper limits of exposure required by the US FDA.

Applications	Derated I_{spta} (mW cm^{-2})	Derated I_{sppa} (W cm^{-2})	MI	TI
All except ophthalmology	720	190	1.9	(6.0)*
Ophthalmology	50	NS	0.23	1.0

The upper limit of 6.0 for TI is advisory. At least one of the quantities MI and I_{sppa} must be less than the specified limit. NS: Not specified.

through exposure to ultrasound is increased and that users must be more aware of the safety issues.

EUROPEAN MEDICAL DEVICES DIRECTIVE

One of the main drivers for the development of international and European specification standards over the last few years has been the European Communities (EC) MDD (93/42/EEC). The MDD requires that all medical devices (except custom made and devices intended for clinical investigation) meet essential requirements for safety and performance, and carry a CE mark before they are placed on the market in the EC. The CE mark is the manufacturer's declaration that the device conforms to these requirements. The MDD includes requirements for the visual display or warning of emission of potentially hazardous radiation, and for the indication of accuracy of equipment with a measuring function. The normal method for a manufacturer to demonstrate that they have complied with these requirements would be for them to follow procedures laid down in international standards. Standards, which are recognised as demonstrating compliance with particular safety requirements, will be listed in the *Official Journal of the European Communities*. These would normally be IEC or ISO standards where such standards exist. This structure in not yet in place for ultrasound and so it is not yet clear exactly what the implications of the MDD are in this field.

INTERNATIONAL STANDARDS

Of the existing international standards, only IEC 61157 (1992) *Requirements for the Declaration of the Acoustic Output of Medical Diagnostic Equipment* makes any safety-related requirements of manufacturers. They must provide specific information relating to the acoustic output of their scanners in water under conditions which produce the maximum temporal-average intensity

(see Appendix 13C for definitions of parameters) and the maximum negative pressure for each mode of operation (B-mode, M-mode, colour-flow, etc.). Some of this information is in the equipment manual. IEC 61157 also sets exemption levels for the declaration of p_-, I_{ob} and I_{spta} as shown below. Equipment, whose output falls below all three of these levels (usually, this applies only to fetal Doppler and peripheral vascular Doppler devices only), need not provide such detailed output information:

Acoustic quantity	Exemption levels
Peak negative pressure at maximum of p_-	<1 MPa
Output beam intensity I_{ob}	<20 mW cm^{-2}
Spatial-peak temporal-average intensity at maximum of I_{spta}	<100 mW cm^{-2}

IEC 60601-2-37, *Medical electrical equipment, Part 2: Particular requirements for the safety of ultrasonic medical diagnostic and monitoring equipment*, effectively implements the AIUM/NEMA ODS methods and requires calculation and display of TI and MI values subject to the same conditions as the ODS. In addition, it places upper limits for the temperature of the transducer surface which is in contact with the patient.

The users' responsibility

The role of the sonographer in managing safety is obviously vital. The user must ensure that they are properly trained and that they keep their knowledge up to date with changing technology and practices. They must choose and use scanners which are appropriate for the type of examination and the condition of the patient. They must follow good practice for reducing the risk to the patient. They must take part of the responsibility for ensuring that the equipment they use is properly maintained and meets necessary standards.

PROPER TRAINING

It is obvious, but worth repeating, that all users need to be trained in and familiar with both the relevant anatomy and physiology for the examinations they make and the strengths and weaknesses of the equipment they use. As new equipment and techniques are developed, further training will be needed to ensure that, for instance, different imaging artefacts are understood and an accurate diagnosis made. The greatest risk to the patient still comes from misdiagnosis and that should never be overlooked.

To complement this, users need also to appreciate the current thinking with respect to hazard posed by the ultrasound exposure itself and should seek training either through their own department, their professional body, the British Medical Ultrasound Society (BMUS) or published literature. Various committees and professional bodies have offered guidance to the sonographer when it comes to assessing the possible risks (AIUM, 1988; WFUMB, 1997). A summary of the various positions taken by national and international bodies has recently been summarised by Barnett *et al.* (2000). EFSUMB publish a clinical safety statement, which is kept under annual review. The current version may be found at www.efsumb.org.

The BMUS published a Statement and Guidelines for safety in 2000, prepared by the BMUS Safety Group and based on the best expert judgements available. These documents are reproduced in Appendix 13A, and are also available at www.bmus.org.

APPROPRIATE EQUIPMENT

If a probe is intended for a specific purpose, it should only be used for that purpose because choice of working frequency, acoustic output levels and field geometry are tailored to the intended use. A probe that is perfectly safe for adult cardiac use may not be safe for an obstetric or neonatal cephalic examination. If possible, use equipment which provides safety information to the user – this will, generally, be in the form of TI and MI display – and take note of this information and your knowledge of the patient when planning and carrying out the scan.

In general, you should be less concerned about examining "normal", non-pregnant adults. You should be more concerned when examining:

- the fetus (or the maternal abdomen near the fetus),
- neonates,
- patients with fever or elevated core temperature,
- patients under anaesthetic or during surgery.

In some types of examination, TI and MI are more likely to underestimate the amount of heating or cavitation. In general, you should be more cautious for

- fetal examination through the full bladder;
- the use of trans-vaginal, trans-rectal or other internal probes;

- trans-cranial examination;
- the use of injected ultrasound-contrast agents.

GOOD SAFETY PRACTICE

Keeping up to date with current thinking on ultrasound, safety and risk minimisation will allow the sonographer to make the best decisions on how to maximise the benefit to the patient while reducing the risk. The previous section on use of appropriate equipment, in conjunction with the list below, gives some simple guidelines:

- Only carry out an examination if there are clinical grounds to do so.

- Make sure you get the information you need to make a good diagnosis. There is more chance of causing harm by misdiagnosis than through heating or cavitation.

- Reduce the amount of time that the probe is in contact with the patient. You can do this by stopping the examination as soon as you have the information you want and by removing the probe during the examination, if you need to talk to the patient or to a colleague and are not able to concentrate on the image on the scanner.

- Generally, Doppler modes (PW, colour or power Doppler) are more likely to cause heating. So, use grey-scale imaging to find the clinical site and only use Doppler modes, if they are necessary and when you have found the site.

- The most cautious approach is to display TIB most of the time. Only display TIS if you are sure that there is no bone, developing bone or cartilage anywhere in the region you are scanning. Only display TIC for trans-cranial examinations.

PROPER MAINTENANCE

The final point is that users are not stuck with the equipment they are given! They can and must play an active role in making sure that the equipment is properly maintained and repaired, and they can actually help develop better and safer equipment by making safety issues an important issue with manufacturers. They can do this both by questioning manufacturers directly (and, of course, a trained and knowledgeable sonographer will be able to ask more challenging questions) and by taking active part in the debates within the BMUS, the professional bodies, the British Standards Institute (BSI) and IEC. It is these debates which, in the long run, produce better international standards with which the equipment bought by individual hospitals and departments will comply.

Is exposure increasing?

An important practical question in discussions of ultrasound safety is whether current clinical practice causes higher ultrasound exposure to the patient population than was so in the past. There are three overlapping but distinct questions.

1. Are the acoustic pressures, intensities or powers used today higher than those used for the same applications in the past, either average or maximum values?

2. Has the introduction of any new scanning modes (such as Doppler imaging or harmonic imaging) or transducers (such as those for trans-vaginal or trans-oesophageal scanning) been accompanied by altered exposure?

3. Has the clinical use of ultrasound altered over the years, by the numbers of scans being carried out, and/or by the exposure dwell time used?

INCREASING OUTPUT FROM DIAGNOSTIC SCANNERS

There is now good evidence of a continuing trend towards higher ultrasound output, which has continued over about three decades. Duck and Martin (1991) reviewed literature surveys from the late 1970s showing this trend, and later surveys (Henderson et al., 1995) confirmed that higher output still was being used, on average, during the 1990s. A summary of present acoustic output for M-, B- and Doppler-modes of operation is given in Tables 13.2 and 13.3 (Barnett and Kossoff, 1998). There may be several causes for the observed increases. The most probable recent cause, however, is the relaxation of regulatory limits applied by the FDA in the US (see above). In particular, the limit for derated I_{spta} for non-cardiovascular scanning, including obstetric scanning, was raised from 94 to $720\,mW\,cm^{-2}$. As a

Table 13.2 Maximum ultrasound exposure in water from B-mode and M-mode operation.

Application	Range	Median
B-mode imaging and M-mode		
Peak rarefaction pressure, p_r (MPa)	0.45–5.54	2.4
Spatial-peak pulse-average intensity, I_{sppa} (W cm^{-2})	14–933	230
M-mode only		
Spatial-peak temporal-average intensity, I_{spta} (mW cm^{-2})	11.2–430	106
Total acoustic power (mW)	1–68	9
B-mode only		
Spatial-peak temporal-average intensity, I_{spta} (mW cm^{-2})	0.3–991	34
Total acoustic power (mW)	0.3–285	75

Table 13.3 Maximum ultrasound exposure in water for pulsed Doppler and Doppler imaging modes.

	Range	Median
Spectral pulsed Doppler		
Peak rarefaction pressure, p_r (MPa)	0.67–5.32	2.1
Spatial-peak pulse-average intensity, I_{sppa} (W cm^{-2})	1.1–771	144
Spatial-peak temporal-average intensity, I_{spta} (mW cm^{-2})	173–9080	1180
Acoustic power (mW)	10–440	100
Doppler imaging		
Peak rarefaction pressure, p_r (MPa)	0.46–4.25	2.38
Spatial-peak pulse-average intensity, I_{sppa} (W cm^{-2})	60–670	275
Spatial-peak temporal-average intensity, I_{spta} (mW cm^{-2})	21–2050	290
Acoustic power (mW)	15–440	90

result, manufacturers are increasingly using the increased allowance to exploit new methods of scanning, with the result that outputs are all tending to move towards the limits set by the FDA.

The introduction of pulsed Doppler during the 1980s and of Doppler imaging during the 1990s were the two most important changes giving rise to increased output. Table 13.3 summarises the exposure associated with these modes. Overall, the greatest intensities are associated with pulsed Doppler operation, although some settings for Doppler imaging can give rise to intensities commonly associated only with pulsed Doppler. These occur when Doppler imaging is used with a narrow colour box, high line density and high frame rate. All forms of Doppler imaging, whether colour-flow imaging or so-called "power Doppler", use the same range of acoustic output.

While Doppler modes are associated with the highest intensities, the highest pulse amplitudes (given by either rarefaction pressure, p_r, or I_{sppa}) for Doppler applications are broadly similar to those used for imaging. On an average, maximum rarefaction pressures are about 2.5 MPa, although extreme examples of pressures reaching over 8 MPa have been reported. Newer imaging applications such as harmonic imaging can be expected to use amplitudes confined to the upper range, since it is only at such pressures that harmonics are generated significantly in tissue.

Other changes in technology have also altered exposure. This is particularly true with the development of higher-frequency probes, and those for intra-luminal use, such as trans-rectal, trans-oesophageal, and trans-vaginal transducers. The output from such transducers is ultimately limited in the USA, and hence elsewhere, by the same regulations which govern all transducers. However, the FDA Regulations do not set limits based on predicted temperature rise in tissue, apart for the ophthalmic use. Since interstitial transducers generally operate at higher ultrasound frequencies, they are capable of causing greater tissue heating while still operating within the regulations, than is true for transducers operating at a lower frequency.

According to the WFUMB, one-quarter of all medical-imaging studies worldwide is now an ultrasound scan (WFUMB, 1997). In England, there were 1.9 million obstetric ultrasound scans in the year April 1997 to March 1998 (DoH, 1998), a reported increase of 10.5% from the previous year. A greater increase of 17.8% in non-obstetric scans was reported, reaching an annual total of 2.88 million. It is clear from these and other data that exposure to ultrasound, quantified in terms of proportion of the population exposed, is growing, and may be expected to continue to grow. Within this group, the majority of scan times will be short, not least because of time pressures within ultrasound clinics. Nevertheless, there are reasons why some patients may be exposed for more extended periods. This may arise because the procedure requires it (e.g. fetal breathing studies, flow studies, or guided interventional procedures) or because there is an increased usage of ultrasound by novice practitioners who are yet to develop mature skills and confidence in ultrasound scanning. In general, it may be concluded that overall exposure of the population to ultrasound for medical diagnostic reasons is currently growing strongly, and may be expected to continue to do so for the foreseeable future.

Safety for specific uses of diagnostic ultrasound

Reviews of the safety of ultrasound often explore the exposure and bioeffects mechanisms but only occasionally review the safety aspects of the tissues being exposed (see e.g. Barnett et al., 1997). Often it is assumed that embryological and fetal exposure are the only concern. Some general recommendations are based upon a rationale specific to exposure in utero. This is true of the World Federation recommendations on heating (Barnett, 1998) which were developed from investigations only into thermal teratology. It is helpful, therefore, to consider separately the safety concerns relating to a few particular uses of diagnostic ultrasound.

Diagnostic ultrasound during the first trimester

Probably the most critical question concerns the exposure of the embryo during the early stages of pregnancy. This is a period of rapid development and complex biochemical change, which includes organ creation and cell migration. There is widespread evidence that during this period the developing embryo is particularly sensitive to external agents, whose effect on subsequent development may range from fatal developmental malformation to minor and subtle biochemical disturbance. It is because of this sensitivity that EFSUMB have advised that "until further scientific evidence is available, investigations should be carried out with careful control of output levels and exposure times". (EFSUMB, 2002). This statement recognises both that there are gaps in our knowledge and understanding of the way in which ultrasound may interact with embryonic tissue, and that any adverse effect may result in developmental problems because of the particular sensitivity of the tissue at this time. Moreover, this sensitivity may be cyclic, with some tissues being sensitive only during particular time-bands of rapid cell development and differentiation. Heat is a teratogen, and any temperature increase from the absorption of ultrasound can disturb subsequent development, if of sufficient magnitude and maintained for sufficiently long. Fortunately, the tissue with the greatest tendency to heat, bone, only starts to condense at the end of the first trimester. In the absence of bone, present evidence suggests that temperature rises above 1.5°C will not occur within embryonic tissue at present diagnostic exposures. While this suggests that significant developmental changes may not occur, the kinetics of biochemical processes are known to be temperature sensitive, and little research has investigated the influence of small temperature changes induced locally on membranes and signal transduction pathways. There is no evidence that cavitation occurs either, since there are no gas bubbles to act as nucleation sites within the uterus. Radiation pressure is exerted on embryonic tissue during exposure however, and certainly amniotic fluid is caused to stream around the embryo during exposure. Acoustic streaming itself seems to present no hazard. Nevertheless, the forces which cause the stream are also experienced by the embryological tissues. If of sufficient magnitude and exposure duration, permanent tissue displacement might occur. There is no evidence that this actually happens at present levels, however. Thus although our present understanding suggests that present practice is safe, there is sufficient uncertainty about the detailed interaction processes to advise caution.

Diagnostic ultrasound during the second and third trimesters

Bone ossification is the main developmental change during the second and third trimesters of pregnancy of significance to ultrasound safety. As bone condenses it forms local regions of high attenuation. Ultrasound energy is absorbed more by the fetal skeleton than by fetal soft tissues, causing preferentially heating. This is important in part because soft tissues alongside this bone will also be warmed by thermal conduction, reaching a higher temperature than expected from ultrasound absorption alone. Neurological tissues are known to be particularly

sensitive to temperature rise, and the development of brain tissue, and of the spinal cord, could be affected if adjacent skull or vertebral bone were heated too much. Within the fetal haematopoietic system, the bone marrow is the main site of blood formation in the third trimester of pregnancy. Abnormal cell nuclei in neutrophils in guinea pigs have been reported after 6 min exposure at 2.5°C temperature elevation. This temperature increase in bone is within the capability of modern pulsed Doppler systems.

Cavitation is unlikely to occur during these later stages in pregnancy in diagnostic fields, as is the case during the first trimester, because of the absence of available nucleation sites. Radiation pressure effects can occur, and streaming will be caused within fluid spaces *in utero*. It seems unlikely that streaming, or other radiation pressure effects have a safety significance at this stage. The development of collagenous structures and an extracellular matrix gives increased strength to fetal tissues.

Obstetric scanning on patients with fever

It is noted in the WFUMB recommendations that "care should be taken to avoid unnecessary additional embryonic and fetal risk from (heating due to) ultrasound examinations of febrile patients". If a mother has a temperature, her unborn child is already at risk of maldevelopment as a result of the elevated temperature. This being so, it is sensible not to increase this risk unnecessarily. This does not mean withholding obstetric scanning from patients if they have a temperature. The methods of limiting exposure, including minimising TI, limiting the duration of the scan and avoiding casual use of Doppler techniques, should be employed with particular vigilance in these cases.

Neonatal scanning

Two particular concerns have been raised to do with neonatal scanning: these are neonatal head scanning and cardiac scanning. The reasons for caution are different for each, so they will be dealt with separately. Often, scanning is carried out when neonates are seriously ill, and the paramount needs for diagnosis should be judged against any potential for hazard and consequent risk.

NEONATAL HEAD SCANNING

The exposure of the neonatal head to diagnostic ultrasound carries with it the same safety issues as for second- and third-trimester scanning. Neuronal development is known to be particularly sensitive to temperature.

Temperature increases of a few degrees can occur in bone when exposed to diagnostic ultrasound. This means that there is the potential for brain tissue close to bone to experience temperature elevations by thermal conduction. The temperature increases may occur either close to the transducer, or within the skull. At the surface, there are two potential sources of heat. Firstly, the ultrasound beam is absorbed by the skull bone. The TIC provides the user with an estimate of this temperature rise. Secondly, transducer self-heating can further increase the surface temperature, whether or not the transducer is applied over bone or the anterior fontanelle. Transducer heating may increase the surface temperature by a few degrees when transducers are operated at the highest powers. The other place which may heat preferentially lies at the inner surface of the skull bone where it is exposed to the ultrasound beam, again giving the potential to heat adjacent neural tissues. In this case, the more appropriate safety index is the TIB.

NEONATAL CARDIAC SCANNING

Neonatal cardiac scanning, including Doppler blood-flow imaging, may expose surrounding pleural tissue. There is good experimental evidence for alveolar capillary damage both in adult small animals, and juvenile larger animals, although there is no evidence for lung damage in humans – even in neonates. The experimental evidence suggests that as pleural tissue matures it thickens and becomes stronger, so preventing capillary rupture. Immature (and hence structurally weak) neonatal pleura may be vulnerable to stress caused by diagnostic ultrasound pulses. The relevant safety index is the MI, and this should be kept to a minimum appropriate to effective diagnosis.

Ophthalmic scanning

The eye is the only tissue identified separately for regulation by the US FDA, and the only case for which TI is used for regulation. The limit for derated time-averaged intensity is $50\,\mathrm{mW\,cm^{-2}}$ (in comparison with $720\,\mathrm{mW\,cm^{-2}}$ for all other applications), and 0.23 for MI (compared with 1.9) – see Table 13.1. The TI limit is 1.0. The reason for the regulatory caution is the particular sensitivity of parts of the eye to potential damage. The cornea, lens and vitreous body of the eye are all unperfused tissues. This means that they dissipate heat only by means of thermal conduction. Furthermore, the lack of blood perfusion limits the ability to repair any

damage arising from excess exposure. The acoustic attenuation coefficient of the lens is about $8\,\mathrm{dB/cm^{-1}}$ at 10 MHz, and since a lens has a greatest thickness of about 4 mm, about one-half of the incident acoustic power may be deposited there. A further specific concern is that the lens lies very close indeed to the transducer under normal scanning conditions. Transducer self-heating becomes an important secondary source of heat under these circumstances. For all these reasons, particular care is exercised in the design of systems specifically for ophthalmic use. If general-purpose scanners are used for eye studies, great care needs to be exercised to reduce to an absolute minimum any chance of lens heating.

Summary and conclusions

Ultrasound has an enviable record for safety. Indeed it is partly its lack of toxicity, which has allowed it to grow to the point where "more than one out of every four imaging studies in the world is an ultrasound study". All the epidemiological evidence points to the conclusion that past and current practice presents no actual risk to the patient, and may be considered as safe. Nevertheless, there is ample evidence that modern scanners, designed in accordance with national and international standards and regulations, can warm tissues by several degrees under some circumstances. If gas bubbles or other pockets of gas lie in the ultrasound field, the tissues may be damaged from stresses from cavitation-like oscillations. Radiation pressure, sufficient to cause acoustic streaming *in vivo*, is exerted on all exposed tissues. These are important facts underpinning both the responsibilities of the manufacturers to produce safe equipment to use, and for the users of ultrasound in managing their scanning practice.

Recent changes to the regulations in the US have resulted in a new generation of scanning equipment which displays safety indices allowing users greater feedback for safety judgements to be made. These changes have also enabled higher output to be used in, e.g. obstetric scanning. Greatest intensities and powers, and the greatest potential heating, occurs when using pulsed Doppler modes. There is considerable overlap between modes, however. Particular safety concerns pertain during all obstetric scanning, during neonatal scanning, during ophthalmic scanning, and when using contrast materials.

APPENDIX 13A

British Medical Ultrasound Society Statement on the safe use, and potential hazards, of diagnostic ultrasound, 2000

Ultrasound is now accepted as being of considerable diagnostic value. There is no evidence that diagnostic ultrasound has produced any harm to patients in the four decades that it has been in use. However, the acoustic output of modern equipment is generally much greater than that of the early equipment and, in view of the continuing progress in equipment design and applications, outputs may be expected to continue to be subject to change. Also, investigations into the possibility of subtle or transient effects are still at an early stage. Consequently, diagnostic ultrasound can only be considered safe if used prudently.

Thermal hazard exists with some diagnostic ultrasound equipment, if used imprudently. A temperature elevation of less than 1.5°C is considered to present no hazard to human or animal tissue, including a human embryo or fetus, even if maintained indefinitely. Temperature elevations in excess of this may cause harm, depending on the time for which they are maintained. A temperature elevation of 4°C, maintained for 5 min or more, is considered to be potentially hazardous to a fetus or embryo. Some diagnostic ultrasound equipment, operating in spectral pulsed Doppler mode, can produce temperature rises in excess of 4°C in bone, with an associated risk of high temperatures being produced in adjacent soft tissues by conduction. With some machines, colour Doppler imaging modes may also produce high temperature rises, particularly if a deep focus or a narrow colour box is selected. In other modes, temperature elevations in excess of 1°C are possible, but are unlikely to reach 1.5°C with equipment currently in clinical use, except where significant self-heating of the transducer occurs.

Non-thermal damage has been demonstrated in animal tissues containing gas pockets, such as lung and intestine, using diagnostic levels of ultrasound (mechanical index (MI) values of 0.3 or more). In view of this, it is recommended that care should be taken to avoid unnecessary exposure of neonatal lung, and to maintain MI as low as possible when this is not possible. In other tissues, there is no evidence that diagnostic ultrasound produces non-thermal damage, in the absence of gas-filled contrast agents. However, in view of the difficulty of demonstrating small, localised, regions of damage *in vivo*, the possibility of this cannot be excluded. The MI, if displayed, acts as a guide to the operator. The use of contrast agents in the form of stabilised gas bubbles increases the probability of cavitation. Single beam modes (A-mode, M-mode and spectral pulsed Doppler) have a greater potential for non-thermal hazard than scanned modes (B-mode, colour Doppler), although the use of a narrow write-zoom box increases this potential for scanning modes.

British Medical Ultrasound Society Guidelines for the safe use of diagnostic ultrasound equipment, 2000

Scope and purpose

These guidelines are intended to assist all those who use diagnostic ultrasound equipment for any purpose in order that they may be able to make informed judgements about ultrasound safety, and in order to protect patients from excessive exposure. The guidelines are based on the best scientific information available at the time of writing, using advice and evidence from international experts. Some specific guidelines, namely Guidelines 7, 8, 10, 11 and 15, are supported by a more detailed rationale. In particular, Guidelines 11 and 15 set out action levels for thermal index (TI) and MI, and these are justified in the rationale. Further background information on the safe use of ultrasound may be found in more extensive texts, including ter Haar and Duck (2000).

Guidelines

1. *Medical endorsement.* Ultrasound should only be used for medical diagnosis, if endorsed by a medical practitioner.[1] See Guideline 15 for non-diagnostic use.

2. *Operator training.* Diagnostic ultrasound procedures should be carried out only by persons, who are fully trained in the use of the equipment, the interpretation of its results and images and in the safe

use of ultrasound, including an appreciation of its potential hazards.

3. *Awareness of machine factors influencing hazard.* Operators should understand the likely influence of the machine controls, the operating mode (e.g. B-mode, colour Doppler imaging or spectral Doppler) and probe frequency on the thermal and cavitation hazards.[2]

4. *Initial power setting.* Machines should be set up so that the default (switch-on) setting of the acoustic output power control is low. If a low-default setting cannot be achieved, a low setting should be selected after switching on. A low setting should be selected for each new patient. The output should only be increased during the investigation, if this is necessary to produce a satisfactory result.

5. *Exposure time.* The overall examination times should be kept as short as is necessary to produce a useful diagnostic result.

6. *Stationary probe.* The probe should not be held in a fixed position for any longer than is necessary, and should be removed from the patient whenever there is no need for a real-time image or spectral Doppler acquisition. For example, using the freeze frame or cine-loop facilities allows images to be reviewed and discussed without continuing the exposure.

7. *Probe self-heating.* Endo-probes (e.g. vaginal, rectal or oesophageal probe) should not be used if there is noticeable self-heating of the probe when operating in air. This applies to any probe, but particular care should be taken if trans-vaginal probes are to be used to investigate a pregnancy during the first 8 weeks after conception.

8. *Pre-existing temperature elevation.* Particular care should be taken to reduce output and minimise exposure time of an embryo or fetus when the temperature of the mother is already elevated.

9. *Sensitive tissues.* Particular care should be taken to reduce the risk of thermal hazard when exposing the following to diagnostic ultrasound:

- an embryo less than 8 weeks after conception;
- the head, brain or spine of any fetus or neonate;
- an eye (in a subject of any age).

10. *Pulsed Doppler.* The use of spectral pulsed Doppler, or colour Doppler mode with a narrow write-zoom box selected, is not recommended for the investigation of any of the targets identified in Guideline 9, unless an estimate of the maximum

likely temperature elevation has been obtained and considered in relation to the anticipated exposure time (see Guideline 11).

11. *Thermal and Mechanical Indices.* For machines which display on-screen TI and MI values,[3] operators should continually monitor their values and use control settings that keep them as small as is consistent with achieving diagnostically useful results. In obstetric investigations, soft tissue thermal index (TIS) should be monitored during scans carried out in the first 8 weeks after conception, and bone thermal index (TIB) thereafter. In applications where the probe is very close to bone (e.g. trans-cranial applications), cranial thermal index (TIC) should be monitored. For eye scanning TIS should be monitored. In other applications, TIB should be monitored.

MI > 0.3 There is a possibility of minor damage to neonatal lung or intestine. If such exposure is necessary, try to reduce the exposure time as much as possible.

MI > 0.7 There is a risk of cavitation if an ultrasound-contrast agent containing gas micro-spheres is being used. There is a theoretical risk of cavitation without the presence of ultrasound-contrast agents. The risk increases with MI values above this threshold.

TI > 0.7 The overall exposure time (including pauses) of an embryo or fetus should be restricted in accordance with Table 13A.1.

TI > 1.0 Eye scanning is not recommended, other than as part of a fetal scan.

TI ≥ 3.0 Scanning of an embryo or fetus is not recommended, however briefly.

Where an on-screen TI or MI is not displayed, try to obtain *worst-case* estimates (considering all possible combinations of control settings) of temperature elevation (ΔT_{max}) and MI (MI_{max}) for the particular

Table 13A.1 Maximum recommended exposure times for an embryo or fetus.

TI	Maximum exposure time (min)
0.7	60
1.0	30
1.5	15
2.0	4
2.5	1

probe and mode in use.[4] If these can be obtained, assume that the MI value is equal to MI_{max} and the TI value is equal to $0.5\Delta T_{max}$ and refer to Table 13A.1.

12. *Doppler for fetal heart monitoring.* The power levels used for fetal heart monitoring (CTG) are sufficiently low, so that the use of this modality is not contraindicated, on safety grounds, even when it is to be used for extended periods.

13. *Peripheral pulse monitoring.* The output from CW Doppler devices intended for monitoring peripheral pulses is sufficiently low, so that their use is not contraindicated, on safety grounds.

14. *Trans-cranial ultrasound investigations.* Trans-cranial ultrasound investigations may require higher acoustic output than other applications. BMUS Safety Guidelines 1–11 should be applied in the use of both imaging and stand-alone Doppler equipment. TIC should be monitored.

15. *Non-diagnostic uses of diagnostic ultrasound equipment.* Examples of non-diagnostic uses of ultrasound equipment include repeated scans for operator training, equipment demonstration using normal subjects, and the production of souvenir pictures or videos of a fetus.

For equipment for which the safety indices are displayed over their full range of values, the TI should always be less than 0.5 and the MI should always be less than 0.3. When the safety indices are not displayed, ΔT_{max} should be less than 1°C and MI_{max} should be less than 0.3. Frequent exposure of the same subject is to be avoided. Guidelines 2–10 should be followed.

Scans in the first trimester of pregnancy should not be carried out for the sole purpose of producing souvenir videos or photographs, nor should their production involve increasing the exposure levels or extending the scan times beyond those needed for clinical purposes.

Notes

1. Routine investigations as part of a clinical protocol are considered to comply with Guideline 1, as do specific investigations requested by a clinician or midwife. Research and "bonding" scans endorsed by a clinician or midwife are also considered to comply.

2. A Medical Physics Department should be able to give advice. There are no universal rules for predicting the effect of machine controls (other than the output power control) on output, since, in an effort to limit outputs, manufacturers often arrange for more

than one parameter to change when a particular control is adjusted. However, the following may be helpful as general guide. In scanning modes, greater heating potential is often associated with multiple or deep transmission focus settings, and the use of write-zoom (particularly with a long, narrow or deep zoom) box. In spectral pulsed Doppler mode, greater heating potential is usually associated with a high pulse repetition frequency (e.g. a high limit on the frequency scale), and a shallow range gate. The likelihood of cavitation is greater for large output settings and lower frequencies. In Doppler modes, the likelihood is increased by selecting short range gates or by selecting a high Doppler frequency scale.

3. The TI is intended to give a rough guide to the likely maximum temperature rise that might be produced after long exposure. Three forms of TI may be displayed, according to the application. TIS assumes that only soft tissue is insonated. TIB assumes bone is present at the depth where temporal intensity is greatest. TIC assumes bone is very close to the front face of the probe. However, note that errors in calculating TI values, and the limitations of simple models on which they are based, means that TI values can underestimate the temperature elevation by a factor of up to two.

The MI is intended to offer a rough guide to the likelihood of the occurrence of cavitation. Its value is constantly updated by the machine, according to the control settings, using the formula $MI = p_{-0.3}/f$, where f is the pulse centre frequency and $p_{-0.3}$ is the maximum value of peak negative pressure anywhere in the ultrasound field, measured in water but reduced by an attenuation factor equal to that which would be produced by a medium having an attenuation coefficient of $0.3\,dB\,cm^{-1}\,MHz^{-1}$.

There should be independent checks that the displayed TI and MI values are accurate. These should be made soon after installation and after hardware or software changes.

4. A Medical Physics Department may be able to make these estimates, using either test objects or measurements of acoustic power and intensity. For abdominal and obstetric applications, the worst-case estimate of temperature elevation should assume a soft tissue and bone model, with the interface lying at the depth where the derated temporal-average intensity is a maximum. For other applications (e.g. the eye or superficial bone), the model used should be appropriate to the particular tissues involved.

Rationale for BMUS safety guidelines

Probe self-heating (Guidelines paragraph 7)

The raised tissue temperature due to probe self-heating is likely to be greater for endo-probes than for surface probes. This is because the adjacent tissue is at an initial temperature of 37°C, or higher in the case of a febrile patient, rather than closer to room temperature as in the case of surface-applied probes. Also, there is no opportunity for heat removal by air convection or radiation, as is the case for probes applied to the patient's skin.

Pulsed Doppler (Guidelines paragraph 8)

Pulsed Doppler techniques generally involve greater temporal-average intensities and powers than B- or M-mode, and hence greater heating potential, due to the high pulse repetition frequencies and consequent high duty factors that are often used. In the case of spectral pulsed Doppler, the fact that the beam is held in a fixed position during an observation leads to a further increase in temporal-average intensity. Colour flow mapping and Doppler power mapping involve some beam scanning, and so, generally, have a heating potential that is intermediate between that of B- or M-mode and that of spectral pulsed Doppler.

Sensitive tissues (Guidelines paragraph 10)

Up to 8 weeks after conception, organogenesis is taking place in the embryo. This is a period when cell damage might lead to fetal anomalies or subtle developmental changes. The brain and spinal cord continue to develop through to the neonatal period.

The presence of bone within the beam greatly increases the likely temperature rise, due to both direct absorption in the bone itself and conduction of heat from bone to adjacent tissues.

The following table identifies the important relevant landmarks in early pregnancy:

Gestation from LMP	Gestation from conception/ fertilisation	Title of conceptus	Major relevant events
0–14 days	Nil	–	–
14–28 days	0–14 days	Zygote	Rapid cell multiplications
29–70 days 4.1–10 weeks	15–56 days 2.1–8 weeks	Embryo	Organogenesis
10–11 weeks	8–9 weeks	Foetus	Ossification of spine starts
13–14 weeks	11–12 weeks	Foetus	Ossification of skull and long bone starts

The eye is particularly vulnerable to thermal hazard since the lens and the aqueous and vitreous humours have no cooling blood supply. This applies to an eye of a subject of any age (e.g. child or adult) as well as a fetus, although a fetal eye is better cooled, due to its liquid environment.

Thermal index values and maximum exposure time recommendations (Guidelines paragraph 11)

TI values are intended to give a rough indication of the likely equilibrium temperature rise that might be produced. However, theoretical (Jago et al., 1999) and experimental (Shaw et al., 1998) studies have shown that, in some circumstances, TI can underestimate the temperature elevation by a factor of up to 2. As a safety precaution, the TI values given in Table 13.A.1 are assumed to be half the actual worst-case temperature elevations. Thus a TI value of 1.0 is considered to correspond to a worst-case temperature elevation of 2.0°C.

Following their review of the literature on the effects of temperature elevation on animal fetuses, the WFUMB (1998) concluded that an ultrasound exposure that elevates human embryonic or fetal temperature by 4°C above normal for 5 min should be considered potentially hazardous. Miller and Ziskin (1989) showed that there is a logarithmic relationship between temperature elevation and the exposure time needed to produce adverse biological effects in animal fetuses. They showed that, for temperatures below 43°C, the necessary exposure time reduced by a factor of 4 for every 1°C increase in temperature elevation. Adopting a maximum "safe" exposure time of 4 min for a temperature elevation of 4°C, and applying the above logarithmic rule, results in the following exposure times:

Temperature elevation (°C)	Maximum exposure time (min)
5	1
4	4
3	16
2	64
1	128

In Table 13A.1 of the Guidelines (paragraph 11), rounded values of these exposure times have been used for exposures up to 15 min. The 64 and 128 min maximum exposure times have been reduced to 30 and 60 min, respectively, as a safety precaution to reflect the present lack of knowledge about possible subtle bioeffects associated with prolonged moderate temperature elevation. No time limit is specified for TI values of less than 0.7, in accordance with the statement in the WFUMB (1998) recommendations on thermal effects that "a diagnostic exposure that produces a maximum temperature rise of no more than 1.5°C above normal physiological levels (37°C) may be used clinically without reservation on thermal grounds".

In examinations of the embryo or fetus in the first 8 weeks after conception, when there is no ossified bone, only soft tissue is exposed and so TIS should be monitored. In all other obstetric applications, TIB is recommended as the particular TI value to monitor. This avoids the complication of constantly switching attention between TIS and TIB according to whether or not bone is being insonated, and introduces a safety factor since TIB values are always greater than or equal to TIS values.

In eye-scanning applications, it is recommended that TIS is monitored as this is the TI used in the study by Herman and Harris (1999), which concluded that, in eye scanning, TIS values should be limited to a maximum of 1.0.

In other applications, it is recommended that TIB to be monitored.

Mechanical index threshold values (Guidelines paragraph 11)

The MI value of 0.3, representing the threshold for the possibility of capillary bleeding in gas-containing organs, such as the lungs and intestines, is taken from the 1992 Statement on Non-human Mammalian *in vivo* Biological Effects of the American Institute of Ultrasound in Medicine (AIUM, 1993).

The MI value of 0.7 is chosen as the threshold for cavitation, following the theoretical study by Apfel and Holland (1991), from which the formula for MI is derived. The model used for this study assumes the availability of micro-bubble nuclei of all sizes. Such micro-bubbles are believed to be produced when the shells of the micro-bubbles of some ultrasound-contrast agents are destroyed by pulses with higher acoustic pressures. There is experimental evidence that cavitation damage occurs in animals when contrast agents are present (Miller and Gies, 1998; Skyba *et al.*, 1998). In tissues not containing such artificially introduced nuclei, cavitation due to diagnostic ultrasound remains a theoretical possibility only, although it is produced in tissue during lithotripsy treatment (ECURS, 1994) and bubble formation has been demonstrated in agar gel

exposed to diagnostic levels of ultrasound (ter Haar *et al.*, 1989)

Non-diagnostic uses of diagnostic ultrasound equipment (Guidelines paragraph 15)

Since evidence suggests that there are thresholds for both cavitation and thermal effects, it might be argued that it is justifiable to use diagnostic ultrasound at sub-threshold levels for any purpose, with or without clinical purpose or endorsement. However, there are, inevitably, uncertainties associated with establishing the values of these thresholds, and in measuring the threshold parameters. For example, while it is generally accepted that temperature rises of less than 1.5°C may be sustained indefinitely without harming the embryo or fetus, there may be subtle effects at lower temperature that have not yet been detected. TI, the parameter used to estimate temperature rise, is known to be a rough approximation only, and makes no allowance for self-heating of the probe. Cavitation has not been observed *in vivo* in the absence of gas bodies. If it did occur, it may be a very localised event and be very difficult to detect. The MI provides no more than a rough guide to the likelihood of its occurrence.

Thus, the use of diagnostic ultrasound at levels close to bioeffects thresholds involves a risk–benefit balance. The maximum levels recommended for non-diagnostic investigations, where there is no clinical benefit, are therefore chosen to provide a lower degree of risk, while still permitting acceptable performance. The lower thresholds of TI (0.5) and MI (0.3) give appropriate extra margins of confidence in safety management for temperature rise and risk of cavitation. The MI threshold of 0.3 is also judged to be appropriate for exposure of gas bodies (lung and intestine). This is because, this threshold is based on relatively little experimental evidence, including exposure of mouse lung at low frequencies, and adequate estimates of safety margins have already been included.

APPENDIX 13B

Useful contacts

1. BMUS Safety Group. See: www.bmus.org.

2. The British Standards Institution (BSI) acts as the focus for the UK's input to the international standards scene. Committees within BSI mirror those within IEC and CENELEC. The particular committees are:

   - *BSI Committee EPL/87* mirrors IEC Technical Committee 87: Ultrasonics. Contact: Mr G Briffa.
   - *BSI Committee CH/111* mirrors the diagnostic and therapeutic ultrasound aspects of IEC Technical Committees TC 62, SC 62B and SC 62D which deal with electrical equipment in medical practice. Contact: Dr P McNeillis.

3. European Federation of Societies for Ultrasound in Medicine and Biology (EFSUMB) has a standing safety committee, the European Committee for Medical Ultrasound Safety (ECMUS). A Clinical Safety Statement, safety tutorials and literature reviews are available freely from the EFSUMB web site: www.efsumb.org.

APPENDIX 13C

Acoustic output parameters and their measurement

Acoustic output parameters

Many different parameters have been defined in order to try and characterise medical ultrasound fields. Due to the complexity of these fields, it is not possible to describe the parameters fully and unambiguously here. Definitions of some terms are given; the more interested reader can find further formal definitions and description in IEC 61102 (1991) and AIUM/NEMA (1992). There are five which seem to be most important to safety: peak negative pressure, pulse-average intensity, temporal-average intensity, total power and acoustic frequency.

PEAK NEGATIVE ACOUSTIC PRESSURE

The peak negative acoustic pressure (also called the peak rarefactional pressure and given the symbol p_r) is simply the most negative pressure that occurs during the pulse: in Figure 13.1, this is about 3.5 MPa. This is an important parameter because it relates to the occurrence of cavitation. Negative acoustic pressure means that the acoustic wave is trying to pull the water molecules apart; the water molecules resist this separation but, if the pressure is sufficiently negative and lasts for long enough, it is possible to produce a small void, a cavitation bubble. If there are pre-existing gas bubbles or dust particles in the water, cavitation occurs more easily. A similar effect can occur in tissue.

TEMPORAL-AVERAGE INTENSITY

We can also consider the intensity of the ultrasound field at a point. Intensity is a measure of the rate at which energy is flowing through a small area around the measurement point. Intensity varies with time as the ultrasound pulse passes the point and for most practical purposes is given by

$$i(t) = \frac{p(t)^2}{\rho c},$$

where c is the speed of sound in the medium and ρ is its density and p is the pressure. From this relationship, we can see that intensity is always a positive (unlike acoustic pressure, which can be positive or negative) and that intensity is highest when the pressure amplitude is highest. The time-averaged value of the intensity at a particular point is called the temporal-average intensity and given the symbol I_{ta}. Imaging scanners,

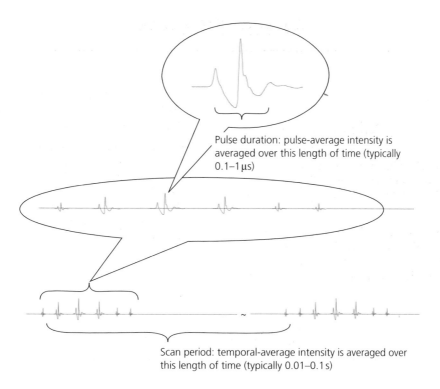

Pulse duration: pulse-average intensity is averaged over this length of time (typically 0.1–1 μs)

Scan period: temporal-average intensity is averaged over this length of time (typically 0.01–0.1 s)

Fig. 13C.1 Representation of temporal-average and pulse-average intensity in a typical imaging scan-frame.

generally, produce a large number of short pulses (approximately 1 μs long) separated by relatively long gaps (perhaps 100 μs long) and these pulses are often directed along different axes so it may take several hundred milliseconds for the pattern of intensity at any point to repeat. This means that the true temporal-average intensity must be averaged over the full scan repetition period or over a time which includes many scan repetition periods (see Figure 13C.1). Note that the time between pulses is actually much longer in relation to the pulse duration than is shown in the figure). I_{ta} is relevant because its spatial distribution is one of the main factors governing temperature rise in tissue. The maximum value of I_{ta} in the field is called the spatial-peak temporal-average intensity I_{spta}. This is one of the parameters on which the acoustic output is regulated in the USA by the Food and Drug Administration (FDA).

PULSE INTENSITY INTEGRAL AND PULSE–AVERAGE INTENSITY

Instead of averaging the intensity over the whole scan repetition period, it is possible to examine only a single pulse. The pulse intensity integral (*PII* or p_i) is calculated by integrating the intensity over the duration of the pulse; p_i is greatest at the focus and this is the position where many measurements are made. Dividing p_i by the duration of the pulse gives a parameter called the pulse-average intensity, I_{pa}; the maximum value in the field is the spatial-peak pulse-average intensity, I_{sppa}, which is also a parameter limited by FDA Regulations.

TOTAL POWER AND OUTPUT BEAM INTENSITY

Total power is the amount of ultrasonic energy radiated by the transducer every second. This is an important parameter for safety because it is relevant to heating and is used to calculate TIs. It is worth noting that, for a typical imaging transducer, the total radiated power is substantially less than the total electrical power supplied to the transducer and most of the electrical energy is converted to heat in the transducer. This "self-heating" is an important factor in determining the hazard to tissues close to the transducer.

Dividing the total power by the output area of the transducer gives the output beam intensity, I_{ob}. This is the mean temporal-average intensity at the transducer face.

201

ACOUSTIC FREQUENCY

As the wave passes a point, the water molecules are squeezed together during the high-pressure periods and stretched apart during the low-pressure periods. The acoustic frequency is essentially the rate at which this squeezing and stretching takes place. In Figure 13.1, the time between consecutive high-pressure periods is about $0.3\,\mu s$ and so the acoustic frequency is approximately $1/(0.3\,\mu s) = 3.3\,MHz$.

Frequency is important to safety because the absorption coefficient of most soft tissues increases with frequency leading to energy being absorbed in a smaller volume and producing higher temperature rises. Additionally, cavitation is more likely to occur at lower frequencies because the periods of negative pressure last for longer and cavitation nuclei have more time to grow.

Calculation of in situ exposure parameters

As ultrasound travels through tissue it is attenuated. That is, some of the energy is lost from the beam by absorption or scatter. This means that the *in situ* intensity (i.e. the intensity at some point in tissue) is less than the intensity measured in water at the same point in the field.

The propagation of ultrasound of the type used in medical imaging is an extremely complex phenomenon and there is no accepted way of deriving truly reliable estimates of the *in situ* exposure levels from the acoustic output measurements made in water. The most widely used method is that of "derating", used in the US FDA Regulations (see later), and the AIUM/NEMA Output Display Standard (AIUM/NEMA ODS). Derating involves multiplying the value of an acoustic property measured in water by a logarithmic attenuation factor. This factor is always frequency dependent and is often distance dependent. The most widely used theoretical attenuation model comes from the AIUM/NEMA ODS and uses a derating factor of $0.3\,dB\,cm^{-1}\,MHz^{-1}$ to estimate exposure in tissue. The assumption is that soft tissue fills the path between the transducer and the point where the exposure level is required. The value of $0.3\,dB\,cm^{-1}\,MHz^{-1}$ is lower than the attenuation of most soft tissues (which is typically closer to $0.44\,dB\,cm^{-1}\,MHz^{-1}$) to allow for the possibility of some fluid in the path (as would be the case for examination of a fetus through the bladder). The value of $0.3\,dB\,cm^{-1}\,MHz^{-1}$ means that at 3 cm from a 3.3 MHz transducer, the derated temporal-average intensity, $I_{ta.3}$, is 3 dB less than (i.e. half of) the value measured in water; the derated peak negative pressure, $p_{r.3}$, is 70% of the

value in water. This derating factor is used in calculating TI and MI, and if you see the term "derated" being used without the derating factor being specified, it is generally this AIUM/NEMA value which has been used.

Other attenuation models have been proposed by the NCRP (1992) using different attenuation factors. These models are less commonly used but generally suggest higher *in situ* values than does the AIUM/ NEMA derating factor.

How do you measure ultrasound?

Two types of device are used to measure the acoustic output of imaging and other medical ultrasonic equipment. The first is the hydrophone; the second is the radiation force balance (sometimes called a power balance, a power meter or a radiation pressure balance).

HYDROPHONES

Hydrophones are underwater microphones. Usually they are made of a piezoelectric material that converts the rapid pressure changes in the ultrasound pulse to an electrical signal which can be measured with an oscilloscope. If the hydrophone is calibrated, the pressure waveform can be calculated from the voltage waveform measured by the oscilloscope. In order to make measurements of real ultrasound fields, the hydrophone element must be small ($<1\,mm$) and it must be mounted in a positioning system that allows it to be moved to different positions in the field. This allows the acoustic quantities to be measured throughout the field and the spatial-peak values determined. In principle, any of the acoustic properties described above can be measured with a hydrophone but this type of measurement is really only possible in a laboratory or medical physics department with substantial experience and equipment for characterising ultrasound fields.

There are two types of hydrophone in general use: the membrane hydrophone and the probe hydrophone. In general, membrane hydrophones are to be preferred because they have a smoother frequency response than probes, especially at frequencies below 4 MHz and are more stable over time. Probe hydrophones, however, are generally cheaper to buy and are available with smaller active elements.

RADIATION FORCE BALANCES

Radiation force balances (RFBs) are much easier to use than hydrophones and are used to measure only one property of the ultrasound field, i.e. the total ultrasonic power radiated by the transducer. RFBs work by measuring the force exerted on a target when it absorbs or reflects an ultrasound beam. The relationship between the measured force and the incident power depends on the design of the balance and so, although this relationship can be calculated approximately, the balance should be calibrated. For most designs of balance in common use, a power of 1 mW produces a force equivalent to approximately 69 μg. Measuring power from diagnostic equipment is complicated by the fact that output powers are relatively low and the fields are focused and scanned. The resulting low forces require considerable sensitivity for the balance design. The focused and scanned nature of the fields means that the relationship between the measured force and the total power can only be determined approximately (in other words, two transducers which generate the same ultrasonic power may produce different readings on the RFB).

References and bibliography (including references for the BMUS Safety Guidelines)

AIUM 1993. *Bioeffects and Safety of Diagnostic Ultrasound.* AIUM, 11200 Rockville Pike, Suite 205, Rockville, Maryland 20852-3139, USA.

Apfel RE and Holland CK. Gauging the likelihood of cavitation from short-pulse, low-duty cycle diagnostic ultrasound. *Ultrasound Med. Biol.* 1991; **17**: 179–185.

Barnett SB (Ed.). WFUMB Symposium on Safety of Ultrasound in Medicine. *Ultrasound Med. Biol.* 1998; **24**(Suppl 1).

Barnett SB and Kossoff G (Eds). *Safety of Diagnostic Ultrasound.* Progress in Obstetric and Gynecological Sonography Series. Parthenon, New York. 1998.

Barnett SB, Rott H-D, ter Haar GR Ziskin MC and Maeda K. The sensitivity of biological tissue to ultrasound. *Ultrasound Med. Biol.* 1997; **23**: 805–812.

Barnett SB, ter Haar GR, Ziskin MC, Rott H-D, Duck FA and Maeda K., International recommendations and guidelines for the safe use of diagnostic ultrasound in medicine. *Ultrasound Med. Biol.* 2000; **26**: 355–366.

Department of Health 1998. KH12 data.

Duck FA and Martin K. Trends in ultrasound diagnostic exposure. Phys. Med. Biol. 1991; **36**: 1423–1432.

ECURS 1994. Guidelines for the safe use of extracorporeal shock-wave lithotripsy (ESWL) devices. *Eur. J. Ultrasound* 1994; **3**: 315–316.

EFSUMB: Tutorial paper. Epidemiology of diagnostic ultrasound exposure during human pregnancy. *Eur. J. Ultrasound* 1996; **4**: 69–73 (efsumb@compuserve.co).

EFSUMB 2002. Clinical safety statement for diagnostic ultrasound (2002). www.efsumb.org/safstat.htm

Henderson J, Willson K, Jago J and Whittingham TA. A survey of the acoustic outputs of diagnostic ultrasound equipment in current use in the Northern Region. *Ultrasound Med. Biol.* 1995; **21**: 699–705.

Herman BA and Harris GR. Theoretical study of steady-state temperature rise within the eye due to ultrasound insonation. *IEEE Trans. Ultrason. Ferroelectr. Freq. Control* 1999; **46**: 1566–1574.

Jago JR, Henderson J, Whittingham TA and Mitchell G. A comparison of AIUM/NEMA Thermal Indices with calculated temperature rises for a simple third trimester pregnancy tissue model. *Ultrasound Med. Biol.* 1999; **25**: 623–628.

Leighton TG. *The Acoustic Bubble.* Academic Press, London. 1994.

Leighton TG. An introduction to acoustic cavitation. In: FA Duck, AC Baker and HC Starritt (Eds) *Ultrasound in Medicine.* Institute of Physics Publishing, Bristol. 1998, 199–223.

Miller DL and Gies RA. Gas-body-based contrast agent enhances vascular bioeffects of 1.09 MHz ultrasound on mouse intestine. *Ultrasound Med. Biol.* 1998; **24**: 1201–1208.

Miller MW and Ziskin MC. Biological consequences of hyperthermia. *Ultrasound Med. Biol.* 1989; **15**:707–722.

NCRP Report 113. *Exposure Criteria for Medical Diagnostic Ultrasound: I. Criteria Based on Thermal Mechanisms.* National Council for Radiation Protection and Measurements, Bethesda, MD 20814, USA, 1992.

Shaw A, Bond AD, Pay NM and Preston RC. A proposed standard thermal test object for medical ultrasound. *UMB* 1999; **25**(4): 121–132.

Shaw A, Pay NM and Preston RC. Assessment of the likely thermal index values for pulsed Doppler ultrasonic equipment – Stages II and III: Experimental assessment of scanner/transducer combinations. *NPL Report CMAM 12, April 1998.* National Physical Laboratory, Teddington, UK.

Skyba DM, Price RJ, Linka AZ *et al.* Microbubble destruction by ultrasound results in capillary rupture: adverse bioeffects or a possible mechanism for in vivo drug delivery? *J. Am. Soc. Echocardiol.* 1998; **11**: 497.

ter Haar G, Duck F, Starritt H and Daniels S. Biophysical characterisation of diagnostic ultrasound equipment – preliminary results. *Phys. Med. Biol.* 1989; **34**: 1533–1542.

ter Haar G and Duck FA (Eds). *The Safe Use of Ultrasound in Medical Diagnosis.* BMUS/BIR, London. 2000.

WFUMB News 1997; **4**(2). *Ultrasound Med. Biol.* 1997; **23**: 974f.

WFUMB Conclusions and recommendations on thermal and non-thermal mechanisms for biological effects. *Ultrasound Med. Biol.* 1998; **24**(Suppl 1): xv–xvi.

Ziskin MC and Petitti DB. Epidemiology of human exposure to ultrasound: a critical review. *Ultrasound Med. Biol.* 1998; **14**: 91–96.

Standards and definitions

AIUM/NEMA UD 3-1992. *Standard for Real-Time Display of Thermal and Mechanical Acoustic Output Indices on Diagnostic Ultrasound Equipment.* American Institute for Ultrasound in Medicine/National Electrical Manufacturers Association, USA. 1992.

IEC 61102. Measurement and characterisation of ultrasonic fields using hydrophones in the frequency range 0.5 MHz to 15 MHz. 1991.

IEC 61157. Requirements for the declaration of the acoustic output of medical diagnostic equipment. 1992.

IEC 61220 Ultrasonics – fields – measurement and characterization of ultrasonic fields generated by medical ultrasonic equipment using hydrophones in the frequency range 0.5 to 15 MHz. 1993.

Medical Devices Directive. 93/42/EEC, *Official J. EC* 1993; **36**: L169.

Preston RC (Ed.). *Output Measurements for Medical Ultrasound.* Springer-Verlag, ISBN 0-540-19692-7. 1991.

14

RECENT AND FUTURE DEVELOPMENTS

WN McDicken and T Anderson

Introduction

Medical diagnostic ultrasound grew out of industrial non-destructive testing and has developed at a steady pace, since its inception. This growth has been witnessed both in instrumentation and in clinical application. Indeed, the technical sophistication and range of clinical application of the field now surpass anything that was foreseen in the early days. The versatility of the tool is such that development is likely to continue into the foreseeable future. If the past is anything to go by, we are not very good at forecasting the future, and no doubt it will hold some significant surprises. New technology is usually quite crude in its initial development, so judgement on its value is best reserved till user-friendly devices are available, and there is ample time for clinical research and assessment.

It is a feature of medical ultrasound that once the student has learned the basic principles, new knowledge can be added in an accumulative manner without the need to start again from square one and a new set of basic principles. In this chapter, some techniques currently in a development phase will be considered.

Contrast agents

Contrast agents are an important feature of all types of medical imaging, where they are used to increase the sensitivity and to alter the image contrast, i.e. to increase the size of the signal from structures and to make them more readily visible in the surrounding tissues. Although various liquids containing particles have been proposed as contrast agents, it is those containing microbubbles that are by far the most successful (Ophir and Parker, 1989).

Microbubbles

It is most fortunate that small thin-shelled microbubbles about the size of red blood cells can be manufactured, since the large difference in density and compressibility of gas compared to tissue makes the bubbles very strong scatterers of ultrasound. The use of bubbles as a contrast agent was first reported by Gramiak and Shah, who developed a suggestion by Joyner (Gramiak and Shah, 1968). However, progress in the field was slow till small encapsulated bubbles were made that could be injected intravenously and survive the passage through the lungs (Feinstein *et al.*, 1984). Prior to this, the gas in unencapsulated bubbles passed out of the blood in the lungs, therefore, they had to be injected into arteries to avoid the lungs, if tissue perfusion was to be studied. Several

manufacturers are now developing microbubble agents; to date, three or four have been marketed and around a dozen are in clinical trials.

Scattering and resonance

The strong scattering that occurs as a result of the gas–tissue interface at bubbles is further enhanced by the resonant oscillation, which occurs when bubbles of a few micron diameter are insonated with ultrasound of frequency in the low-megahertz range. Resonance is enhanced vibration of a structure, which occurs when there is some relationship between a dimension of the structure and the wavelength of the incident ultrasound. Recall that a transducer crystal can be made to resonate, if its thickness is equal to half of the ultrasound wavelength. It is pure coincidence that for microbubbles with diameters of a few micron (the size of a red blood cell), the resonant frequencies are the same as the ultrasound frequencies employed in diagnostic ultrasound.

The resonant frequency of an unencapsulated bubble is given by

$$\text{resonance frequency } (f) = \frac{3.3}{r},$$

where r is the radius of the bubble in micron and f is the frequency in megahertz. Hence, a bubble of 2 μm diameter has a resonant frequency of 3.3 MHz. The situation is complicated by the fact that the manufacturing process results in a range of bubble diameters in a sample, e.g. 2–8 μm, and that the ultrasound pulse contains a range of frequencies. Nevertheless, the resonance phenomenon is considered typically to increase echo signal strength by a factor of 1000.

Typical microbubble agents

Table 14.1 presents data on some of the more common contrast agents that are being actively evaluated. It can be noted that the thin shell, or capsule, is often a protein or fat membrane and that the gas can be air, but more recently gases of large molecular weight have been preferred to extend the lifetime by slowing down diffusion of the gas from the bubble. The bubble diameters need to be no larger than that of red blood cells to permit passage through capillaries. The most difficult aspect of the specification of agents is the variety of ways in which manufacturers quote doses. There is no standard method of dose specification, although typically around 10,000,000 microbubbles are used in each injection. As things stand, the best approach is to follow the manufacturers' instructions precisely. This is also

Table 14.1 The characteristics of some currently manufactured lung-crossing contrast agents designed for intravenous injection.

Left heart agent	Manufacturer	Type of agent	Capsule	Gas	Bubble size	Dose (Concentration)
LEVOVIST	Schering	Lipid stabilised bubble	Palmitic acid	Air	3–5 μm	0.8–3.2 g
SONOVIST (SHU 563A)	Schering	Solid microspheres	Cyano-acrylate	Air	Mean 2 μm	0.1–1 μl/kg 200 ×10^8 μbubbles/ml
DEFINITY (DMP-115)	ImaRx/Du Pont	Encapsulated bubble	Lipid	Perfluoropropane	Mean 2 μm	3–5 μl/kg (10 ×10^8 μbubbles/ml)
OPTISON	Mallinckrodt	Encapsulated microsphere	Albumin	Octafluoropropane	Mean 3.7 μm	1 ml @ fundamental 0.5 ml @ second harmonic (5–8 × 10^8 μbubbles/ml)
SONOVUE™ (BR1)	Baracco	Stabilised bubble	Phospholipids	SF$_6$	2–3 μm (90% <8 μm)	5–40 μl/kg (1–5 ×10^8 μbubbles/ml)
SONAZOID (NC100100)	Nycomed	Information not available	Surfactant membrane	Fluorocarbon	Median 3.2 μm	3 μl/kg of suspension for bolus imaging (1% gas volume/ volume suspension)
ALBUNEX (Infoson in Europe)	Nycomed (Europe) Mallickrodt (USA)	Encapsulated bubbled	Albumin	Air	Mean 4 μm Range 2–10 μm	0.025–1.0 ml/kg (3–5 × 10^8 μbubbles/ml)

important from the point of view of preserving the integrity of the bubbles. Since, the microbubbles are often fragile entities, the handling protocol has to be strictly adhered to.

Bubble–ultrasound interaction

So far we have noted that the echo signal is created by scattering of ultrasound from bubbles, which may well be resonant. It is worth considering the interaction of an ultrasound pulse with a bubble in more detail, since different types of interaction can give rise to different types of image. Figure 14.1 illustrates the different types of bubble–ultrasound interaction that typically occurs as the pressure amplitude of the incident ultrasonic wave is increased. It was noted in Chapter 2 that when an ultrasound wave interacts with a small target, such as a red blood cell, whose dimensions are much smaller than the wavelength, it is scattered off in all directions. The same happens when the target is a small bubble. Consider the situation when the amplitude of the wave is quite low, 0.05 MPa in Figure 14.1. Here, the bubble oscillates in a symmetrical fashion about its centre and the same frequency of ultrasound as that incident is scattered in all directions (we are assuming that the bubble is not in overall translational motion which would produce a change of frequency due to the Doppler effect). When the amplitude of the wave is increased (0.1 MPa in Figure 14.1), the bubble starts to oscillate in a distorted fashion and higher-harmonic frequencies as well as the fundamental incident frequency are in the scattered ultrasound. At even higher wave amplitudes (1.0 MPa in Figure 14.1), the bubble may leak or even disintegrate instantaneously. This introductory account of the interaction of ultrasound and bubbles shows that different phenomena take place at different acoustic pressure amplitudes, these phenomena can be exploited to give different types of image.

Imaging technique versus pressure amplitude

At a low-ultrasound output power, which usually gives low-pressure amplitude, e.g. 0.05 MPa, scattering of bubbles gives a strong echo signal, which can be used to enhance a grey-shade B-mode or a colour Doppler image. It can also be used to increase the power of the signal displayed in spectral Doppler. A number of applications of contrast agents are dependent on simple enhancement of the power of the echo signals either from small blood vessels or perfused tissue. However, in many applications, there is a need for even greater increases in sensitivity. At higher output power (pressure amplitude, e.g. 0.1 MPa), the harmonics in the signal from the bubbles can be used to discriminate between bubbles and tissue. Some harmonic frequencies can be present in the signal from tissue (see Harmonic Imaging, Chapter 4), but they are weaker than the harmonics in the signals from bubbles. The electronic circuitry in the scanner can separate the harmonic component of the echoes from the fundamental component and create a harmonic image with it (Burns, 1996). Figure 14.2 illustrates the increase in sensitivity of harmonic contrast imaging over conventional contrast B-mode imaging. In this case, the endocardial wall of the left ventricle of the heart is better defined in the harmonic case, an aid to observing wall motion in stress testing. At higher output (e.g. 1.0 MPa), when the bubble capsule is destroyed, a free bubble may be created, which scatters even more strongly than the thin-walled microbubble. A strong signal is obtained giving an enhancement that normally lasts for just a few scanning frames, since the unencapsulated gas dissolves quickly into the tissue or blood. This type of imaging is normally called transient or intermittent imaging, since time is normally allowed between scan sweeps to enable the contrast agent to be replenished (Porter and Xie, 1995). A similar technique

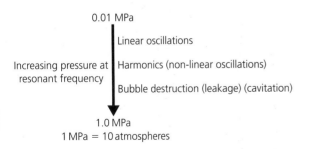

Fig. 14.1 The changing behaviour of a microbubble with increasing ultrasound pressure amplitude.

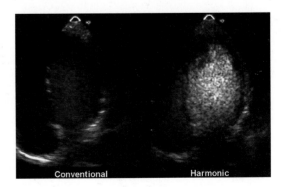

Fig. 14.2 Increased sensitivity of harmonic contrast imaging over B-mode contrast imaging (courtesy of Philips).

RECENT AND FUTURE DEVELOPMENTS

using colour Doppler imaging depends on rapid disintegration of the bubbles, which puts random phase changes into the returning echoes. The Doppler circuitry interprets these phase-changed echoes as having Doppler shifts, and hence creates Doppler images at the location of the agent. This technique is called stimulated acoustic emission (SAE) imaging (Hauf *et al.*, 1997).

Pulse inversion imaging

Pulse inversion imaging is another new modality, which has recently been introduced to increase the sensitivity

of detection of contrast agent in the body (Simpson and Burns, 1997). In this method, every second transmitted pulse is an inverted version of the previous one (see 1 and 2 in Figure 14.3). The echoes from tissue cancel out when those resulting from pairs of transmitted pulses are added. The echoes from bubbles do not cancel out, since harmonic frequencies generated at the bubbles move the position of the peaks in the echoes (see 3 and 4 in Figure 14.3). Using signal processing, the harmonic parts of the echo signal can be separated out and further processed to produce a grey-shade B-mode or Doppler image (Figure 14.4). Pulse inversion imaging appears

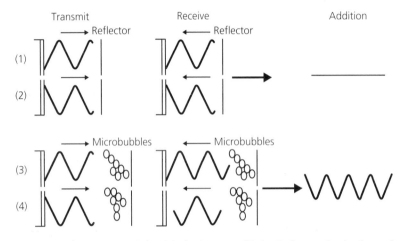

Fig. 14.3 Pulse inversion signal processing. Pulse 2 is the inverse of Pulse 1, the received echoes, therefore, cancel when they are added. Pulse 4 is the inverse of Pulse 3; however, harmonics in the echoes from the bubbles alter the echo shapes and complete cancellation does not occur.

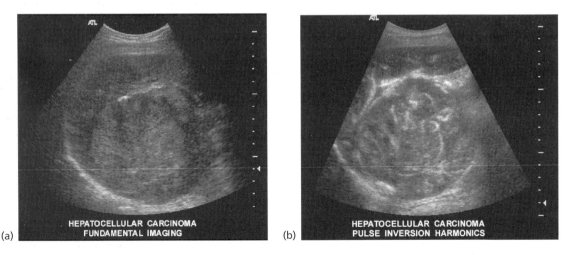

Fig. 14.4 (a) Tumour image with no contrast agent. (b) Tumour image with contrast agent and pulse inversion processing, vascularity of tumour now evident (courtesy of Philips).

to be most successful in the detection of microbubbles in small vessels, where the bubbles are moving slowly, and hence do not move far between successive transmitted pulses. Pulse inversion is performed at relatively low-pressure amplitudes, where the bubbles are not destroyed.

Bolus versus infusion

To date, contrast agents are primarily being researched to enhance the detection of tumours, observe perfusion of the myocardium and enhance the visualisation of small blood vessels. The injection of a bolus of agent may produce strongly localised scattering with a corresponding difficulty in seeing beyond it, due to the strong attenuation of the beam. One approach to avoid this attenuation is to use a slow infusion of agent rather than a bolus. This reduces the sudden attenuation seen with a bolus; on the down side is the extended time of a study and the gradual build-up of background signal from a diffuse distribution of agent in neighbouring tissues.

Quantification

It is desirable to quantify the passage of contrast agent through an organ as is done in Nuclear Medicine with radiopharmaceuticals. The aim is to produce a wash-in/wash-out curve (Figure 14.5). Unfortunately, as we have noted above, the ultrasound beam can destroy the agent making quantification difficult. Indeed, the situation is even more complex, since different phenomena can be happening in different parts of the beam due to the different pressure amplitudes. Although true quantification looks like being very difficult, it may be possible to identify some parameters of the curve, such as the rise time or the area under the curve, which can be tested by clinical trial to see if they can provide diagnostic information.

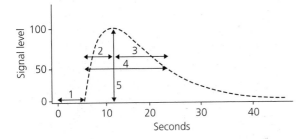

Fig. 14.5 Parameters of a wash-in/wash-out curve for microbubbles passing through tissue. 1: time after venous injection for bubbles to arrive at site of interest. 2: time to reach peak signal level. 3: time for signal level to fall from peak to half peak level. 4: width of curve at half peak value. 5: peak signal level.

Contrast agents in practice

The characteristics of a B-mode grey-shade image suitable for contrast studies are similar to the non-contrast case; however, prior to injection of contrast the tissues of interest should be displayed in the darker shades of grey to help the observation of the uptake of agent. It may also be necessary to wait several seconds or even minutes for the level of agent to reach its maximum value in the tissue of interest. Obviously, a well thought out protocol has to be established for each contrast technique, paying particular attenuation to the way the agent is handled. For each application, a decision has to be made as to whether a bolus or infusion technique is more appropriate. Of particular importance is the need to work-up techniques that give reproducible results. With regard to machine settings, one approach to this is given below:

1. Fix the machine controls, which influence the pressure amplitude in the transmitted field, i.e. output power, pulse repetition frequency, focus. This fixes the "active" factors in the interaction of ultrasound and bubbles.

2. Use the "passive" (reception) factors to vary the sensitivity of the machine to account for different patient builds, i.e. vary gain, time–gain compensation, LGC.

Other factors, such as transducer and frequency, should be fixed during the work up of the technique.

Almost all successful diagnostic techniques involve the detection of echo signals, which are then processed to give grey-shade B-mode or Doppler images, contrast agents add a whole new aspect to these established techniques. We have already seen that agents with different properties are being developed, that the interaction of agents and the ultrasound beam can be varied and that imaging instrumentation is being designed for specific types of contrast imaging. The field is still in the process of being introduced to clinical practice, new developments can be expected. In the future, we may see bubbles that are biologically active, and which bind to specific tissue sites or that can be disrupted to deliver drugs or genetic material.

Three-dimensional imaging

Principles of 3D imaging

Just as we can create a two-dimensional (2D) image of a plane through tissue by sweeping an ultrasound beam through the plane and collecting the echoes at each beam direction, we can create a three-dimensional (3D) image by sweeping a beam through a volume of tissue (Fenster *et al.*, 1995). It worth remembering, however, that with real-time 2D imaging techniques, the operator is often building up a mental 3D image, so 3D scanners will have to offer more than that to become established as a clinical tool. 3D imaging is possible for both grey-shade B-mode and Doppler imaging. Power Doppler tends to be more favoured than velocity Doppler imaging, since the former is less angle-dependent, and hence produces a more complete 3D image. The designer of a 3D scanner is faced with two problems, the collection and storage of a large amount of echo data and the display of a 3D image on a flat screen. Fortunately, the availability of cheap computer memory is reducing the problem of data storage, the optimum type of display will only be determined when user-friendly machines are tested in clinical practice. However, display of 3D images is intrinsically difficult, since external structures tend to obscure internal ones. Interactive techniques, whereby the user can remove part of the image to see further into the structures, may prove to be of value. Another attraction of 3D scanning is that scan planes, which cannot be directly accessed by the transducer beam, due to say bone or gas, can be extracted from the stored echo data and displayed. A further challenge is to create a real-time 3D image, since it takes a significant amount of time to collect the echoes from all of the beam directions in a 3D scan. Attempts at real-time 3D imaging are just beginning to appear on the market.

Free-hand 3D imaging

One common approach to 3D scanning is called "free-hand scanning" (Barry *et al.*, 1997). Here, a conventional 2D transducer is moved by hand, so that the scan plane sweeps through a volume (Figure 14.6a) and an image registration system records the position of the scan plane in 3D space at each instant. We are fortunate that such systems exist, which operate with the necessary accuracy, e.g. recording scan plane position to within 1 mm. In the most widely used type of registration system, a transmitter of radio waves is placed next to the bedside and a small receiver is attached to the transducer. The size of the signal picked up by coils in the receiver is used to work out the position of the scan plane in 3D space. This information together with the echo information is used to build-up the 3D image. An advantage of this approach is that the volume scanned can be quite large, e.g. to include the whole of a fetus at term or an extended vascular tree (Figure 14.7). The amount of skill required of the operator is being assessed in clinical trials. This approach is quite demanding of the image processing in the scanner, since the 2D images are not recorded at equally spaced intervals or even in the same orientation. New scanning skills require to be developed by the operator.

Mechanical drive 3D imaging

Another common approach to 3D imaging is to systematically alter the position of the 2D scan plane using a mechanical drive (Figure 14.6b) (Fenster *et al.*, 1995). This way a selected volume of the tissue is repeatedly scanned and 2D frames are collected at regularly spaced intervals. The most even scanning pattern is that obtained by collecting parallel 2D images; however, the problem of non-constant image spacing due to non-parallel collection is not severe. To date, the main problems of mechanical drive systems are the bulk of the transducer assembly and the relatively slow operation. In theory, it is possible

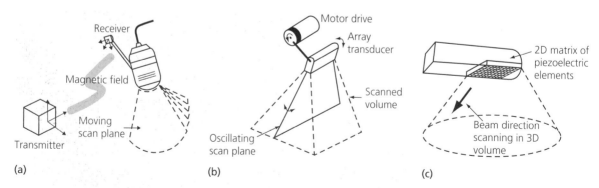

Fig. 14.6 Common 3D scanning mechanisms. (a) Free-hand scanning with electromagnetic position registration device. (b) Mechanical oscillation of an array transducer. (c) 2D array of piezoelectric transducer elements with phasing of excitation pulses to produce a 3D scan without transducer motion.

to perform a real-time 3D scan with a mechanical drive; in practice, with a single moving beam, it is difficult to collect the echoes from a scanned volume sufficiently quickly and vibrations from the rapidly moving transducer can be problematic.

Electronic array 3D imaging

The main hope for fast or real-time 3D imaging lies with the development of 2D transducer arrays (Figure 14.6c) (Shattuck *et al.*, 1984). Just as a conventional 1D phased array can direct a beam at different angles in a 2D scan plane, a 2D array can direct a beam in directions throughout a 3D scan volume. Several simultaneous beams can be generated with such an array helping to solve the speed of echo collection problem. Since the number of elements in a 2D array is large, e.g. 4000 compared to 128 in a 1D array, the amount of electronic signal handling and processing is a major challenge. Nevertheless, the first commercial system has appeared containing almost 2000 array elements in a circular aperture and capable of a scanning rate of 45 volumes per second.

3D in practice

3D imaging is at an early stage of development. Only time will tell if it is of genuine clinical value or is a technologically driven solution looking for a problem.

The methods of using 3D scanners have still to be worked out and will no doubt depend on the application. Examples of such methods are free-hand scanning of a large volume in the case of fetal weight measurement and small volume real-time scanning of a heart valve. Measurement techniques and growth charts are still in their infancy. The use of images from non-standard sections through a scanned volume may find application in specific clinical problems.

Tissue motion

Tissue motion techniques

Grey-shade B-mode and M-mode as means of detecting tissue motion have been described in Chapter 4, and are firmly established, particularly, in cardiology. These methods are normally used to observe the overall motion of a tissue structure, such as a heart wall or valve. To get more information on the internal tissue motions of organs, methods based on Doppler imaging (Doppler Tissue Imaging, DTI), duplex spectral Doppler and speckle tracking of the echo pattern of tissue parenchyma are being developed (Anderson and McDicken, 1999).

Doppler tissue imaging

The DTI mode is a modification of the more common colour Doppler imaging used for blood flow. It can be implemented by lowering the wall thump filters to record low velocities and reducing the sensitivity to remove the blood signal leaving only the stronger tissue signal in the image (Figure 14.8) (McDicken *et al.*, 1992). DTI is now a feature of many machines and the operator activates it directly by selecting the DTI mode

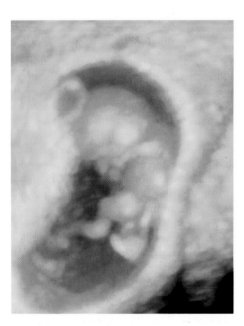

Fig. 14.7 Detailed 3D image of a 9-week fetus (courtesy of Medisonics and Juan Carlos Pons, Venezuela).

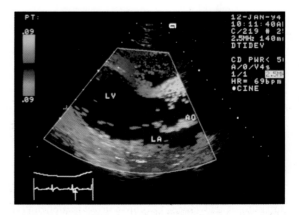

Fig. 14.8 DTI of longitudinal section through heart.

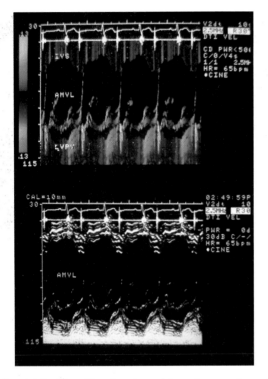

Fig. 14.9 Top, Doppler tissue M-mode scan through interventricular septum, mitral valve leaflet and left ventricular posterior wall. Bottom, grey-shade M-mode scan corresponding to Doppler tissue M-mode.

rather than by manipulating the wall filter and sensitivity. The DTI M-mode is analogous to the grey-shade M-mode, the ultrasound beam is fixed in a direction of interest through the tissues and the velocities at different depths are presented on the screen on a vertical line, which is swept across the screen (Figure 14.9) (Fleming *et al.*, 1996).

Duplex spectral doppler

Duplex spectral Doppler is the same as that used for blood flow, except that the sample volume is placed at a site of moving tissues rather than blood (Kostis *et al.*, 1972). The spectrogram produced is interpreted in the same way as that for blood flow.

Speckle tracking

Speckle tracking exploits the power of modern computers to quickly compare consecutive frames during real-time B-mode scanning. The changes in position of

the speckle pattern are considered to be directly related to the changes in the position of the soft tissue or blood (Bohs and Trahey, 1991; Hein and O'Brien, 1993; Evans and McDicken, 2000). Tracking the speckle pattern in a 2D image gives the two components of velocity in the scan plane. However, since the lateral resolution in an image is typically two or three times poorer than the axial resolution, the accuracy of velocity measurement in the lateral direction is also poorer. In theory, speckle can be tracked in 3D images to provide all three velocity components. Speckle tracking is easier to implement than vector Doppler, since it makes use of echo information from standard imaging techniques, but errors in the velocity components acquired are larger.

Sonoelasticity

This approach looks at the response of tissue to an externally applied force and attempts to derive knowledge of the elasticity of the tissue. This technique is often called "sonoelasticty" (Lerner *et al.*, 1990). A number of methods are being developed to image the elastic properties of tissue, and they could become a useful adjunct to conventional imaging (Gao *et al.*, 1996). It is known that tissues have different elasticity and, in particular, the properties malignant tissues are often significantly different from those that surround them. Sonoelasticity is at an early stage of development; at present, images are of relatively low resolution.

Tissue motion in practice

Imaging tissue motion using the Doppler effect is essentially still at a research phase. It can be difficult to interpret the large amount of velocity information in a real-time DTI image. Often, a slow replay via a cineloop is used or individual images are interpreted in terms of the mean velocity occurring at each point at the time of recording. As for Doppler blood flow images, it should be remembered that what is displayed is the velocity component along the beam direction at each point. Although the DTI M-mode presents velocities along only one beam direction, it has the attraction of high temporal resolution along the horizontal time axis of the display, and it can be recorded simultaneously with physiological signals, such as the ECG and phonocardiogram. As well as application in cardiology, there is interest in high-frequency DTI for the study of the motion of artery walls.

Having obtained the velocity information for each pixel in an image, it is possible to generate other images displaying related information. For example, the velocity gradients in the image or the extension (strain) of the tissue throughout the field of view may be displayed (Fleming *et al.*, 1996; Heimdal *et al.*, 1998).

High-frequency imaging

Throughout the development of diagnostic ultrasound, there has been a desire to obtain higher-resolution images by using higher frequencies. As transducer and machine sensitivity have improved, the frequencies employed for the abdomen and thorax have moved gradually from 2.5 to 5 and even 7 MHz. With increased use of internal transducers, requiring less penetration, 7 MHz found wider application (Lees and Lyons, 1996). Imaging of superficial structures saw the introduction of 10 MHz devices, e.g. for scanning blood vessels or neonates. In recent years, there has been an upsurge in interest in even higher-frequency transducers, in the range 10–20 MHz, presumably due to the manufacturers' ability to make devices, which give surprisingly good resolution. There is particular interest in studying the range 0–2 cm from the skin surface in applications, such as musculo-skeletal (Gibbon, 1996), vascular (Allan *et al.*, 2000) and breast imaging (Cosgrove and Eckersley, 2000). All of the techniques described at low frequencies can be implemented at high frequencies; the main challenge is the manufacture of high-frequency transducers of adequate sensitivity (Foster, 2000).

High-frequency transcutaneous scanning

Figure 14.10 illustrates a high-resolution musculo-skeletal image, obtained at 8 MHz, in which detail of less than 0.2 mm can be observed. Use of even higher frequencies makes possible resolution in the few tens of micron range, admittedly with limited penetration, e.g. 3 mm at 30 MHz in skin.

It should be appreciated that the subject of high-frequency ultrasound, say in the range 20–200 MHz, is very much in its infancy, its potential in medicine and biology is far from fully appreciated. The term "ultrasonic microscopy" is often used to describe very high-frequency imaging (Saido and Chubachi, 2000).

At the most basic level, there is little data on the ultrasonic properties of tissue at high frequencies, and there are still many challenges in the manufacture of transducers, particularly array transducers. Not surprisingly, single element transducers have been the easiest to push to high frequencies, some progress has also been made with linear arrays. Phased arrays with their particularly small

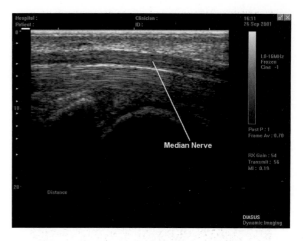

Fig. 14.10 High-frequency (10 MHz) imaging of superficial structures showing sub-millimetre resolution in median nerve (courtesy of Dynamic Imaging).

elements are proving most difficult. To date, only a few centres have worked on high-frequency Doppler devices. Likewise, although high-frequency ultrasound at around 25 MHz has been shown to scatter quite strongly from current contrast agents, these agents have not been designed for this type of application.

Invasive transducers, in general, can be considered as part of the class of high-frequency devices, although trans-vaginal, transrectal, transosophageal and intraoperative probes usually work in the range 5–10 MHz, where the technology has been mastered. Advances in these types of probe involve changes in shape and size to enable new procedures. High-frequency catheter scanners for imaging arteries (intravascular ultrasound (IVUS) catheters) are described below.

High-frequency imaging in practice

The physics and engineering of high-frequency scanners are the same as low-frequency devices, so the techniques for use are very similar. It is always worth checking the scale of the image on the display screen, since there is plenty of room to present a magnified image that may be several times the life size. Obviously, with such high frequencies, the penetration is just a few millimetres; however, many structures are of these dimensions or less. Fresh thinking is leading to new applications. Although one of the main attractions of diagnostic ultrasound is its non-invasive nature, there are applications where the quality of result justifies invasive techniques. The real-time aspect of image production and blood flow detection plus the large range of transducer types make the technology well suited to invasive methods.

Intravascular ultrasound imaging

Another area of much research and some clinical application is in the assessment with catheter transducers of atheromatous plaque before and after treatment. Here, the transducer can get to within a few millimetres of the structures whose shape can be clearly defined and whose constituents can possibly be characterised (Bom and Roelandt, 1989).

Intravascular ultrasound catheters

Such IVUS transducers commonly operate at 20–30 MHz, but experimental units have been made up to 100 MHz. The simplest catheter transducer takes the form of a single crystal mounted on the end of a wire inside a thin plastic sheath. The beam from the crystal is directed perpendicular to the axis of the wire, and by rotating the wire about this axis a 360° scan is performed. More recently, the transducer has taken the form of an electronic array in which 64 elements are arranged around a cylindrical surface enabling a radial beam to be swept again through 360°. The electronic array removes the problem of the rotating wire sticking with related distortion in the image. At present, the rotating crystal devices still have slightly better image quality and can be manufactured at higher frequencies. Figure 14.11 presents an image of plaque formation in a coronary artery. Pull-back devices are supplied with catheter scanners enabling a series of parallel and equally spaced images to be recorded from which the plaque volume can be calculated.

Intravascular ultrasound Doppler

Doppler techniques employ catheters with a single crystal whose beam points along the blood vessel are used with spectral frequency analysis to note the changes in arterial haemodynamics as a result of physical therapy, such as angioplasty or drug therapy (Doucette *et al.*, 1992). At present, Doppler imaging along a vessel has only been demonstrated with prototype devices, since the beams of most IVUS catheters are directed at 90° to the direction of blood flow.

Intravascular ultrasound in practice

To date, IVUS techniques are mostly employed as tools for research, where they are very valuable, since they

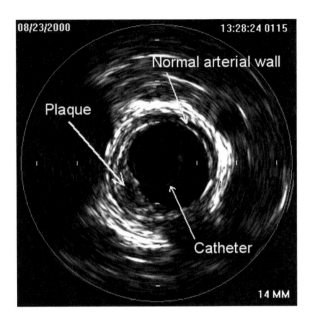

Fig. 14.11 The 30 MHz IVUS image of plaque in artery (courtesy of Jomed).

can be located close to the vascular sites of interest. The cost of catheters, which can only be used once in clinical practice due to the fear of infection, is a significant problem. In future, cheaper devices may be produced.

Techniques with clinical potential

At any time, a number of techniques look as though they could become part of the medical ultrasound armamentarium, though until they are thoroughly assessed clinically, it is difficult to forecast what their final role will be.

Tissue characterisation

Tissue characterisation has been a holy grail of diagnostic ultrasound for many years, yet for most of the envisaged areas of application, there is still no clinical package on commercial machines. It would appear that the complexity of tissue and the beam degradation between the transducer and the site of interest have been underestimated. Research is still being pursued in a few fields. These tend to be where there is well-defined tissue between the transducer and the tissue of interest as in eye tumours and plaque formation in arteries. Another technique is to try to characterise change in tissue, e.g. in the myocardium over the cardiac cycle or before and after therapy. Assessment of tissue vascularity by Doppler or contrast agents is another type of characterisation

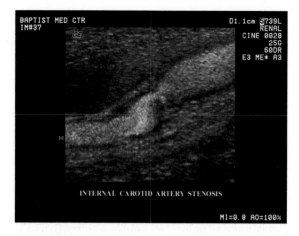

Fig. 14.12 B-flo image of blood in vessel (courtesy of General Electric).

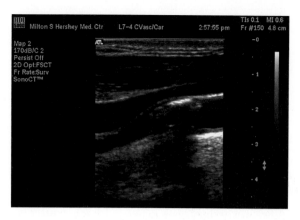

Fig. 14.13 SonoCT image of carotid artery (courtesy of Philips).

though again care has to be taken not to take an over-simplified view. The main contributions that ultrasonics makes to tissue characterisation are still via the interpretation of grey-shade images or by the guidance of biopsy needles. The technology of needle guidance is still being developed to make it more precise.

B-flo

B-flo is a name given by GE Ultrasound to a technique they have introduced for the real-time imaging of blood motion. This technique depicts the changing speckle pattern of moving blood, which can be observed when very high sensitivity is used (Figure 14.12). The technical details are not available for commercial reasons; however, the echo production at high sensitivity is said to be based on pulse-coding techniques (Chapter 1). In pulse coding, the transmitted pulse has a pattern to its structure and that pattern is identified in the returning ultrasound to identify genuine echoes amongst spurious signals and noise, in other words the signal-to-noise ratio is improved. The idea has been around for some time, but the GE Ultrasound version is the first that has successfully appeared in clinical equipment. This machine preserves the sharply defined vessel walls at high sensitivity and shows the blood speckle contained within the vessels.

Complex speckle patterns are observed, which appear to show the flow of blood and often non-laminar flow around complex structures. A pulsing in the brightness of the blood signal amplitude is also seen. Interpretation of moving speckle patterns can be difficult and more work is required in this area. At this stage of development,

there is no way of measuring the velocity of the blood. The final role of B-flo and its place relative to other techniques, such as power and velocity Doppler imaging, still has to be determined.

SonoCT

In the familiar X-ray CT imaging, narrow X-ray beams are passed through the body in many directions, and by measuring the total attenuation along each beam path, an image of the attenuating properties can be produced. The same is possible with ultrasound; however, ultrasound beams are blocked by gas and bone, so the method has proven difficult to implement. In theory, ultrasound can offer more types of image than X-rays, since quantities such as tissue velocity can also be used to create images. Occasionally, manufacturers call a technique CT ultrasound when a lot of computation is involved in producing an image. Such images are not necessarily analogous to X-ray CT. Recently, the ATL Corporation has launched sonoCT. It is not clear just how close this is to the conventional X-ray type, but at least computational processes are employed to bring into sharp registration ultrasonic images derived from scanning the tissues from several directions (Figure 14.13). In time, this processing may be close to that used in conventional X-ray CT.

Portable scanners

The concept of very portable scanners has recently seen a revival. The power of modern computer chips and capacity of memory mean that a great deal of processing can be performed in a small unit, as is commonly seen in laptop computers. Though representing clever engineering, the high quality of grey-shade B-mode and Doppler images from portable scanners is not altogether surprising. There is no fundamental compromise in the principles employed to produce either the real-time B-mode or the Doppler images. These scanners represent a challenge to our thinking as to how and where diagnostic ultrasound should be applied. They are another good illustration of the versatility of the technology, and how it is well suited to use in medicine.

Clinical assessment of new technology

When new technology is introduced, it is important not to judge its value too quickly. Most of the established techniques have only reached that status after many years of struggle by workers in the field. It may also be that their clinical applications only became apparent several years after they were introduced. Often, the initial difficulties are a result of the technology not being particularly user friendly. Technology usually appears in a fairly primitive form, and it is then refined as a result of user experience or as a result of advances in other fields, such as computing or materials science. The rate of advance in one field is difficult to predict probably, because it depends on advances in others. Good examples of this at present are 3D imaging and contrast agents. An important role of the clinical user in this process, apart from the obvious one of identifying new applications, is to persevere with new technology and to highlight difficulties in practice.

References

Allan PL, Dubbins PA, Pozniak MA and McDicken WN. *Clinical Doppler Ultrasound*. Churchill Livingstone, London. 2000.

Anderson T and McDicken WN. Measurement of tissue motion. *Proc. Instn. Mech. Engrs.* 1999; **213**: 181–191.

Barry CD, Allott CP, John NW, Mellor PM, Arundel PA, Thomson DS and Waterton JC. Three-dimensional freehand ultrasound imaging: image reconstruction and volume analysis. *Ultrasound Med. Biol.* 1997; **23**: 1209–1224.

Bohs LN and Trahey GE. A novel method for angle independent ultrasonic imaging of blood flow and tissue motion. *IEEE Trans. Biomed. Eng. BME* 1991; **38**: 280–286.

Bom N and Roelandt J. *Intravascular Ultrasound*. Kluwer Academic Publishers, Dordrecht. 1989.

Burns PN. Harmonic imaging with ultrasound contrast agents. *Clin. Radiol.* 1996; **51**(Suppl 1): 50–55.

Cosgrove DO and Eckersley RJ. Breast. *Ultrasound Med. Biol.* 2000; **26**(Suppl 1): S110–S115.

Doucette JW, Corl D, Payne HM, Flynn AE, Goto M, Nassi M and Segal J. Validation of a Doppler guidewire for intravascular measurement of coronary artery flow velocity. *Circulation* 1992; **85**: 1899–1911.

Evans DH and McDicken WN. *Doppler Ultrasound: Physics, Instrumentation and Signal Processing*, 2nd edition. Wiley, Chichester. 2000.

Feinstein SB, Shah PM, Bing RL, Meerbaum S, Corday E, Chang B-L, Santillan G and Fujibayashi Y. Microbubble dynamics visualized in the intact capillary circulation. *J. Am. Coll. Cardiol.* 1984; **4**: 595–600.

Fenster A and Downey DB. 3-D ultrasound imaging: a review. *IEEE Eng. Med. Biol.* 1996; **15**(6): 41–51.

Fenster A, Tong S, Sherebrin S, Downey DB and Rankin RN. Three-dimensional ultrasound imaging. *Soc. Photo-optical Instrument. Eng. Proc.* 1995; **2432**: 176–184.

Fleming AD, Palka P, McDicken WN, Fenn LN and Sutherland GR. Verification of cardiac Doppler tissue images using grey-scale M-mode images. *Ultrasound Med. Biol.* 1996; **22**: 573–581.

Foster FS. Transducer materials and probe construction. *Ultrasound Med. Biol.* 2000; **26** (Suppl 1): S2–S5.

Gao L, Parker KJ, Lerner RM and Levinson SF. Imaging of the elastic properties of tissue – a review. *Ultrasound Med. Biol.* 1996; **22**: 957–977.

Gibbon WW. *Musculoskeletal Ultrasound: The Essentials*. Greenwich Medical Media, London. 1996.

Gramiak R and Shah PM. Echocardiography of the aortic root. *Invest. Radiol.* 1968; **3**: 356–366.

Hauff P, Fritzsch T, Reinhardt M, Weitscheis W, Luders F, Uhlendorf V and Heldmann D. Delineation of experimental tumours in rabbits by a new ultrasound contrast agent and stimulated acoustic emission. *Invest. Radiol.* 1997; **32**: 94–99.

Heimal A, Stoylen A, Torp H and Skjaerpe T. Real-time strain rate imaging of the left ventricle by ultrasound. *Amer. Soc. Echocard.* 1998; **11**: 1013–1019.

Hein IA and O'Brien WD. Current time-domain methods for assessing tissue motion by analysis from reflected ultrasound echoes – a review. *IEEE Trans. Ultrason. Ferroelec. Freq. Contr.* 1993; **40**: 84–102.

Kostis JB, Mavrogreogis EM, Slater A and Bellet E. Use of the range-gated, pulsed ultrasonic Doppler technique for continuous measurement of velocity of the posterior heart wall. *Chest* 1972; **62**: 597–604.

Lees WR and Lyons EA (Eds). *Invasive Ultrasound*. Martin Dunitz, London. 1996.

Lerner RM, Huang SR and Parker KJ. Sonoelasticity images derived from ultrasound signals in mechanically vibrated tissues. *Ultrasound Med. Biol.* 1990; **16**: 231–239.

McDicken WN, Sutherland GR, Moran CM and Gordon LN. Colour Doppler velocity imaging of the myocardium. *Ultrasound Med. Biol.* 1992; **18**: 651–654.

Ophir J and Parker KJ. Contrast agents in diagnostic ultrasound. *Ultrasound Med. Biol.* 1989; **15**: 319–333.

Porter TR and Xie F. Transient myocardial contrast after initial exposure to diagnostic ultrasound pressures with minute doses of intravenously injected microbubbles: demonstration and potential mechanisms. *Circulation* 1995; **92**: 2391–2395.

Saido Y and Chubachi N. Microscopy. *Ultrasound Med. Biol.* 2000; **26**(Suppl 1): S30–S32.

Shattuck DP, Weinshenker MD, Smith SW and von Ramm OT. Explososcan: a parallel processing technique for high speed ultrasound imaging with linear phased arrays. *J. Acoust. Soc. Am.* 1984; **75**: 1273–1282.

Simpson DH and Burns PN. Pulse inversion Doppler: a new method for detecting nonlinear echoes from microbubble contrast agents. In: SC Schneider, M Levy and BR McAvoy (Eds), *Proceedings of the 1997 IEEE Ultrasonics Symposium*, IEEE, Piscataway, NJ. 1997, 1597–1600.

APPENDICES

A. THE DECIBEL

The dB is the unit, which is normally used to describe the relative amplitude of echoes in ultrasound systems. In practice, the absolute amplitude of an echo signal (expressed in volts) is rarely of interest. It is more useful to know how echoes compare with one another. The ratio of the two amplitudes can be expressed in decibels (dB). As the dB is used only for ratios, there are no other units involved (e.g. mW, MPa). The dB is a logarithmic scale, so in very simple terms, if the ratio is 1000:1 or 1,000,000:1, rather than writing out lots of zeros, the dB scale effectively counts the zeros, rather like expressing these numbers as 10^3 or 10^6.

The Bel is simply $\log_{10} R$, where R is the ratio. Hence a ratio of 1000:1 is 3 Bel, and a ratio of 1,000,000:1 is 6 Bel. In practice, the unit of 1 Bel (ratio of 10) is often too large and it is more useful to use the decibel which is one-tenth of a Bel. Hence, the ratio R in dB is given by R (dB) $= 10 \log_{10} R$ dB.

The dB, as defined above, is used to express only ratios of power or intensity. For example, as an ultrasound pulse propagates through tissue and is attenuated, the ratio of the intensities within the pulse at two different depths can be expressed in dB. The ratio of the intensities

$$\frac{I_2}{I_1}(dB) = 10 \log_{10}\left(\frac{I_2}{I_1}\right) \ dB. \tag{A.1}$$

As described in Chapter 2, the intensity of a pulse is proportional to the square of the acoustic pressure, i.e.

$I \propto p^2$. So the ratio of two intensities

$$\frac{I_2}{I_1} = \frac{p_2^2}{p_1^2} = \left(\frac{p_2}{p_1}\right)^2.$$

That is, the intensity ratio is equal to the pressure ratio squared. The intensity ratio in dB can be expressed in terms of the pressure ratio:

$$\frac{I_2}{I_1}(dB) = 10 \log_{10}\left(\frac{p_2}{p_1}\right)^2.$$

This equation can be rewritten as

$$\frac{I_2}{I_1}(dB) = 20 \log_{10}\left(\frac{p_2}{p_1}\right) dB. \tag{A.2}$$

Equation (A.2) is used whenever two amplitudes (pressure, voltage) are compared, whereas Equation (A.1) is used to compare power or intensity levels. An intensity ratio of 10 equates to 10 dB and a ratio of 2 to 3 dB. For pressure or voltage ratios of 10 and 2, the corresponding numbers are 20 and 6 dB, respectively.

A further important advantage of the dB scale is that it simplifies the combination of ratios. As the dB is a logarithmic unit, instead of multiplying the two ratios together, the corresponding values in dB are simply added. For example, an intensity ratio of 20 (2×10) equates to 13 dB (3 dB + 10 dB). A pressure ratio of 40 ($2 \times 2 \times 10$) equates to 32 dB (6 dB + 6 dB + 20 dB).

B. THE BINARY SYSTEM

A number in the decimal system consists of several digits, each representing a quantity of units, 10s, or 100s, etc. For example, the decimal number 6473 represents 6 thousands plus 4 hundreds plus 7 tens plus 3 units. The value of 1 count in each column is a power of 10, i.e. $1 \times 100 = 10^2, 1 \times 1000 = 10^3$. The maximum count of a 4-digit number is 9999. When counting from zero, the digit in the right-hand column (units) is increased until it reaches 9, and on the next count it returns to 0, while the digit in the 10s column is increased by 1. Each column carries over into the next to the left after a count of 9.

The binary system operates in an identical fashion but the value of one count in each column is a power of 2, e.g. 2^3, 2^2, 2^1, 2^0. In decimal terms, the values of the digits are 8, 4, 2, and 1, and the maximum count in each column is 1. So the maximum value for a 4-digit number is 1111 which is 15 in decimal. Counting from 0, the digit on the right (2^0 column) changes from 0 to 1. On the next count, it goes back to 0 and the digit to the left (2^1 column) goes from 0 to 1. In the binary system, a digit is referred to as a bit (short for binary digit). So 1111 is a 4-bit number.

INDEX

by skin
ECHO for neonates